Stroke

YOUR QUESTIONS ANSWERED

For Churchill Livingstone

Commissioning Editor: Ellen Green
Project Manager: Alison Ashmore
Design Direction: Jayne Jones and Keith Kail

Stroke

YOUR QUESTIONS ANSWERED

Graeme J. Hankey

MBBS MD FRCP(Lond) FRCP(Edin) FRACP

Consultant Neurologist and Head of Stroke Unit,
Royal Perth Hospital, Australia.

Clinical Professor, Department of Medicine,
The University of Western Australia.

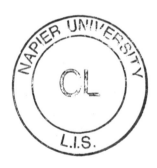

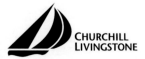

CHURCHILL
LIVINGSTONE

EDINBURGH LONDON NEW YORK OXFORD PHILADELPHIA ST LOUIS SYDNEY TORONTO 2002

CHURCHILL LIVINGSTONE
An imprint of Elsevier Limited

First published 2002
Reprinted 2004

ISBN 0 443 07146 2

British Library Cataloguing in Publication Data
A catalogue record for this book is available from the British Library

Library of Congress Cataloging in Publication Data
A catalog record for this book is available from the Library of Congress

Note
Medical knowledge is constantly changing. As new information becomes available, changes in treatment, procedures, equipment and the use of drugs become necessary. The authors and the publishers have taken care to ensure that the information given in this text is accurate and up to date. However, readers are strongly advised to confirm that the information, especially with regard to drug usage, complies with the latest legislation and standards of practice.

 your source for books, journals and multimedia in the health sciences

www.elsevierhealth.com

The publisher's policy is to use paper manufactured from sustainable forests

Printed in China

Contents

Preface

Stroke affects 0.2% of the entire population, and more than 1% of people older than 65 years, each year. Stroke is fatal in up to one-third of cases, making it the third most common cause of death in developed countries, after coronary heart disease and cancer. Among survivors of stroke, who comprise at least 0.8% of the general population, at least half are permanently disabled, making stroke a major cause of long-term physical, cognitive, emotional, social and vocational disability.

A general practitioner (GP) with a list of 2000 people is therefore likely to see at least one new acute stroke patient every 3 months and to be continually caring for at least 16 stroke survivors at any one time, half of whom are likely to be dependent on someone else to carry out their activities of daily living. The GP has a primary and pivotal role in all phases of stroke prevention and care – primary prevention, diagnosis, acute management, and ongoing rehabilitation, community care and secondary prevention of recurrent major vascular events. Furthermore, the role is dynamic, evolving and increasing, as new concepts in stroke prevention and management emerge.

However, only recently, stroke was still a 'Cinderella' of medicine and progress continued to be hindered by ignorance, nihilism and negativity both within and outside the medical profession. This has all changed in the past decade. Tremendous advances in understanding the pathogenesis of stroke, coupled with the advent of superb, non-invasive diagnostic techniques and evidence from randomised clinical trials of effective strategies to treat and prevent stroke, have seen stroke medicine establish itself as one of the frontiers of medicine and a 'hands-on', multidisciplinary subspecialty in its own right.

This book aims to be a succinct source of answers, based on the best available current evidence, to questions that are commonly asked by GPs about the definitions, epidemiology, causes, clinical features, investigations, management and outcome of stroke. Although it has been written primarily for GPs, it also hopes to address many questions also asked about stroke by general physicians, neurologists in training, medical students, stroke patients, carers of stroke patients and the general public.

The book is divided into 16 chapters, each with a list of relevant key references for further reading. The first two chapters define what is meant by a stroke and the size of the problem for stroke patients, their carers and the community. Chapters 3–15 address, in turn, the five key questions that should be answered in the diagnosis and management of all stroke patients:

- Is it a stroke? (Chapter 3)
- Where is the stroke lesion? (i.e. which part of the brain and what arterial territory are affected?) (Chapter 4)
- What is the cause of the stroke? (i.e. is it an infarct or a haemorrhage, and what is the cause of the infarct or haemorrhage?) (Chapters 6–8)
- What is the prognosis for survival and handicap? (Chapter 9)
- What can be done to optimise patient outcome and prevent a recurrent stroke? (Chapters 10–15)

Chapter 16 discusses stroke in special populations (e.g. children, pregnant women).

Information for patients and carers is provided at the end of the relevant chapters and postal and internet addresses of stroke organisations are provided in an Appendix.

Graeme J. Hankey
Perth, Australia

How to use this book

The *Your Questions Answered* series aims to meet the information needs of GPs and other primary care professionals who care for patients with chronic conditions. It is designed to help them work with patients and their families, providing effective, evidence-based care and management.

The books are in an accessible question-and-answer format, with detailed contents lists at the beginning of every chapter and a complete index to help find specific information.

ICONS
Icons are used in the book to identify particular types of information:

 highlights important information

 highlights side-effect information.

PATIENT QUESTIONS
At the end of relevant chapters there are sections of frequently asked patient questions, with easy-to-understand answers aimed at the non-medical reader. These questions are also listed at the end of the book.

Terminology and definitions (what is a stroke?)

1

1.1 What is a stroke?

A stroke is a clinical syndrome characterised by an acute loss of focal brain function lasting more than 24 hours or leading to (earlier) death, which is thought to be due to either spontaneous haemorrhage into or over the brain substance (primary intracerebral haemorrhage or subarachnoid haemorrhage respectively – haemorrhagic stroke) or inadequate blood supply to a part of the brain as a result of low blood flow, thrombosis or embolism associated with diseases of the blood vessels, heart or blood (ischaemic stroke/cerebral infarction).[1]

This definition embraces stroke due to cerebral infarction, primary intracerebral haemorrhage (PICH), intraventricular haemorrhage and most cases of subarachnoid haemorrhage (SAH). By convention it does not include subdural haemorrhage, epidural haemorrhage or intracerebral haemorrhage, or infarction caused by trauma, infection or tumour; nor does this definition embrace patients with retinal infarction, despite the fact that retinal and cerebral infarction share many common causes and a similar prognosis for recurrent major vascular events.

The definition also excludes patients with SAH who are conscious and have a headache but no abnormal focal neurological signs (neck stiffness is not invariable and does not occur for several hours). It therefore needs to be recognised that the sudden onset of headache, with or without meningism, and otherwise no focal or global neurological dysfunction, can be a SAH.

1.2 What are the origins of the word 'stroke'?

'Stroke' was originally short for 'stroke of apoplexy'. 'Apoplexy' is derived through French and Latin from the Greek word *apoplexia*, meaning a sudden loss of feeling and motion, as if struck by a thunderbolt. *Apoplexia* is derived from *apoplessein* ('to disable by a blow'); from *plessein* ('to strike') and *apo* (meaning 'off' or 'from', in this case indicating 'completely').[2]

1.3 What is a transient ischaemic attack?

A transient ischaemic attack (TIA) of the brain or eye is a clinical syndrome characterised by the acute loss of focal brain or monocular function lasting less than 24 hours. It is thought to be due to inadequate blood supply to a part of the brain or eye as a result of low blood flow, thrombosis or embolism associated with diseases of the blood vessels, heart or blood.[3]

A TIA of the brain is therefore the same as an ischaemic stroke, as defined above, but the symptoms resolve within 24 hours.

The 24-hour time limit for the duration of symptoms was decided by a World Health Organization committee in 1978 on purely arbitrary grounds, having more to do with the earth's rotation than biology (see below). Abnormal but functionally unimportant focal neurological signs such as reflex asymmetry or an extensor plantar response may persist for longer than 24 hours (in about 5% of patients) and cranial computed tomography (CT) or magnetic resonance imaging (MRI) evidence of infarction may be present. (NB. A small brain haemorrhage can rarely cause transient focal neurological symptoms but the cause is brain haemorrhage, not ischaemia.)

1.4   Why distinguish between a TIA and stroke?

There is no need to distinguish between a TIA and mild ischaemic stroke when considering prognosis and treatment. This is because the only factor that distinguishes TIA from mild ischaemic stroke is *quantitative* – the duration of the symptoms of focal neurological dysfunction (i.e. less or more than 24 hours) – even though most TIAs last minutes rather than hours. Otherwise, patients with TIA and mild ischaemic stroke are *qualitatively* the same; they are of similar age and sex, have a similar prevalence of coexistent vascular risk factors (and probably therefore pathogenesis) and share the same long-term prognosis for serious vascular events. For practical management (i.e. secondary prevention and rehabilitation), it is therefore probably more useful to distinguish patients with reversible ischaemic attacks, who recover in minutes, days or weeks, from those with major disabling ischaemic stroke and a permanent disability.

However, the distinction between TIA and mild ischaemic stroke is important in differential diagnosis, in case-control studies and in measuring stroke incidence. This is because:

- the differential diagnosis of focal neurological symptoms lasting minutes (e.g. seizure, migraine) is quite different from that of attacks lasting several hours to days (e.g. intracranial haemorrhage, tumour, and encephalitis)
- incidence studies of cerebrovascular disease are likely to achieve less complete case ascertainment for TIA than stroke because patients who experience brief attacks (i.e. TIA) are more likely to ignore or forget them and less likely to report them to a doctor than patients who suffer more prolonged or disabling events (i.e. stroke). Nonetheless, it is important to check up on any TIAs that are reported because sometimes a mild stroke is incorrectly labelled as a 'TIA'

- the reliability of the clinical diagnosis of stroke is much better than for TIA
- for case-control studies there is less change in haemostatic factors and no survival bias among TIA patients.

1.5 Are brain imaging appearances needed to distinguish between a TIA and a stroke?

The brain CT and MRI scan appearances of presumed ischaemic lesions in the relevant part of the brain in patients presenting with transient focal neurological symptoms lasting less than 24 hours (TIA) should not change the diagnosis of TIA to stroke. It is the *duration of symptoms* that is relevant to the distinction.

1.6 What is a brain attack?

Now that we have entered an era where patients with an acute cerebrovascular event are being assessed and treated within just a few hours (e.g. with thrombolysis to rescue ischaemic brain tissue), it has become impractical to use the above time-based definitions of TIA and stroke for patients, as they are being seen in this acute phase. For example, when seeing a patient at 2 hours after the onset of an acute loss of blood supply to a part of the brain, it is not possible to know 'whether the attack will turn out to be a TIA or a stroke', as is commonly asked now by students.

In this situation, where the patient is being assessed within 24 hours from onset of symptoms and a focal neurological deficit persists, it is possible that ultimately the diagnosis will be a TIA, a stroke or indeed another, non-vascular, disorder such as a migraine, partial seizure, subdural haematoma, brain tumour or encephalitis (see below). It is suggested that these patients are considered to be having a 'brain attack' because it reminds clinicians about issues such as the accuracy of the diagnosis and scope of the differential diagnosis, which almost certainly differ somewhat from patients with completed stroke (i.e. persistent symptoms after more than 24 hours), and the fact that 'time is brain' (i.e. every moment counts in unravelling the cause, restoring blood flow to the ischaemic brain and improving patient outcome).

1.7 Why has the term 'cerebrovascular accident' been abandoned?

Stroke is not an accident – there is always an underlying cause, which, if recognised earlier and avoided or controlled, might have delayed or prevented the onset of stroke.

PATIENT QUESTIONS

1.8 What is a stroke?

A stroke is a type of injury to the brain. It is characterised by the sudden loss of function of a particular part of the body because of a sudden interruption in the flow of blood to a part of the brain.

The word 'stroke' was originally short for 'stroke of apoplexy' and 'apoplexy' is derived from the Greek word meaning to be struck down, as if by a thunderbolt.

1.9 Why does a stroke occur?

A stroke occurs when there is a sudden interruption to the flow of blood to part of the brain.

This is usually caused by a blockage in a blood vessel (artery) carrying blood to the brain. The blockage stops the blood getting to the part of the brain supplied by that artery, which damages it, because the brain needs a constant supply of oxygen and glucose (sugar) for it to function properly, and the oxygen and glucose is normally delivered to the brain constantly in the blood stream. Therefore, if the blood supply (and thus oxygen and glucose supply) to a part of the brain is shut off for more than a few minutes, then that part of the brain ceases to function properly. If the disturbance in blood supply to a part of the brain is not corrected after a few hours, that part of the brain may die (cerebral/brain infarction), and permanently cease to function. This is called an ischaemic stroke (see below).

Less commonly, an artery bursts and blood spurts out into the brain tissue or over the surface of the brain, causing a bruise in, or over, the brain, This is called a haemorrhagic stroke. A bleed into the brain tissue is called an intracerebral haemorrhage, and a bleed over the surface of the brain is called a subarachnoid haemorrhage (see below). Because the blood spurts out of the ruptured artery under high pressure (equivalent to the blood pressure), it tears some of the brain tissue (which is normally soft) and forms a mass of blood (a haematoma; like a big blood clot), which squashes the normal surrounding brain, preventing it from receiving any nourishing blood supply from other blood vessels. The rim of brain surrounding the haematoma may therefore die.

1.10 What is a transient ischaemic attack?

A transient ischaemic attack (TIA) is a mini-stroke. Like an ischaemic stroke, it is characterised by the sudden loss of function of a particular part of the body because of a sudden lack of blood flow to a part of the brain. The symptoms of a TIA, and its causes, are therefore the same as those of an ischaemic stroke. However, unlike an ischaemic stroke, the symptoms of abnormal function of a part of the body and brain recover completely within 24 hours. This is because the blockage of the artery clears itself very quickly, before the ischaemic brain tissue has died (infarcted).

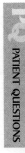
PATIENT QUESTIONS

1.11 Why are transient ischaemic attacks important?

Transient ischaemic attacks are important because they are a 'tap on the shoulder' for the patient, notifying them that they are at increased risk of a future stroke (and heart attack) but that, with appropriate treatment, their risk of having a major disabling or fatal stroke or heart attack can be reduced.

Epidemiology (how big is the problem of stroke?)

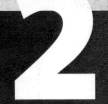

2.1 What is the incidence rate of stroke and transient ischaemic attack?

The incidence of new cases of first-ever stroke, is about 200 per 100 000 per year (i.e. 0.2% of the population) in the few Caucasian populations studied.[1] Transient ischaemic attacks (TIAs) are about one-quarter as common as stroke, affecting about 50 per 100 000 population each year[2] (*Table 2.1*).

TABLE 2.1 The approximate incidence of various neurological disorders and how often a new case will be seen by a general practitioner (GP) with a list size of 2000 people[3]

Neurological disorders	Incidence/100 000 per annum	Number of years between consecutive new cases
Stroke	200	0.3
Carpal tunnel syndrome	100	0.5
First epileptic (non-febrile) seizure	50	1.0
Transient ischaemic attack	50	1.0
Bell's palsy	25	2.0
Essential tremor	24	2.1
Parkinson's disease	20	2.5
Primary brain tumour	15	3.3
Secondary brain tumour	14	3.6
Subarachnoid haemorrhage	10	5.0
Giant cell arteritis	6	8.3
Multiple sclerosis (Scotland)	6	8.4
Trigeminal neuralgia	4	13
Meningococcal meningitis	3	17
Transient global amnesia	3	17
Guillain–Barré syndrome	2	25
Intracranial vascular malformation	2	25
Motor neurone disease	2	25
Neuralgic amyotrophy	2	25
Progressive supranuclear palsy	1	50
Idiopathic intracranial hypertension	1	50
Myasthenia gravis	1	50
Polymyositis/dermatomyositis	1	50
Hemifacial spasm	0.8	63
Multiple system atrophy	0.6	83
Gilles de la Tourette's syndrome	0.5	100

TABLE 2.1 (*Cont'd*)

Neurological disorders	Incidence/100 000 per annum	Number of years between consecutive new cases
Pneumococcal meningitis	0.5	100
Herpes simplex encephalitis	0.2	250
Creutzfeldt–Jakob disease	0.1	500
Tetanus	0.1	500
Subacute sclerosing panencephalitis	0.03	1667
New variant Creutzfeldt–Jakob disease (UK)	0.02	2500

Stroke incidence rises rapidly with age: only about a quarter of cases occur below the age of 65, and about a half below the age of 75 (*Fig. 2.1*). Consequently, the absolute number of stroke patients is likely to increase in the future, because of the ageing of most populations, despite uncertainty over whether stroke incidence is rising, falling or remaining static. Men and women are affected in roughly equal numbers.

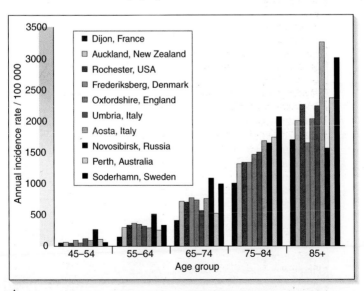

Fig 2.1 Incidence of stroke (ischaemic and haemorrhagic combined) among 10 different communities in age groups 45 years and older. Adapted with permission from Sudlow & Warlow 1997.[1]

Stroke incidence appears to be higher, up to twice as common, in Russia, Eastern Europe and China, particularly when compared with Dijon, in France, which has the lowest incidence.

2.2 What is the prevalence of stroke?

The prevalence of stroke is probably somewhere between 5 and 12 per 1000 population (i.e. 1% of the population) but this figure depends on the age and sex structure of the population (*Table 2.2*).[4] In women and men aged

TABLE 2.2 The approximate prevalence of various neurological disorders and how frequently they are present in an average general practice of 2000 people[3]

Neurological disorder	Prevalence/100 000	No. cases
Migraine	10000	200
Chronic tension headache	3000	60
Carpal tunnel syndrome	3000	60
Stroke	800	16
Alzheimer's disease	800	16
Epilepsy (active)	500	10
Essential tremor	300	6
Parkinson's disease	160	3
Multiple sclerosis	50	1
Benign intracranial tumour	50	1
Migrainous neuralgia (cluster headache)	40	1
Trigeminal neuralgia	40	1
Bell's palsy	25	0.5
Neurofibromatosis (type 1)	13	0.3
Cerebral metastases	10	0.2
Myasthenia gravis	10	0.2
Hemifacial spasm	10	0.2
Narcolepsy syndrome	10	0.2
Huntington's disease	8	0.2
Myotonic dystrophy	7	0.1
Syringomyelia	7	0.1
Motor neurone disease	5	0.1
Malignant brain tumour	5	0.1
Duchenne muscular dystrophy	4	<0.1
Fascioscapulohumeral dystrophy	3	<0.1
Mitochondrial cytopathy	2	<0.1
Friedreich's ataxia	2	<0.1
Progressive supranuclear palsy	1.4	<0.1
Chronic inflammatory demyelinating neuropathy	2	<0.1
Tuberous sclerosis	1	<0.1
Wilson's disease	0.4	<0.1

65–74 years, the prevalence of stroke is 25 and 50 per 1000 respectively.[5–7] Stroke prevalence also depends on incidence and survival.

2.3 Does race/ethnic group influence stroke incidence and prevalence?

ASIAN (SOUTHERN) POPULATIONS

Although there are no reliable data concerning stroke incidence and prevalence, the prevalence of coronary heart disease, central obesity (i.e. high waist-to-hip ratio), insulin resistance, non-insulin-dependent diabetes and hypertension are more common in south Asian populations in the UK than in Asia, and stroke mortality is higher.[8] This seems to be partly the result of genetic susceptibility (high serum lipoprotein (a) levels) in these people, potentiated by dietary and lifestyle-induced changes in lipid levels.

JAPANESE AND CHINESE POPULATIONS

Stroke, particularly primary intracerebral haemorrhage (PICH), appears to be more common in Japan and China than in western countries. In addition, intracranial arterial disease is more common than extracranial disease in the Japanese and Chinese compared with Caucasian populations.[9]

MAORIS AND PACIFIC ISLANDERS

In New Zealand, Maoris have a higher stroke incidence than Europeans, possibly because of differences in risk factors and health-related behaviours.[10]

BLACK POPULATIONS

In the USA and the UK, the prevalence and possibly also incidence of ischaemic and haemorrhagic stroke appear to be higher in black than white populations, possibly because of a higher prevalence of hypertension, diabetes, obesity and sickle-cell trait in Blacks.[11]

2.4 Does the time of day influence stroke incidence?

Ischaemic stroke occurs most frequently in the hour or two after waking in the morning, but it is uncertain whether this applies to intracranial haemorrhage.[12] It is rare for subarachnoid haemorrhage to occur during sleep, but rather during strenuous activities.

2.5 Does the season influence stroke incidence?

Although primary intracerebral haemorrhage is perhaps more likely to occur on cold days, there is little (if any) seasonal variation, at least in temperate climates.[13,14]

However, stroke mortality and hospital admission rates are higher in winter than summer. This might be because the complications of stroke (e.g. pneumonia) are more likely to be fatal in the winter and because it might be more difficult to look after stroke patients at home in cold weather.

2.6 What is the mortality rate of stroke?

The mortality rate of stroke varies from about 20 to 250 per 100 000 population per year (*Table 2.3*). This is because stroke mortality is determined by many factors, such as the incidence of stroke and its aetiological subtypes, the severity and case-fatality of stroke, and the age

TABLE 2.3 Age-standardised stroke mortality (per 100 000 population) between 40 and 69 years of age in 27 countries in 1985[15]

Country	Men Rank	Rate	Women Rank	Rate
Bulgaria	1	249	1	156
Hungary	2	229	2	130
Czechoslovakia	3	177	4	103
Romania	4	172	3	129
Yugoslavia	5	145	5	101
Singapore	6	136	6	92
Japan	7	107	11	60
Scotland	8	99	7	77
Finland	9	98	13	57
Poland	10	96	10	62
Hong Kong	11	94	9	64
Austria	12	90	16	48
Northern Ireland	13	84	8	67
Ireland	14	72	12	59
England and Wales	15	71	14	54
Germany	16	68	19	39
Belgium	17	64	18	41
New Zealand	18	62	15	50
France	19	60	26	28
Australia	20	60	17	45
Denmark	21	55	20	38
Norway	22	55	22	35
Sweden	23	48	24	30
Netherlands	24	47	23	31
United States	25	45	21	35
Canada	26	39	25	28
Switzerland	27	38	27	21

and gender of the population affected by stroke. For example, stroke subtypes with a very low case fatality (e.g. lacunar infarction) contribute little to mortality statistics, whereas subtypes with a high case fatality (e.g. total anterior circulation infarction) do.

Because stroke mortality rises rapidly with age, any assessment of mortality must account for age, and any comparisons in mortality must be age-standardised or, perhaps better, restricted to certain age groups where the diagnosis of stroke is most likely to be correct (age 55–64 years) or where the number of strokes is largest (65–74 years). However, even after adjusting for age, the age-standardised death rate attributed to stroke varies sixfold among developed countries[15] (*Table 2.3*). Very little is known about stroke mortality in the developing world, nor about the relative distribution of stroke subtype mortality among different countries anywhere in the world.

Stroke mortality also varies substantially within countries, and even within large cities such as London. However, part of the variation is probably not real. One reason is because stroke mortality is measured in different places at different times. Because stroke mortality is declining so quickly in many countries (*see Q. 2.8*), the differences may be overestimated (or underestimated) if mortality during different years is compared. Furthermore, some of the variation in mortality could be due to differences, both in time and place, in how death certificates are completed and coded, as well as uncertainties about the population denominators in terms of both age and sex. Indeed, the rate of over- and under-reporting of stroke on death certificates is unacceptably high, even in places such as Framingham that are dedicated to measuring stroke mortality.[16] Despite these potential sources of artefact, the very large observed differences in stroke mortality are probably real, particularly the very high rates reported in eastern Europe and Japan and the very low rates in North America and some, but not all, western European countries (*Table 2.3*).

2.7 What is the overall burden of stroke?

Global significance of stroke as a source of ill-health

- Throughout the world, stroke is the third most common cause of death (after coronary heart disease and all cancers), causing about 4 million deaths in 1990, three-quarters of them in developing countries.[17]
- In the USA in 1994, stroke was the second most common cause of death, the fourth greatest cause of disability-adjusted life years, the fifth highest consumer of days in hospital, the fifth most prevalent major disorder and the eighth most commonly occurring disorder (incidence)[18]
- Stroke accounts for 12% of all deaths in England and Wales, and is the most important single cause of severe disability in people living in their own home.

2.8   Have stroke incidence and mortality changed over time?

Stroke mortality is declining in most places where it has been measured, with the exception of eastern Europe. Indeed, the decline in stroke mortality in some countries is even more rapid than that of coronary heart disease mortality. However, in other countries, such as Australia, there has been a deceleration in the decline (*Fig. 2.2*).

The reason for the decline in stroke mortality is unclear; it may reflect a decline in the incidence of stroke (all types of stroke or just those that are more likely to be fatal, such as haemorrhagic stroke), an improvement in case fatality (survival) after stroke, or an improvement in the accuracy of classifying stroke as a cause of death (e.g. less misclassification of sudden deaths as stroke).[19]

If the incidence of stroke really is declining, the reasons are likely to be environmental and so potentially modifiable (e.g. improved diet, less smoking, greater awareness and control of blood pressure, etc.), rather than genetic.[19]

2.9   Is the burden of stroke likely to decrease or increase?

The burden of stroke is likely to remain substantial for the foreseeable future, if it does not increase. If the incidence of stroke does not fall by at least 2% per year, every year, then the absolute number of incident stroke cases is likely to increase, given the ageing of the population. In developed countries, any increasing burden is likely to fall more on the acute hospital services than on rehabilitation facilities, because strokes are more likely to be fatal in very elderly and disabled people than in younger and fitter patients.[20]

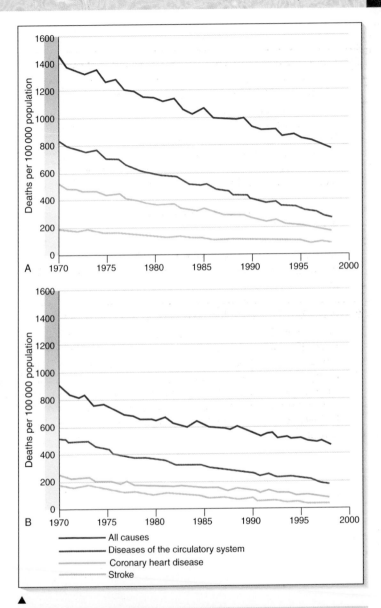

Fig 2.2 Trends in death rates per 100 000 population from all causes (black line), diseases of the circulatory system (dark green line), coronary heart disease (grey line), and stroke (pale green line) for Australian men (**A**) and women (**B**), 1970–98, age-standardised to the Australian population at 30 June 1991. Adapted from Chief Medical Officer's report 1999–2000, Department of Health and Aged Care, Chief Medical Officer Professor Richard Smallwood, Commonwealth of Australia, 2000, pp. 25–26; Copyright Commonwealth of Australia, reproduced with permission.

Diagnosis of stroke and transient ischaemic attack (is it a vascular event?)

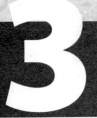

DIAGNOSIS OF STROKE

SYMPTOMS AND SIGNS

3.1   What are focal neurological symptoms and signs?

These are clinical features (*see Box 3.1*) that arise from a disturbance in an identifiable focal area of the brain, for example unilateral weakness (corticospinal tract) or clumsiness (cerebellum), unilateral sensory loss (spinothalamic tract), speech disorder (dominant hemisphere) and double vision (oculomotor pathways). They are caused by focal cerebral ischaemia or haemorrhage.

BOX 3.1   Focal neurological and ocular symptoms

Motor symptoms

Weakness or clumsiness of one side of the body, in whole or in part
    (hemiparesis)
Simultaneous bilateral weakness (paraparesis, quadriparesis)*
Difficulty swallowing (dysphagia)*
Imbalance (ataxia)*

Speech or language disturbances

Difficulty understanding or expressing spoken language (dysphasia)
Difficulty reading (dyslexia) or writing (dysgraphia)
Difficulty calculating (dyscalculia)
Slurred speech (dysarthria)*

Sensory symptoms

Somatosensory

Altered feeling on one side of the body, in whole or in part
    (hemisensory disturbance)

Visual

Loss of vision in one eye, in whole or in part (transient monocular
    blindness or amaurosis fugax)
Loss of vision in the left or the right half or quarter of the visual field
    (hemianopia, quadrantanopia)
Bilateral blindness
Double vision (diplopia)*

Vestibular symptoms

A spinning sensation (vertigo)*

Behavioural or cognitive symptoms

Difficulty dressing, combing hair, cleaning teeth, etc.; geographical
    disorientation; difficulty copying diagrams such as a clock, flower or
    intersecting cubes (visual–spatial–perceptual dysfunction)
Forgetfulness (amnesia)*

---

* As an isolated symptom, this does not necessarily indicate transient focal cerebral ischaemia, because there are many other potential causes.

3.2   What are non-focal neurological symptoms and signs?

Non-focal symptoms (*Box 3.2*) are not neuroanatomically localising: for example, light-headedness, faintness, 'dizziness', generalised weakness, and drop attacks.

BOX 3.2   Non-focal neurological symptoms

Generalised weakness and/or sensory disturbance
Light-headedness
Faintness
'Blackouts' with altered or loss of consciousness or fainting, with or without impaired vision in both eyes
Incontinence of urine or faeces
Confusion
Any of the following symptoms, if isolated*

- A spinning sensation (vertigo)
- Ringing in the ears (tinnitus)
- Difficulty swallowing (dysphagia)
- Slurred speech (dysarthria)
- Double vision (diplopia)
- Loss of balance (ataxia).

* If these symptoms occur in combination, or with focal neurological symptoms, they may indicate focal cerebral ischaemia.

Non-focal symptoms alone should not be interpreted as a transient ischaemic attack (TIA) or stroke because they are seldom due to focal cerebral ischaemia or haemorrhage.

However, the neurological symptoms are not always easy to categorise. Sensory and motor disturbances in a pseudoradicular pattern (such as a wrist drop or tingling in two or three fingers) may reflect focal neurological dysfunction; so may cognitive changes such as amnesia, but these can be difficult to characterise and quantify, particularly when transient. Vertigo, confusion and dysarthria may reflect either focal or non-focal pathology, depending on whether other definitely focal neurological symptoms occur concurrently and whether they occur in the right milieu.

3.3   What are the clinical features (symptoms and signs) of TIA and stroke?

The clinical features of a TIA and stroke are the symptoms and signs of a sudden loss of function of a focal part of the brain (i.e. focal neurological dysfunction; *Table 3.1*). They are determined by the site of the brain that has been damaged by ischaemia or haemorrhage, the extent of the damage and,

> **TABLE 3.1 Neurological symptoms during a transient ischaemic attack (TIA)[1]**
>
> | Symptom | Proportion (%)* |
> | --- | --- |
> | Unilateral weakness, heaviness or clumsiness | 50 |
> | Unilateral sensory symptoms | 35 |
> | Slurred speech (dysarthia) | 23 |
> | Transient monocular blindness | 18 |
> | Difficulty speaking (dysphasia) | 18 |
> | Unsteadiness (ataxia) | 12 |
> | Dizziness (vertigo) | 5 |
> | Homonymous hemianopia | 5 |
> | Double vision (diplopia) | 5 |
> | Bilateral limb weakness | 4 |
> | Difficulty swallowing (dysphagia) | 1 |
> | Crossed motor and sensory loss | 1 |
>
> * Percentage of TIA patients from the Oxfordshire Community Stroke Project (*n* = 184) who experienced each symptom. Many patients had more than one symptom (e.g. weakness as well as sensory loss) and no patients had isolated dysarthria, ataxia, vertigo, diplopia or dysphagia

for patients with TIA, the activities in which the patient was engaged at the time of the TIA. The latter is particularly relevant for patients with a TIA because the neurological symptoms during a brief episode of ischaemia can only reflect what the patient was doing at the time. As many hours of wakefulness are spent in an alert state with eyes open, a keen sensorium, an upright posture and often speaking or reading, it is not surprising that most of the symptoms that patients with TIA experience are a loss of speech and/or a loss of motor, somatosensory and/or visual function on one side of the body. Other, more transient activities, such as swallowing and calculation, are less frequently reported as being affected during a TIA.

3.4 How are focal neurological symptoms and signs elicited quickly and accurately?

- The key points to elicit about focal neurological symptoms are shown in *Box 3.3*.
- As patients may use different terms to describe a symptom, often because of differences in their language or culture, it is important to establish that your interpretation is the same as the patient's. A common example is the interchangeable use of terms such as 'heaviness' and 'numbness' by patients to describe motor and sensory deficits. If you are unsure exactly what the patient means, ask the patient, 'Try to describe what you mean in another way', or paraphrase their description by asking, 'What do you mean by that?'.

> **BOX 3.3 Key points to elicit about focal neurological symptoms**
>
> - *Nature* – was the deficit of the motor, somatosensory, visual and/or other system?
> - *Quality* – was there a loss of function (e.g. weakness or numbness) or a gain of function (e.g. jerking, parastesiae)?
> - *Anatomical distribution* – did the deficit involve the face, arm or leg; or face, arm *and* leg?
> - *Onset* – was it sudden, stuttering or gradual?
> - *Evolution* – e.g. did the deficit recover, stabilise or progress?

- When a patient complains of loss of vision in one eye, the visual loss may be monocular or binocular (e.g. a homonymous hemianopia). If the visual loss was transient, it is important to ask the patient if they had closed each eye in turn during the attack and, if so, if they could be sure whether the blindness involved only one eye, or a part of both eyes. If the visual loss is persistent (i.e. still present), it is crucial to test the visual fields. Although conventional confrontation methods can be difficult, if not impossible, in patients who are drowsy, dysphasic or cognitively impaired, other methods may help determine whether or not there is an abnormality, such as stimulating the patient to look in each direction by doing something 'interesting' in different fields of vision, e.g. getting the patient to follow the examiner's face rather than a finger or a pen.
- Papilloedema is very uncommon in acute stroke; if it is present, suspect other conditions such a brain tumour, subdural haematoma or cerebral venous sinus thrombosis.
- The best screening tests of motor function in the arm and leg are a 'pronator' drift of the outstretched arm from the horizontal with the eyes closed and rapid tapping of the foot against the examiner's hand respectively, but neither test is very specific. The most sensitive clinical test of corticospinal function is probably impairment of fine finger movements (e.g. repetitively tapping the index finger and thumb together) or rapid hand movements.
- Assessing the anatomical extent of the weakness and its functional consequences (i.e. can the patient grip, or walk?) is more important than grading the severity using a motor scale.
- Examination of the sensory system is a notoriously unreliable part of the neurological examination but sensory symptoms are usually quite accurate (particularly for pain and temperature, less so for proprioception), even when there is no deficit identified on examination.

■ Irrespective of the motor and sensory deficit identified by examining the patient in bed, it is essential to see if the patient can sit up, get off the bed and walk – provided there is no risk to patient or clinician. Patients with no motor or sensory deficit on examination in bed may still be unable to walk because of severe gait ataxia, or neglect; cerebellar signs may be missed if the patient's gait is not tested. Indeed, cerebellar infarction may also be misdiagnosed as 'labyrinthitis', or even as upper gastrointestinal disease if nausea and vomiting (secondary to vertigo) are prominent.

■ Disorders of speech and disorders of language are not synonymous: some patients may have slurred speech with normal language function (i.e. a disorder of articulation – dysarthria), while others may have normal articulation (and even speech) with abnormal language function causing difficulty in reading and writing. Because dysphasia is a disturbance of understanding and/or expression of spoken and/or written language, it is important to recognise that reading and writing (as well as speech) are also important language functions that should be assessed. The assessment of language function may be difficult or impossible in those with severe deafness and/or confusion. In these patients, it is important to beware of diagnosing dysphasia, particularly if other symptoms and signs suggest isolated non-dominant hemisphere dysfunction.

■ Visual–spatial-perceptual dysfunction is often best detected by asking the patient to draw a clock and to copy a drawing of intersecting pentagons, and observing how the patient responds to the environment and carries out tasks around the ward, such as interacting with others (does the patient neglect the left hemispace, for instance?), dressing (e.g. putting on a shirt and taking it off), eating, reading a newspaper and writing a sentence.

■ Clinicians assessing stroke patients should be able to identify cognitive disorders in general terms, without having to resort to detailed assessment batteries in order to facilitate diagnosis, localisation of the lesion and basic management. Few cognitive functions are absolutely specific for a single area of the brain and few tests are absolutely specific for a single aspect of higher cerebral function. The terms short- and long-term memory are used loosely by clinicians and often rather differently by neuropsychologists. In patients with stroke, it may be easier to distinguish anterograde amnesia from retrograde amnesia and to observe how the patient is responding to nursing and rehabilitation instructions (are they learning and carrying over new information from day to day?).

3.5 How sudden is the onset of focal neurological symptoms in patients with transient ischaemic attack and stroke?

Most symptoms of an ischaemic event in the brain arise suddenly and are maximal at onset, without intensification or spread. The onset is usually so abrupt that the patient can describe exactly what they were doing at the time of onset. Occasionally, the symptoms may worsen gradually or in a stepwise fashion, but nonetheless their onset is usually sudden. If the patient cannot recall the precise onset of the symptoms but is nevertheless quite aware of them, the diagnosis of TIA and stroke is in doubt.

3.6 Can anything precipitate a transient ischaemic attack or stroke?

The onset of symptoms of TIA and stroke is seldom associated with a precipitating event. Although the circadian variation in stroke onset (with more strokes occurring during the morning, especially between 08.00 and 10.00 hours, than later) suggests some form of predisposition, it remains unexplained. Nevertheless, it is important to ask patients exactly when the symptoms began and what they were doing at the time. This is because symptoms of low flow to the brain or eye ('haemodynamic' TIA/stroke) can be precipitated by a change in posture, neck turning, exposure to bright or white light, a hot bath, a heavy meal (postprandial hypotension), exercise, sexual activity, hypotensive drugs, a general anaesthetic, cardiac arrest or cardioversion, in people with severe carotid and vertebrobasilar occlusive disease and a compromised collateral cerebral and ocular circulation. These symptoms sometimes need to be distinguished from symptoms of hypoglycaemia (precipitated by a large carbohydrate meal) and seizures (provoked by exposure to bright flashing lights).

Vigorous physical activity and coitus have also been associated with haemorrhagic stroke, particularly subarachnoid haemorrhage (SAH). However, apart from isolated case reports, there is no evidence that vigorous physical activity, coitus or stress precipitate TIAs and ischaemic stroke.

Occasionally, the aura of a previously experienced and otherwise unremarkable attack of migraine with aura persists for days or longer, the computed tomography (CT) scan is normal or shows infarction, and the cause is attributed to arterial occlusion that may be due to vasospasm. The simultaneous occurrence of a TIA/stroke and a migraine attack may be:

- coincidental and due to *chance* (both conditions are common; the prevalence of migraine in the general population is about 10% and ischaemic cerebrovascular disease is about 0.8%);
- *causal* (migraine may predispose to cerebral ischaemia by leading to platelet activation, arteriolar constriction and dehydration, or cerebral ischaemia may trigger off a migraine attack);

- a *misdiagnosis* (e.g. carotid or vertebral artery dissection may cause headache and a neurological deficit due to thromboembolism that is misinterpreted as migraine); or
- a syndrome suggestive of stroke or migraine that is a *manifestation of another disease* such as mitochondrial encephalomyopathy with lactic acidosis and stroke-like episodes (MELAS) or an arteriovenous malformation.

The last trimester of pregnancy and the puerperium is a time when otherwise healthy young women may be predisposed to stroke as a result of paradoxical embolism from the venous system of the legs or pelvis, intracranial haemorrhage due to eclampsia, a ruptured arteriovenous malformation, or intracranial venous sinus thrombosis.

DIAGNOSIS OF TRANSIENT ISCHAEMIC ATTACK

3.7 How is the diagnosis of TIA made?

Symptoms indicating a TIA

The diagnosis of TIA is clinical, and rests on the description by the patient or an eye-witness of symptoms:

- of *loss of focal* neurological or monocular function (*Table 3.1*)
- of *sudden onset*
- that are *maximal at onset*, without spread or intensification
- that are thought to be due to *inadequate blood supply* to the brain or eye as a result of arterial thrombosis or embolism, associated with disease of the arteries, heart or blood
- that resolve within 24 hours.

Useful websites can be found at the following locations:

http://www.strokeaha.org
http://www.dcn.ed.ac.uk/spgm

The report of an eye-witness is of great importance, particularly if there is any impairment of recall or consciousness and if the symptoms and signs have resolved.

3.8 How reliable and accurate is the clinical diagnosis of TIA by general practitioners?

The clinical diagnosis of TIA by general practitioners (GPs) is not very accurate. In the Oxfordshire Community Stroke Project (OCSP), 512 patients were referred by their GP or attending hospital doctor with a

---

TABLE 3.2 Diagnsis of suspected TIA by general practitioners in the community (*n* = 512)[1]

	No. of patients (%)
TIA	195 (38)
Not TIA	317 (62)
Migraine	52 (10)
Syncope	48 (9)
Possible TIA*	46 (9)
'Funny turn'[†]	45 (9)
Isolated vertigo	33 (6)
Epilepsy	29 (6)
Transient global amnesia	17 (3)
Lone bilateral blindness[+]	14 (3)
Isolated diplopia	4 (0.8)
Drop attack[§]	3 (0.6)
Intracranial meningioma	2 (0.4)
Miscellaneous[¶]	24 (5)

* Possible TIA was diagnosed in patients in whom the clinical features were not sufficiently clear to make a diagnosis of definite TIA or anything else.
[†] 'Funny turn' was used to describe transient episodes of only non-focal symptoms not due to any identifiable condition (e.g. isolated and transient confusion).
[+] Lone bilateral blindness was later considered to be a TIA, after following these patients and noting their similar prognosis to patients with definite TIA.
[§] Suddent, transient loss of postural tone causing a fall to the ground.
[¶] For example, hypoglycaemia, entrapment neuropathy, demyelination, subdural haematoma, psychogenic.

---

diagnosis of possible TIA of whom 317 (62%) were considered by the OCSP neurologists *not* to have had a TIA but to have suffered from something else[1] (*Table 3.2*). In another study, 30% of the patients originally classified by their doctors as having TIAs were reclassified as not having TIAs when their records were reviewed by a stroke specialist.[2] However, the accuracy of the diagnosis of TIA by GPs is being compared in these instances only with the diagnosis of TIA by a neurologist. So, how accurate is the diagnosis of TIA by a neurologist? (*See Q. 3.9*)

3.9 How reliable and accurate is the clinical diagnosis of TIA by neurologists?

The problem of accurately diagnosing TIA is not unique to general practitioners and hospital doctors. Experienced neurologists also show considerable interobserver variability in the diagnosis of TIA. Kraaijeveld et al[3] investigated the interobserver agreement for the diagnosis of cerebral TIA among eight senior and interested neurologists from the same department, who interviewed 56 patients with suspected TIA in alternating

TABLE 3.3 Interobserver variation in the diagnosis of TIA

| | Neurologist 1 | | |
	TIA, Yes	TIA, No	Total
Neurologist 2			
TIA, Yes	36	4	40
TIA, No	4	12	16
Total	40	16	56
Observed agreement			86%
Agreement expected by chance			59%
Agreement over and above chance (κ statistic)			65% (0.65)

Eight neurologists; 56 patients with possible TIA.

pairs. The diagnosis was based on internationally accepted criteria. The agreement rates were corrected for chance (kappa statistic). Both neurologists agreed that 36 patients had a TIA and 12 had not, but they disagreed about 8 patients ($\kappa = 0.65$; for perfect agreement $\kappa = 1.0$) (*Table 3.3*). Therefore, the interobserver reliability of the diagnosis of TIA is not very good.

3.10* Why is the clinical diagnosis of TIA unreliable?

The clinical diagnosis of TIA is unreliable because there is no diagnostic test, and the diagnosis depends entirely on the history – i.e. on an accurate:

- recollection and communication of the symptoms by the patient (which is a difficulty if the patient delays going to the doctor after an attack or is forgetful – a particular problem in the elderly)
- interpretation of the symptoms by the doctor (several studies have shown that clinicians differ in the interpretation of even isolated elements of the history,[2,4]) and
- application of the symptoms to the diagnostic criteria for TIA (which lack detail) (*see Q. 3.7*).

The likelihood and accuracy of the diagnosis of a TIA increases with the abruptness of the onset of symptoms, the certainty that the neurological symptoms were focal, and the age and vascular risk factor profile of the patient. If the patient is young and free of vascular risk factors, the probability of a TIA is small.

3.11 What are the differential diagnoses of TIA of the brain?
MIGRAINE AURA (WITH OR WITHOUT HEADACHE)
- Young to middle-aged patients
- Positive symptoms (visual scintillations, tingling)

■ Spread of symptoms to adjacent areas over minutes
■ Symptoms resolve gradually and usually within 20–60 minutes
■ Headache (often unilateral and pulsatile) and nausea usually accompany or follow the neurological symptoms
■ Past or family history of migraine is common
■ Vascular risk factors are uncommon
■ Recurrences are usually stereotyped and may be reduced with migraine prophylaxis.

PARTIAL (FOCAL) EPILEPTIC SEIZURES
■ Positive symptoms (e.g. limb jerking, tingling)
■ Symptoms arise over seconds to 1–2 minutes (not abruptly)
■ Symptoms spread or march to adjacent areas over several seconds
■ Symptoms usually resolve quickly within a few minutes but can be prolonged for hours
■ Antecedent partial seizure symptoms may be present (e.g. epigastric discomfort, nausea)
■ Impaired awareness (i.e. complex partial seizure) or secondary generalisation with a tonic–clonic convulsion or loss of consciousness may occur
■ Persistent focal neurological signs may be present after symptoms resolve
■ Recurrences are usually stereotyped and respond to antiepileptic drugs.

TRANSIENT GLOBAL AMNESIA
■ Abrupt onset of loss of anterograde episodic memory for verbal and non-verbal material
■ Usually accompanied by repetitive questioning
■ Resolves within 24 hours (and usually a few hours) leaving a dense amnesic gap for the duration of the attack
■ No clouding of consciousness, loss of personal identity or ability to recognise familiar individuals or places, other focal neurological symptoms, or epileptic features
■ Recurrent attacks are exceptional
■ The diagnosis is all but impossible if there is no witness available.

LABYRINTHINE DISORDERS
(Benign recurrent vertigo, benign paroxysmal positional vertigo, acute labyrinthitis)

■ Vertigo is the only neurological symptom (with secondary nausea and ataxia).

METABOLIC DISORDERS
(Hypoglycaemia, hyperglycaemia, hypercalcaemia, hyponatraemia)

■ Hypoglycaemic attacks may recur at regular times and can be excluded with appropriately timed tests of blood glucose levels.

HYPERVENTILATION, ANXIETY OR PANIC ATTACKS, SOMATISATION DISORDER

■ Consider reproducing the symptoms (e.g. forced hyperventilation).

INTRACRANIAL STRUCTURAL LESION
(Meningioma, tumour, giant aneurysm, arteriovenous malformation, chronic subdural haematoma)

■ Usually cause recurrent stereotyped events; exclude with CT or MRI of the brain.

ACUTE DEMYELINATION (MULTIPLE SCLEROSIS)
■ Usually subacute onset in young adults; exclude with MRI of the brain.

SYNCOPE
■ A non-focal neurological symptom
■ Often a precipitating circumstance.

DROP ATTACKS
■ Usually in middle-aged women
■ Onset when standing or walking
■ Legs give way and patient falls to the ground with otherwise preserved neurological function and consciousness throughout
■ Recovery is immediate unless the patient is injured.

MONONEUROPATHY/RADICULOPATHY
■ Lower motor neurone signs.

MYASTHENIA GRAVIS
■ Fatiguability.

CATAPLEXY
■ Brief muscle weakness precipitated by excitement or emotion (e.g. laughter).

3.12   What are the differential diagnoses of TIA of the eye (amaurosis fugax)?

RETINAL DYSFUNCTION

Vascular

- ■ *Retinal migraine* – gradual 'build-up' of transient monocular visual impairment that is usually incomplete and associated with 'positive' visual symptoms (e.g. scintillations) lasting up to 1 hour. A pulsatile headache or orbital pain may coexist.
- ■ *Anterior-middle cranial fossa dural arteriovenous malformation* – may rarely cause transient monocular blindness (TMB), probably because of transient lowering of retinal arterial pressure associated with shunting of blood away from the ophthalmic artery to the malformation.
- ■ *Central or branch retinal vein thrombosis* – may present with attacks of TMB but the funduscopic appearance is characteristic, with engorged retinal veins and multiple retinal haemorrhages (*Fig. 3.1*).

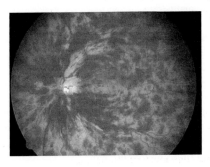

Fig 3.1 Fundus of a patient with central retinal vein thrombosis showing the characteristic engorged retinal veins and multiple retinal haemorrhages. Reproduced with permission from Warlow et al. *Stroke: a practical guide to management.* 2nd edn. Oxford: Blackwell Science Ltd; 2000.

- ■ *Retinal haemorrhage* – if small or located in the periphery of the retina may cause sudden loss of vision in one eye.

Non-vascular

- ■ *Paraneoplastic retinopathy* – painless, brief (seconds to minutes) episodes of monocular dimming of the central field of vision, and overwhelming visual glare and photosensitivity when exposed to bright light. Ophthalmoscopy usually reveals an attenuated calibre of retinal arterioles; electroretinography demonstrates abnormal cone- and rod-mediated responses; and antiretinal antibodies may be present in the serum. Progressive visual loss evolves, during which time a small-cell carcinoma of the lung often declares itself.
- ■ *Phosphenes* – flashes of light and coloured spots that are induced by eye movement in a dark environment and occur in the absence of

luminous stimuli. They may occur following mechanical pressure on the normal eyeball (stimulating the retina), in a healthy dark-adapted closed eye after a voluntary eye movement/saccade (flick phosphene), or with disease of the visual system at any site (e.g. recovery phase of optic neuritis).

■ *Lightning streaks of Moore* – brief, recurrent, stereotyped vertical flashes of light in the temporal visual field of one eye, elicited by eye movement. Common in elderly people when in a dark environment. They are a photopsia (subjective sensation of sparks or flashes of light), which may be caused by collapse of the posterior vitreous with its detachment from the retina (with age), and triggered by the transient mechanical forces of eye movement. Benign.

■ *Chorioretinitis.*

OPTIC NERVE DISORDERS

Vascular

■ *Anterior ischaemic optic neuropathy* due to arteritis (e.g. giant-cell), atherothrombosis or malignant arterial hypertension – may cause abrupt onset of TMB but usually the visual disturbance is permanent and in the form of an altitudinal field defect (loss of either the upper or lower half of the field of one eye) rather than 'as if a curtain has descended or ascended over the whole eye', because the optic nerve is supplied by an upper and lower division of the posterior ciliary artery. Shortly after the onset of blindness, funduscopy may reveal distended veins, a swollen optic disc (or part of the disc), variable pallor of the disc, flame-shaped haemorrhages at or near the disc and, occasionally, cotton wool spots *(Fig. 3.2)*. Systemic upset, tender temporal arteries and a raised erythrocyte sedimentation rate (ESR) are clues to arteritis, and an increased blood pressure and ophthalmoscopic features of retinal arteriolar disease, optic disc oedema and retinal haemorrhages point to the diagnosis of malignant hypertension.

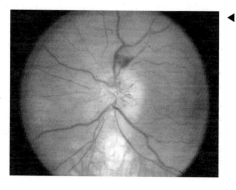

◄ **Fig 3.2** Fundus of a patient with anterior ischaemic optic neuropathy showing swelling and variable pallor of part of the optic disc, flame-shaped haemorrhages near the disc, distended veins and cotton-wool spots. Reproduced with permission from Warlow et al. *Stroke: a practical guide to management*. 2nd edn. Oxford: Blackwell Science Ltd; 2000.

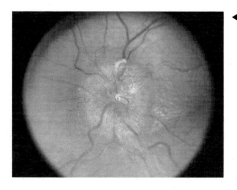

Fig 3.3 Fundus of a patient with papilloedema showing swelling and congestion of the optic nerve head, loss of the physiological optic cup and distension of the retinal veins. Reproduced from Warlow et al. *Stroke: a practical guide to management.* 2nd edn. Oxford: Blackwell Science Ltd; 2000.

Non-vascular

■ *Papilloedema (Fig. 3.3)* – patients with papilloedema from any cause may experience transient visual blurring or obscuration, with or without photopsia. The visual loss in chronic papilloedema is often postural, occurring as patients rise from bed or chair, and may involve either eye alone or both eyes together. The explanation may be transient optic nerve ischaemia caused by a relative decrease in orbital blood flow secondary to raised cerebrospinal fluid (CSF) pressure in the subarachnoid space around the optic nerve with an increase in pressure in the veins draining the optic nerve head.

■ *Optic neuritis and Uhthoff's phenomenon* – patients with optic nerve demyelination (most commonly due to multiple sclerosis) may experience transiently decreased vision in one or both eyes, usually after exercise or exposure to heat (Uhthoff's phenomenon).

■ *Dysplastic coloboma.*

EYE AND ORBIT

Transient changes in the ocular media or intraocular pressure can cause transient monocular visual disturbance but the most common causes (listed below) can usually be excluded from the ophthalmological examination.

■ Anterior (aqueous humour) chamber and posterior chamber (vitreous) haemorrhage

■ Raised intraocular pressure (glaucoma) – may cause transient monocular visual impairment but is usually associated with recurrent attacks of pain in the eye and forehead, which may be precipitated by sitting in the dark, mydriatics or emotional upset. Other features include cloudiness of the cornea, discoloration of the iris, a dilated pupil and circumcorneal injection. An arcuate scotoma and pallid cupped disc are characteristic of narrow-angle glaucoma, which is often familial. Tonometry is necessary to confirm raised intraocular pressure

■ Reversible diabetic cataract
■ Lens subluxation
■ Orbital tumour (e.g. optic nerve sheath meningioma) – may cause gaze-evoked loss of vision but the time course of the blindness is limited to the duration of gaze in the affected direction: the visual acuity usually returns to normal within about 30 seconds of the eye returning to the primary position of gaze. The loss of vision possibly relates to compression of blood vessels surrounding or supplying the optic nerve.

3.13 What is the role of CT imaging of brain in the differential diagnosis of TIA?

The main purpose of cranial CT or MRI in patients with suspected TIA is to detect an underlying structural intracranial lesion, e.g. arteriovenous malformation, meningioma, subdural haematoma (*Fig. 3.4*), which may present like a TIA. It is not to detect low-density lesions (presumed infarcts) or to exclude primary intracerebral haemorrhage (PICH), as in patients with stroke (*see Q. 3.23*), because definite PICH only very rarely causes focal neurological symptoms lasting less than 24 hours.

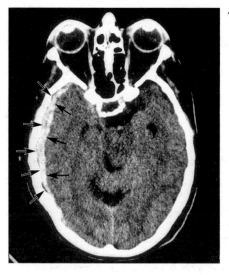

◀ **Fig 3.4** Plain cranial CT scan showing a rim of high signal adjacent to the right temporal and occipital cortex due to a subdural haematoma (arrows).

3.14 What is the yield of CT brain imaging in patients with suspected TIA?

Limited data indicate that the yield of CT for detecting structural lesions is about 1% in patients with suspected TIA.[5] With such a low yield, routine CT imaging of every patient who has had a single TIA must be considered very carefully. The small minority of 'TIA' patients with structural intracranial lesions who will be missed by not performing CT will probably continue to have symptoms (and so return to the doctor) and their outcome is unlikely to be altered by a short delay in diagnosis.

It seems that the small yield of structural brain lesions from CT is almost always in patients with carotid territory 'TIAs' and there is some evidence that performing CT in patients with vertebrobasilar territory TIAs and transient monocular blindness is a waste of resources.[6]

Data on the cost-effectiveness of CT and MRI in patients with TIA are very few and there is a need for a methodologically sound, prospective, multicentre study of this question, particularly in view of the considerable cost implications of a policy of 'CT or MRI for all suspected TIA patients'.

3.15 Which patients with suspected TIA should have CT brain imaging?

Brain imaging by CT should probably be reserved for patients:

- with more than one suspected TIA of the brain, particularly if they are in the carotid territory
- being considered for carotid endarterectomy (to avoid operating on someone with a symptomatic meningioma, for example).[7]

3.16 Should patients with TIA have a plain or a contrast CT brain scan?

Computed tomography for patients with a suspected TIA should initially be a non-contrast study.

3.17 When is a contrast CT or MRI brain scan indicated in patients with a TIA?

Contrast CT or MRI and MR angiography is indicated if a brain tumour, giant aneurysm or arteriovenous malformation (AVM) is suspected as the cause of transient focal neurological symptoms (*Fig. 3.5*). MRI is also indicated for patients who continue to have suspected vertebrobasilar TIAs despite optimal medical therapy, and in whom cranial CT is unhelpful and a structural abnormality in the posterior fossa is still suspected. Although more expensive, MRI of the posterior fossa (and also the cerebral hemispheres) is superior to CT for detecting infarcts and, of more relevance for management, demyelinating and structural lesions. However, even MRI is not 100% sensitive in detecting brainstem infarcts.

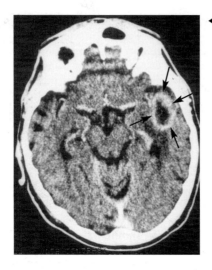

◀ **Fig 3.5** Cranial CT scan with contrast showing a contrast-enhancing rim around a brain tumour in the left temporal lobe of a patient who presented with sudden transient speech disturbance that was initially misdiagnosed as a TIA. The patient was originally considered for left carotid endarterectomy because carotid ultrasonography (performed before CT) revealed 70% stenosis of the left internal carotid artery, which was initially misinterpreted as being the cause of the symptoms.

3.18 What is the role of EEG in patients with suspected TIA?

Electroencephalography (EEG) is indicated in patients with suspected TIA when the clinical diagnosis of TIA is in doubt and partial (focal or localisation-related) seizures are a possibility (e.g. transient positive neurological symptoms that progress, with or without loss of consciousness).[8] About 35% of all patients with epilepsy consistently have epileptiform discharges on the waking interictal EEG, 50% do so on some occasions with repeated sleep-deprived recordings, and about 15% never do. These figures vary according to the type of epilepsy; among patients who present with a first seizure, epileptiform abnormalities on the EEG are present in a higher proportion with idiopathic generalised seizures than with partial seizures.

The results of EEG should be interpreted cautiously.

Besides the modest sensitivity of EEG in distinguishing epileptic seizures from non-epileptic events such as TIA (i.e. only a modest proportion of patients with epilepsy have an abnormal EEG), further difficulty arises as a result of the poor specificity of EEG abnormalities (all too frequently patients with non-epileptic events such as TIA are reported to have an abnormal EEG).

DIAGNOSIS OF STROKE

3.19 How is the diagnosis of stroke made?

> **Symptoms and signs in the diagnosis of stroke**
>
> Like the diagnosis of TIA, the diagnosis of stroke is also clinical and depends crucially on an accurate history, taken from the patient, carer or witness. To decide whether the symptoms and signs are due to a vascular event of the brain, ensure that:
>
> - the neurological symptoms and signs are *focal* (i.e. neuroanatomically localising) rather than non-focal
> - the focal neurological symptoms are *negative* in quality (i.e. loss of function) rather than positive (i.e. muscle paralysis rather than jerking, numbness rather than pins and needles, blindness rather than visual hallucinations)
> - the onset of the focal neurological symptoms was *sudden*
> - the focal neurological symptoms were *maximal at onset* (i.e. evolving over minutes in all of the affected body parts) rather than progressive (evolving over hours to days and migrating from one body part to another).

Useful websites can be found at the following locations:

http://www.strokeaha.org
http://www.dcn.ed.ac.uk/spgm

If all these criteria are met, the likelihood of a vascular disturbance (ischaemia or haemorrhage) of brain function is high. The likelihood is even greater if the 'milieu' is appropriate (e.g. an elderly patient with prolonged exposure to several vascular risk factors). About 80% of stroke patients have at least one vascular risk factor, and most are elderly; stroke is uncommon (but not that rare) in young people.

The exception to these criteria is the minority of patients with SAH who present with headache but have no focal neurological symptoms or signs (neck stiffness is not invariable and may not occur for several hours). As the clinical features of SAH may differ substantially from those of intracerebral haemorrhage and infarction, they are discussed separately (*see Q. 3.47*).

3.20 How accurate is the clinical diagnosis of stroke?

The clinical diagnosis of stroke is accurate about 80–85% of the time, depending on the time since stroke onset and the experience of the examiner.[9,10]

3.21 What are the common pitfalls in the clinical diagnosis of stroke?

The clinical diagnosis of stroke is often most difficult in the hyperacute phase (e.g. within 6 hours of onset) when symptoms and signs may change rapidly. This and other difficulties in the diagnosis are shown in *Box 3.4*.

BOX 3.4 Pitfalls in the diagnosis of stroke

■ Assessment is taking place within 6 hours of onset (i.e. in the hyperacute phase)
■ Onset of symptoms is uncertain (e.g. because of coma, dysphasia, confusion, lack of witnesses)
■ Neuroanatomical localising value of the symptoms is uncertain (e.g. confusion, amnesia, coma)
■ Symptoms are positive in nature (e.g. movement disorders such as hemiballismus caused by lesions of the subthalamic nucleus of Luys in the midbrain)
■ Symptoms are progressing (rather than recovering) over hours or even days
■ Patient does not recognise that there is a problem at all (e.g. patients with isolated visual–spatial–perceptual dysfunction such as hemispatial neglect or geographical disorientation – the so-called 'inobvious stroke').

In these situations the clinical diagnosis of stroke is less certain and further investigations are usually required quite urgently to exclude alternative diagnoses that may require different and immediate treatment (e.g. hypoglycaemia, non-convulsive epileptic seizures, brain infection, subdural haematoma) (*see Q. 3.22*).

3.22 What are the differential diagnoses of stroke?

Differential diagnosis of stroke (in order of frequency of occurrence in general practice)

■ Metabolic/toxic encephalopathy (hypoglycaemia, non-ketotic hyperglycaemia, hyponatraemia, Wernicke–Korsakoff syndrome, hepatic encephalopathy, alcohol and drug intoxication)
■ Functional/non-neurological (e.g. hysteria)
■ Epileptic seizure (postictal Todd's paresis) or non-convulsive seizures
■ Hemiplegic migraine
■ Structural intracranial lesion (e.g. subdural haematoma, brain tumour, arteriovenous malformation).

- Encephalitis (e.g. herpes simplex virus) or brain abscess
- Head injury
- Peripheral nerve lesion(s)
- Hypertensive encephalopathy
- Multiple sclerosis
- Creutzfeldt–Jakob disease.

3.23 What is the role of CT brain imaging in the diagnosis of stroke (vs not-stroke)?

- To exclude non-vascular intracranial pathology (e.g. subdural haematoma, brain tumour) as the cause of the focal neurological symptoms and signs.
- To confirm the presence of recent cerebral infarction, or intracerebral or SAH which is relevant to the clinical presentation.

3.24 What is the yield of early CT of the brain in identifying a relevant stroke lesion?

Early CT imaging of the brain, done within the first few days of stroke, identifies intracerebral haemorrhage in all cases, SAH in about 95–97% and cerebral infarction in about two-thirds. The yield for cerebral infarction may be lower because:

- the CT has been done early
- the infarct is too small to be imaged in this way
- the infarct is obscured by artefact (particularly in the posterior fossa)
- the resolution of the CT is not very good.

However, even within 5 hours of symptom onset, CT will show abnormalities of cerebral infarction in about 50% of cases.[11]

3.25 Does a normal CT scan mean that the patient has not had a stroke?

No. The absence of a visible infarct on CT does not mean that the patient has not had a stroke. A patient with a clinical diagnosis of stroke and an early CT brain scan that is either normal or shows a relevant hypodense lesion, consistent with infarction (*see Qs. 3.28–3.32*), is classified as having an ischaemic stroke.

3.26 What do primary intracerebral haemorrhage and subarachnoid haemorrhage look like on CT?

Intracerebral and subarachnoid blood appear immediately as a white area of high density on CT in the brain (*Fig. 3.6*) or subarachnoid space (*Fig. 3.7*) respectively.

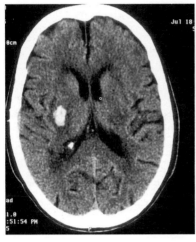

▲

Fig 3.6 Plain cranial CT scan showing a round area of high density (whiteness) in the right posterior putamen (basal ganglia), representing an acute haemorrhage.

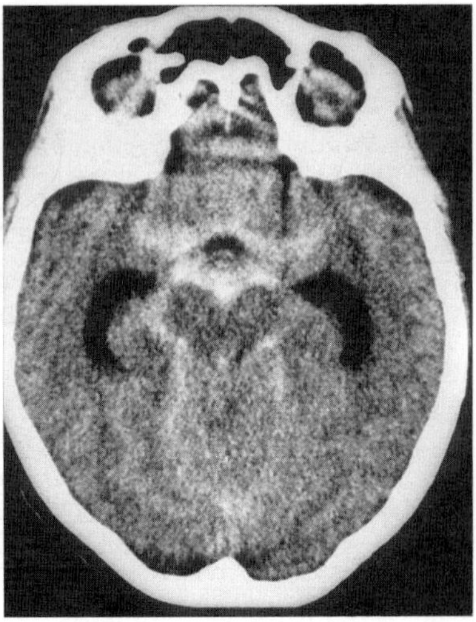

▲

Fig 3.7 Plain cranial CT scan showing high density (whiteness) due to blood in the subarachnoid space around the base of the brain.

3.27 Does the appearance of the haemorrhage evolve with time on CT brain scan?

Yes. With time, the CT appearance of a white, hyperdense area of haemorrhage becomes less dense and, after a few days to a few weeks (depending on its size), it becomes isodense with surrounding brain tissue ('fogging') and may be difficult to see. It is the smaller haemorrhages that may become isodense within days.[12] Thereafter the haemorrhage becomes hypodense and may be mistaken for an old infarct (*Fig. 3.8*). This is one of the main reasons why CT must be done early, within the first few days of stroke: to identify intracerebral haemorrhage reliably if it has occurred.

3.28 What does a very recent cerebral infarct look like on CT brain imaging?

In the hyperacute stage of an ischaemic stroke (i.e. within the first few hours), the CT brain scan often appears normal. However, within 3 hours of onset of middle cerebral artery territory infarction there are usually subtle changes in the ischaemic brain parenchyma, which are easily

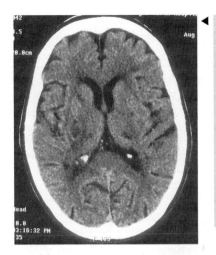

Fig 3.8 Plain cranial CT scan of the patient in *Figure 3.6*, performed 14 days after the initial CT scan, now showing only a small area of low intensity, which looks like infarction but actually represents resolution of haemorrhage, in the right posterior putamen. A follow-up scan was performed because the original tomogram was missing, and the radiologist described the lesion as an infarct in the right posterior putamen. This emphasises the importance of performing CT early in patients with suspected stroke, within the first week (and preferably within the first hours to days), in order to document the pathology clearly and optimise diagnosis and treatment.

overlooked by the inexperienced or untrained observer. These include loss of outline (obscuration) of the lentiform nucleus and loss of visualisation of the insular ribbon, due to loss of normal grey–white matter differentiation (at the basal ganglia–white matter and cortex–white matter interfaces)[13] (*Fig. 3.9*). Other features include effacement of the overlying cortical sulci and compression of the lateral ventricle due to focal brain swelling caused by cerebral oedema, and hypodensity. Indeed, loss of grey–white matter

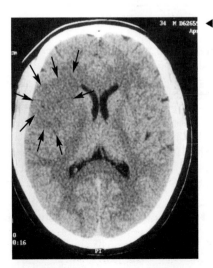

Fig 3.9 Plain cranial CT scan performed 3 hours after onset of acute right frontal lobe ischaemic stroke, showing loss of outline (obscuration) of the right lentiform nucleus, loss of visualisation of the insular ribbon, effacement of the overlying cortical sulci and compression of the lateral ventricle due to focal brain swelling.

differentiation, loss of basal ganglia outline and loss of the insular ribbon are all forms of hypodensity, in which the ischaemic grey matter first becomes hypodense with respect to the normal grey matter.

3.29 What is the hyperdense artery sign on CT brain imaging?

The hyperdense artery sign is another early, but indirect, radiological sign of ischaemic stroke. In some patients, the occluded intracranial cerebral artery (e.g. middle cerebral artery or basilar artery) may appear more hyperdense than the other intracranial arteries owing to acute thrombosis or embolism in the artery[14] (*Fig. 3.10*). However, the reliability of this sign is uncertain. It may be valid in young patients, in whom the arteries tend to be less calcified, but elderly patients frequently have calcified artery walls, particularly around the carotid siphon, which may produce a similar appearance. Of course, evidence of calcification persists on rescanning, but not the hyperdense artery sign, which disappears in a few days.[15]

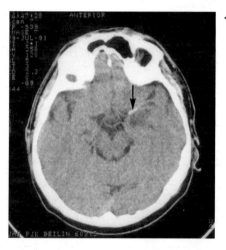

◀ **Fig 3.10** Plain cranial CT scan showing a linear area of high density, representing blood clot (thrombus), in the origin of the left middle cerebral artery.

Therefore, the hyperdense artery sign is probably a reasonably reliable indicator of an occluded cerebral artery when the hyperdensity is visible at a distance from the carotid siphon, for example in the proximal middle cerebral artery (MCA) or its branches, and particularly in younger patients.[16,17] An absent sign is certainly not a reliable indicator of a patent artery.

3.30 Does the appearance of a cerebral infarct on CT evolve with time?

Yes. As the infarct 'progresses' during the first few days, it becomes more clearly demarcated and more hypodense (black) and well defined. The ischaemic white matter becomes hypodense with respect to normal white matter, and the abnormal grey matter becomes even more hypodense, so that overall the whole lesion appears darker than the surrounding brain.[18]

Swelling of the infarct is usually maximal around days 3–5 and this gradually subsides during the second and third week. However, occasionally infarct swelling can occur very rapidly, within the first 24 hours, to cause brain herniation, but generally only with very extensive infarcts. The amount of infarct swelling and the rate at which it appears vary between patients, for reasons that are not well understood.

Small infarcts probably appear later than large ones, because there is less tissue altering its density, so that lacunar infarcts are less likely to show up in the first 24 hours and sometimes do not do so at all. Small infarcts in the brainstem and cerebellum are particularly difficult to visualise with CT because of artefacts arising from the petrous bones; this is probably less problematic with modern scanning technology and thinner scan sections.[19]

3.31 What is 'fogging' on CT brain images?

The so-called 'fogging effect' usually occurs during the second week after stroke onset, when the hypodense infarct on CT gradually increases in density, sometimes becoming isodense.[20] The infarct is then indistinguishable from normal brain and may be overlooked at this time.[21] It is less pronounced in large infarcts, but may lead to underestimation of infarct size. It does not occur in all infarcts and the timing of occurrence after stroke onset may vary. The 'fogging effect' may last for up to 2 weeks and then the infarct becomes progressively more hypodense.

3.32 What does an old cerebral infarct look like on CT?

Old brain infarcts are usually atrophic, very hypodense (similar to CSF) and sharply demarcated from surrounding normal brain (*Fig. 3.11*).

Although these features generally make it possible to 'age' infarcts, it is not always possible to tell with absolute certainty how old an infarct is. It is important to bear this in mind when trying to ascribe particular clinical symptoms to lesions seen on CT.

3.33 What features of a low-density lesion on CT distinguish arterial infarcts from other pathologies?

Brain infarcts caused by arterial occlusion are usually easy to diagnose from their site, shape and density, in association with appropriate clinical features. However, other pathologies can occasionally produce similar appearances, which may be confusing.

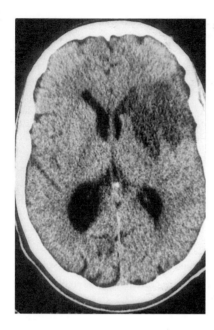

◀ **Fig 3.11** Plain cranial CT scan showing an old brain infarct as a discrete area of low density in the territory of supply of a branch of the upper division of the left middle cerebral artery.

VENOUS INFARCTS

Venous infarcts, although uncommon, are frequently misdiagnosed as arterial infarcts, intracerebral haemorrhages or tumours on CT. Many are overlooked because the possibility of venous infarction is not even considered. They are typically of low density and may be wedge-shaped, like arterial infarcts, but the key differentiating features are:

- they often do not quite fit the usual site of an arterial infarct
- they are much more swollen for their size than an equivalent-sized arterial infarct
- there may be swelling in the hemisphere beyond the low-density area
- they often contain haemorrhage.

The haemorrhage is typically in the centre of the low-density area and may be patchy and finger-like in distribution, whereas in arterial infarcts the haemorrhage is usually around the edges. The high density of a thrombosed cortical vein or sinus may also be visible (hyperdense vein sign). After intravenous contrast, there may be an 'empty delta' sign in the venous sinus and serpiginous enhancement at the edges of the infarct (*Fig. 3.12*).

VIRAL ENCEPHALITIS

Viral encephalitis due to herpes simplex virus is usually focal and typically involves the medial temporal lobes. However, it is sometimes more

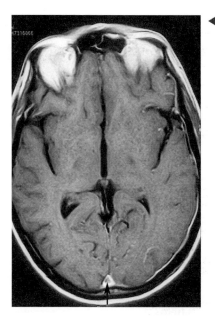

Fig 3.12 MRI brain scan, T1-weighted image, with gadolinium contrast, showing contrast as a white hyperdensity in the torcula (venous sinus) and a filling defect, due to thrombus, as a black, low density in the torcula (arrow), in a patient with cerebral venous sinus thrombosis.

widespread, affecting the frontal and temporal lobes, or temporal–parietal lobes, and can look exactly like an infarct (*Fig. 3.13*). In these cases the clues to encephalitis are usually associated clinical features of subacute

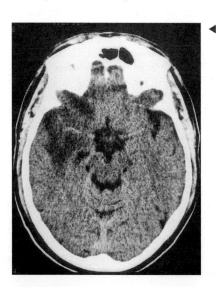

Fig 3.13 Plain cranial CT scan showing an area of low density in the right inferior frontal and anteromedial temporal lobes that was originally diagnosed as a right middle cerebral artery territory infarct but later confirmed as herpes simplex virus encephalitis.

(as opposed to acute) onset, fever and progression (if not treated with aciclovir) rather than improvement. It is essential that the CT scan is reviewed with all the clinical information and, if in doubt, other diagnostic tests are done, such as EEG, CSF and MRI.

PURULENT CEREBRITIS

Purulent cerebritis can look like an infarct, although the lesion is usually not wedge-shaped and involves more white matter than cortex; the clinical picture should allow the distinction to be made.

TUMOURS

Occasionally, a metastasis to the cerebral cortex may mimic an infarct on CT, particularly if there is a lot of white matter oedema. However, metastases are lower in density than an infarct, and administration of intravenous contrast may reveal an enhancing cortical nodule (*Fig. 3.5*). If there is still doubt, repeat the CT scan a few weeks later, because infarcts usually get smaller whereas tumours usually stay the same size or increase in size.

3.34 Does intravenous contrast help?

The only indication for performing CT with intravenous contrast in a patient with suspected stroke is when the plain (non-contrast) CT scan, and clinical features, are suggestive of a structural intracranial lesion mimicking a stroke, such as a brain tumour, abscess or AVM. These lesions enhance with contrast (*Fig. 3.5*).

If the patient has indeed had an ischaemic stroke, the contrast usually has little effect on the appearance of the infarct in the first week after onset. However, in the second and third weeks more striking contrast enhancement occurs, frequently corresponding with the time of maximal blood–brain barrier breakdown and positivity of radioisotope scans. The mechanism is probably a combination of blood–brain barrier breakdown, neovascularisation and impaired autoregulation, and the resulting appearance on CT is referred to as 'luxury perfusion'.[22] The tendency to enhance with contrast gradually resolves over the following few weeks.

3.35 What does haemorrhagic transformation of the infarct look like on CT brain scan?

Recent haemorrhage in the infarct produces areas of increased density relative to both normal brain and infarcted tissue, and presumably contributes to any swelling (*Fig. 3.14*).

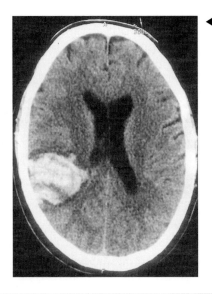

Fig 3.14 Plain cranial CT scan showing an area of patchy high signal (whiteness) due to patchy haemorrhage, with an area of low attenuation (darkness) due to infarction in a wedge-shaped distribution involving the cortex and subcortex of the right parietal lobe. This is commonly caused by embolic occlusion of a branch of the middle cerebral artery. The source of the embolus is frequently the heart or the proximal large arteries (e.g. aortic arch, extracranial internal carotid artery). The patient's earlier CT scan, showing fresh infarction, is *Fig. 6.1.*

3.36 Are there any advantages of MRI over CT brain imaging in the diagnosis of stroke?

Magnetic resonance imaging of the brain is more sensitive than CT for detecting cerebral infarction, particularly small deep infarcts (e.g. lacunar infarcts) and those occurring in the posterior fossa. Furthermore, certain MRI techniques, such as diffusion-weighted imaging (DWI), are very sensitive in highlighting the recent ischaemic lesion and may be particularly helpful when conventional MRI (e.g. T2-weighted imaging) shows several areas of abnormality. However, even MRI can be normal in clinically definite stroke.[24]

3.37 When is an MRI scan of the brain preferable to CT in patients with suspected stroke?

The choice of CT or MRI will depend on local availability, cost and effectiveness. If CT is available, it should be performed as soon as possible in all patients because it is the best technique for diagnosing or excluding early intracerebral haemorrhage and is essential to image suspected SAH; MRI is no substitute and can fail to image SAH. MRI will more often confirm the site of cerebral infarction suspected clinically but, as yet, this is rarely necessary; the immediate priority is to exclude intracerebral haemorrhage.[25] So MRI is not necessarily better than CT. Furthermore, CT is an excellent technique for ill, confused patients – as many stroke patients are – and MRI is a more difficult technique to apply. Circumstances in which brain MRI is preferable to CT are shown in *Box 3.5.*

BOX 3.5 Circumstances where MRI is preferable to CT

■ When more than 10 days has elapsed since stroke onset, CT shows a low-density area that could have been infarction or resolving haemorrhage and it is essential to know whether the stroke was ischaemic or haemorrhagic
■ When CT is negative and it is crucial to be able to localise the infarct (this happens only very occasionally); MRI is more likely to image the lesion
■ Arterial dissection is a suspected cause of cerebral infarction.

3.38 What does a recent cerebral infarct look like on MRI?

The earliest changes of cerebral ischaemia detected by *routine* MRI (i.e. not with spectroscopy, perfusion or diffusion imaging; *Fig. 3.15*) at various times after stroke onset are:

■ *Minutes*: loss of the normal flow void in the symptomatic artery within minutes of onset (the MR equivalent of the hyperdense artery sign on CT)
■ *3 hours*: swelling of the ischaemic brain on T1-weighted images, but without signal change on T2-weighted images
■ *8 hours*: signal changes on T2-weighted images
■ *16 hours*: signal change on T1-weighted images.[26,27]

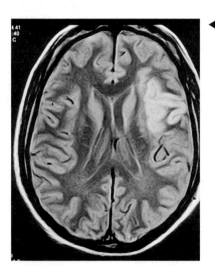

◀ **Fig 3.15** MRI brain scan. T2-weighted image showing an area of high signal (whiteness) in the left frontal lobe in a patient with an acute ischaemic stroke.

Large infarcts are often visible on routine T1- and T2-weighted imaging within 6 hours, but small cortical and subcortical infarcts may never become visible. Infarcts of any size are more often and more quickly visible on fluid-attenuated inversion recovery (FLAIR) and DWI, but currently these are not in widespread routine use.

3.39 Does the appearance of infarction on MRI evolve with time?

As with CT, MRI also shows that the infarct swells.

In the second week after infarct onset, MRI T2-weighted images often show a diffuse increase in signal (brightness) of gyri overlying the infarct, probably as a result of neovascular capillary proliferation or loss of autoregulation in leptomeningeal collaterals. It remains visible for up to 8 weeks after onset. A similar appearance is seen on CT, attributed to areas of breakdown of the blood–brain barrier, and corresponds to the gyriform petechial haemorrhages seen at autopsy.

Infarcts do not usually show enhancement with intravenous contrast until the second week after the stroke. Thereafter they generally show marked contrast enhancement around the edges (and within the infarct if sufficient contrast is administered) for several weeks after the stroke.

3.40 Is there a fogging effect on MRI (as there is with CT)?

Yes, probably. In the second to third week after onset, some infarcts increase in signal on T1-weighted MRI, decrease in signal on T2-weighted images, and become isodense with normal brain on MRI (as they may do on CT – the 'fogging' effect). As the infarcts may have lost most of their mass effect at this stage, they may be difficult to identify.

3.41 What is the cause of the fogging effect on MRI?

It is probably due to diffuse petechial haemorrhage from leaky capillaries, with diapedesis of red blood cells.[28] On CT, the red blood cells cause a diffuse increase in Hounsfield numbers, raising the low density of the lesion to that of normal brain parenchyma.

3.42 What are the late appearances of infarction on MRI?

After several weeks, the infarcted brain appears as an area with similar signal characteristics to CSF, i.e. bright on T2 and dark on T1, with an ex vacuo effect on the surrounding brain. Other long-term effects of ischaemic stroke seen on MRI include wallerian degeneration, visible as atrophy and low intensity in the white matter of the brainstem, and the late effects of any haemorrhagic transformation.

3.43 Can MRI differentiate new from old infarcts?

Yes. Diffusion-weighted imaging (*see Q. 3.44*) is an MRI technique that shows recent infarcts as an area of increased signal for up to several weeks after the stroke[29] (*Fig. 3.16*).

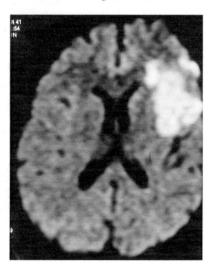

◀ **Fig 3.16** MRI brain scan. Diffusion-weighted image showing an area of high signal (whiteness) in the left frontal lobe in a patient with an acute ischaemic stroke.

3.44 What is diffusion-weighted MRI?

Diffusion-weighted imaging signals reflect the mobility of water molecules within tissues (e.g. brownian motion). In ischaemic tissues, energy failure leads to impairment of cell membrane function (e.g. the sodium–potassium ATP pump), which results in movement of water into the cell (cytotoxic oedema).[30] Intracellular water restricts diffusion and produces high signal on DWI images.

The major potential advantage of DWI in acute ischaemic stroke is the rapid appearance of abnormal signal soon after onset of blood flow impairment. In animal models, affected cerebral tissues exhibit high signal within 14 minutes of vessel occlusion. In stroke patients, initial studies have shown alteration of water diffusibility in the suspected infarcted tissue, which varied both within the lesion and over time.[31]

3.45 What is perfusion-weighted MRI?

Perfusion-weighted MRI aims to measure the patency of, and degree of blood flow through, the cerebral microcirculation. This can be achieved by examining the magnetic properties of flowing blood ('arterial spin tagging') or a bolus of contrast agent, such as gadolinium, which has been injected intravenously.

3.46 What is the role of EEG in the differential diagnosis of stroke?

In patients with suspected stroke EEG helps to determine whether there is a seizure focus when the clinical diagnosis is in doubt (e.g. in those with suspected postictal paresis or suspected non-convulsive status epilepticus who may present with the sudden onset of a confusional state) and the CT scan is normal or shows a lesion that is not typical of an infarct or PICH. It is also helpful if there is any suspicion of Creutzfeldt–Jakob disease or herpes encephalitis (e.g. clinical deterioration with new neurological signs, particularly myoclonus and cognitive decline, or hemiparesis, dysphasia and fever).

The EEG is not useful for diagnosing stroke: stroke is a clinical diagnosis and has no specific EEG features.[32]

The usual EEG findings in acute stroke are a localised reduction of normal cortical rhythms and a major surrounding slow-wave abnormality with individual waves of less than 1 Hz. Focal EEG slowing, however, is not specific; it indicates only the presence and side of the lesion. Although the EEG may help distinguish between small deep (lacunar) and cortical infarction, the clinical features and brain CT or MRI are more effective tools for doing this.[33,34]

SUBARACHNOID HAEMORRHAGE

3.47 What are the clinical features of subarachnoid haemorrhage?

Clinical features of subarachnoid haemorrhage

■ Headache is the cardinal clinical feature of SAH and is the only symptom in about one-third of patients. It usually arises suddenly, 'like a blow on the head' or 'an explosion inside the head', reaching a maximum within seconds.[35] It is the most severe headache the patient has ever had and is initially generally diffuse and poorly localised. However, after minutes to hours the headache spreads to the back of the head, neck and back as blood tracks down into the spinal subarachnoid space. Previous similar headaches, due to presumed previous, unrecognised 'warning leaks' are most uncommon. The 30–40% of patients who lose consciousness immediately complain of headache within seconds to minutes of regaining consciousness.

■ Altered consciousness – at least 60% of patients; 30–40% of patients lose consciousness immediately

■ Epileptic seizures – about 10% of patients.

- ■ Nausea and vomiting: common at the outset
- ■ Photophobia
- ■ Neck stiffness: takes 3–12 hours to develop (usually 6–12 hours)
- ■ Confusional state/delirium: the presenting syndrome in less than 5% of cases
- ■ Brudzinski's sign – forward flexion of the neck evokes flexion at the hip and knee
- ■ Limitation of straight leg raising
- ■ Kernig's sign – passive extension of the knee with the hip flexed elicits pain in the back and leg and resistance to hamstring stretch
- ■ Intraocular preretinal subhyaloid haemorrhage, usually near the optic disc (*Fig. 3.17*)
- ■ Focal neurological signs (uncommon) – oculomotor (IIIrd cranial) nerve palsy suggests posterior communicating artery aneurysm; dysphasia and hemiparesis suggest intracerebral extension of the SAH; bilateral VIth nerve palsy suggests raised intracranial pressure (a false localising sign)
- ■ Fever – but the pulse rate remains disproportionately low (compared with fever due to infection in which the pulse rate also rises).

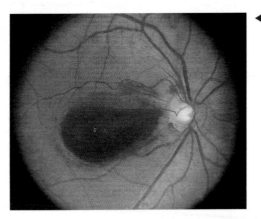

◄ **Fig 3.17** Fundus showing a subhyaloid haemorrhage in a patient with subarachnoid haemorrhage. Reproduced with permission from Warlow et al. *Stroke: a practical guide to management.* 2nd edn. Oxford: Blackwell Science Ltd; 2000.

3.48 What are the differential diagnoses of SAH?

The sudden, unexpected onset of a severe headache is caused by a SAH in about 60% of cases, another serious condition (e.g. cerebellar or intraventricular haemorrhage) in about 5% of cases, and more benign conditions (e.g. 'thunderclap headache', benign orgasmic or exertional cephalalgia, tension headache and 'crash' migraine, which uncharacteristically can sometimes start suddenly rather than gradually) in about 35% of cases (*Box 3.6*).

BOX 3.6 Differential diagnosis of sudden unexpected headache

With neck rigidity	**Without neck rigidity**
Subarachnoid haemorrhage	Migraine
Acute painful neck conditions	Thunderclap headache
Meningitis/encephalitis	Benign orgasmic cephalalgia
Cerebellar stroke	Benign exertional headache
Intraventricular haemorrhage	Pituitary apoplexy
Pituitary apoplexy	Reaction whilst on monoamine
Recent head injury*	oxidase inhibitors
	Phaeochromocytoma
	Expanding intracranial aneurysm
	Carotid or vertebral artery
	dissection
	Intracranial venous thrombosis
	Occipital neuralgia
	Acute obstructive hydrocephalus

* Recent head injury is a common pitfall in the diagnosis of subarachnoid haemorrhage. If a patient presents unconscious following a head injury and CT brain imaging shows blood in the subarachnoid space (± intracerebral space) it can be difficult to be sure in some patients whether the primary diagnosis is a subarachnoid haemorrhage causing loss of consciousness and head injury, or vice versa, with the head injury causing the subarachnoid haemorrhage and loss of consciousness.

Indeed, common manifestations of common headache syndromes (e.g. sudden onset of migraine) are probably more frequent than common manifestations of uncommon headache syndromes (e.g. sudden headache of SAH). Therefore, although a large minority of individuals with a sudden severe headache have not had a SAH, they must all be investigated to exclude it. Not uncommonly, the history of onset of headache is unclear, and the differential diagnosis is even wider.

3.49 How is the diagnosis of SAH made?

The diagnosis of SAH is frequently suspected from the clinical history and examination, but requires confirmation by CT (*Fig. 3.7*), which is positive in at least 95% of cases of SAH when performed within 1–2 days of onset.

If SAH is suspected but the CT scan appears normal, it is important to look carefully at the interpeduncular cistern, the ambient cisterns, the quadrigeminal cistern, the region of the anterior communicating artery and posterior inferior cerebellar artery, the posterior horns of the lateral ventricles and the cortical sulci (*Fig. 3.18*). If blood is present in these sites, it

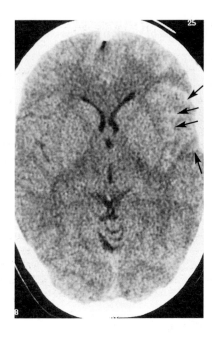

Fig 3.18 Plain cranial CT scan showing high attenuation, due to blood, in the subarachnoid space overlying the cortical sulci of the left cerebral hemisphere.

may be isodense or slightly hyperdense, and hence the normally hypodense cisterns and sulci may be difficult to see and seem 'absent'.

If the early CT scan is still considered 'negative', as it will be in 3–5% of cases of SAH, a lumbar puncture is required to identify the characteristic yellowish colour (xanthochromia) of the centrifuged CSF due to the breakdown products of haemoglobin (oxyhaemoglobin and bilirubin).

3.50 When should lumbar puncture be performed in patients with suspected SAH and negative CT findings?

Lumbar puncture should be done only after at least 12 hours have elapsed since the onset of headache to enable a reliable distinction to be made between a traumatic tap and haemorrhage in the subarachnoid space. This is because it takes up to 12 hours for red cells to lyse and haemoglobin to be broken down to oxyhaemoglobin and bilirubin, which after centrifugation of the CSF results in a yellowish colour of the supernatant (xanthochromia) and on spectrophotometry can be recognised by characteristic absorption bands.[36] Because xanthochromia is the only reliable proof that haemorrhagic spinal fluid has not resulted from the trauma of the puncture itself,[36] it is crucial that the CSF is not examined within 12 hours of onset of headache; no xanthochromia within 12 hours does not exclude SAH and a repeat CSF cannot be performed at a later date because it may not be able to distinguish xanthochromia due to SAH from that due to any trauma from the initial CSF tap. Although a decreased red blood cell concentration in serial samples taken at the same procedure occurs more often in traumatic punctures than in intracranial haemorrhage, it can still occur in patients with intracranial haemorrhage and, conversely, a constant number of red cells can be seen with traumatic taps. So the time-honoured 'three tube method' should be abandoned in favour of looking for xanthochromia, which is invariably found in the CSF of patients with SAH if it has been taken between 12 hours and 2 weeks after onset. At 3 weeks after SAH, xanthochromia is still found, but in only 70% of patients, and after 4 weeks it is found in only 40%.[37]

3.51 What are the common pitfalls in the diagnosis of SAH?

Because SAH is uncommon, with an annual incidence of six per 100 000, GPs encounter it only once in every 8 years on average, and therefore rarely think of it. When they do, it is usually in a patient with sudden onset of severe headache (because this is the cardinal clinical feature of SAH), but only one in eight patients whose only symptom is sudden severe headache will have SAH; the other seven have mostly innocuous conditions such as migraine.

Other reasons for misdiagnosis of SAH include:

- Failure to appreciate the spectrum of presentations of SAH – the diagnosis has to be considered with atypical presentations such as coma, seizure, delirium and focal stroke
- Failure to understand the limitations of CT of the brain – no extravasated blood is seen in about 2–5% of patients with SAH having CT within 12 hours of onset, or in 50% of those imaged with CT at 1 week
- Failure to perform lumbar puncture at the appropriate time and correctly interpret CSF findings.[38,39]

PATIENT QUESTIONS

3.52 What are the symptoms of TIA and stroke?

Every stroke is different, and people who have strokes are affected in different ways. The symptoms of stroke depend on the part of the brain that is affected by a lack of blood flow and the size of the damaged area. They also vary in severity from complete recovery within 24 hours (a TIA) to a prolonged, and even persistent, deficit due to permanent damage to a part of the brain (stroke).

The symptoms of stroke usually come on suddenly, and are noticed suddenly. However, if they come on during sleep they are not noticed until the affected person wakes up. It is the suddenness of the onset of the symptoms that usually stamps them as being due to a stroke, as opposed to a condition such as migraine or brain tumour. So, if the symptoms come on slowly, and also gradually get worse over a few days, weeks or months, they are unlikely to be due to stroke. The common symptoms of stroke are described below.

Muscle weakness or paralysis

Stroke may cause a lack of muscle strength in any group of muscles in the body, but most commonly causes weakness of the muscles of the face, hand, arm and leg on one side (hemiparesis). Weakness on the right side of the body (right hemiparesis) is due to impaired function of the left side of the brain (by ischaemia/infarction or haemorrhage into the brain). Weakness on the left side of the body is due to impaired function of the right side of the brain. At least half of patients with stroke have some form of hemiparesis.

Mild weakness may sometimes involve only a difficulty in controlling movement, rather than a difficulty of actual movement.

The common symptoms of stroke include:

Loss of sensation (feeling)

Stroke may cause a loss or alteration of feeling in any part of the body but, like weakness, most commonly causes a loss of feeling (numbness) of the skin of the face, hand, arm and leg on one side of the body (hemisensory loss or hemianaesthesia). Sensory impairment on the right side (hemianaesthesia) is due to impaired function of the left side of the brain (by infarction or haemorrhage into the brain). Sensory impairment on the left side of the body is due to impaired function of the right side of the brain. About half of patients with stroke have some form of hemianaesthesia.

Difficulty with speech

Stroke may cause slurred speech by causing weakness or incoordination of the muscles of the face, mouth and throat. As a result, it is difficult to articulate sounds. This is called dysarthria. Speech content is normal, however. Stroke may also cause difficulty with speech (dysphasia) in the form of difficulty:

- Understanding what is said to you, like listening to a foreign language (receptive dysphasia)

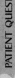

- Finding the right words and speaking fluently (expressive dysphasia)
- Understanding what is written (i.e. difficulty reading – dyslexia)
- Writing (dysgraphia).

Dysphasia (disturbance of language) is caused by impaired function of the side of the brain that is dominant for language. The left side of the brain (hemisphere) is dominant for language in almost all individuals who are right handed. The right side of the brain is dominant for language in about half of individuals who are left handed, the other half having a dominant left hemisphere like right-handed people.

Consequently, a stroke involving the left side of the brain (left hemisphere) commonly gives rise to a loss of speech and a loss of muscle strength and feeling on the right side of the body. This is because a part of the left side of the brain controls speech (in most individuals) and an adjacent part of the left side of the brain controls movement on the right side of the body. The same major blood vessel supplies blood to these areas and, if blocked, causes loss of function of both parts of the left hemisphere of the brain.

Visual symptoms

Stroke and TIA can cause a loss of vision in the whole visual field of one eye (monocular blindness), in half of the visual field of each eye (homonymous hemianopia), or double vision (diplopia).

Loss of vision in one eye that comes on suddenly and resolves within 24 hours (often 5–10 minutes) is usually due to a transient ischaemic attack of the eye (a temporary lack of blood supply to one eye) and is commonly called amaurosis fugax.

A homonymous hemianopia is a loss of vision to one side, so that the patient cannot see anything to the one side (either the left side or the right side) with either eye.

It can be difficult to tell the difference between transient/brief episodes of monocular blindness and homonymous hemianopia unless the patient closes each eye in turn during the episode of blindness and notes whether all of the vision in one eye, or the left or right half of the vision in both eyes, is affected.

Double vision occurs when one eye is looking in one direction and the other eye is looking in another direction, so that the brain receives images of two different objects at the same time from the two eyes looking in different directions. Double vision occurs when the visual axis of both eyes are different, in the vertical, horizontal or indeed any plane. This is usually caused by damage to one of the nerves that control the muscles that move the eyeball in certain directions.

Dizziness

Stroke and TIA involving the nerves originating in the balance organ in the inner ear (labyrinth) may cause a feeling of spinning called vertigo. When the world around appears to be moving (when it actually is not), this makes us feel nauseated (sometimes with vomiting) and unsteady on our feet (ataxic).

Headache

Stroke and TIA do not usually cause headache. However, headache may arise if the membrane covering the brain (the meninges) or the blood vessels in the brain are stretched or irritated.

The meninges may be stretched by swelling of a part of the brain, as occurs soon (minutes to hours) after a large bleed into the brain, or a few days after a large infarct, when swelling (oedema) of the brain is maximal. Bleeding over the surface of the brain (subarachnoid haemorrhage) characteristically causes a very severe headache, because the blood directly irritates the pain-sensitive meninges that cover the brain.

Occasionally a stroke may be caused by a tear in the inside lining of the wall of an artery (dissection) to the brain, which may lead to blockage of the artery (and ischaemic stroke) and also cause quite severe pain in the head or neck, wherever the arterial wall is torn.

Vomiting

Vomiting after stroke is not common, but can be caused by:

■ Other symptoms of the TIA or stroke, such as vertigo. Vertigo is a sensation of rotation or spinning such that the individual feels as if he or she – or the world around them – is spinning around. This may occur if a TIA or stroke involves the nerves in the brainstem that receive information from the balance organ (labyrinth) in the inner ear. Vertigo causes both a feeling of nausea and vomiting, and also unsteadiness when walking (ataxia).
■ Direct involvement of the 'vomiting centre' in the base of the brain (medulla)
■ Raised pressure inside the head (commonly due to a large bleed or infarct of the brain) which is transmitted to the 'vomiting centre' in the base of the brain (medulla).

Drowsiness or unconsciousness

Stroke and TIA do not commonly cause a loss of consciousness. However, as with vomiting, drowsiness and loss of consciousness can be caused by:

■ Complications of the stroke (e.g. an epileptic seizure), although the drowsiness is usually transient, recovering after a few minutes to hours
■ Direct involvement of the 'consciousness centre' in the brainstem (midbrain, pons) by a strategically located bleed or infarct
■ Raised pressure inside the head (commonly due to a large bleed or infarct of the brain) which is transmitted directly or indirectly to the 'consciousness centre' in the upper brainstem (mid brain, pons).

Localisation of the lesion (where is the damage?)

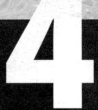

4

Once the diagnosis of a transient ischaemic attack (TIA) or stroke has been established, the next step is to localise the part of the brain (or eye) and the part of the vascular system that has been affected. This depends on a basic knowledge of neuroanatomy, cerebrovascular anatomy and common clinical stroke syndromes.

CAROTID AND VERTEBROBASILAR TERRITORY ISCHAEMIA

4.1 What is the main arterial supply to the brain?

> ### Blood supply to the brain
> The blood supply to the brain is delivered by the two internal carotid and two vertebral arteries (*Fig. 4.1*), which anastomose at the base of the brain to form the circle of Willis (*Fig. 4.2*). The carotid artery system supplies the anterior two-thirds of the brain (hence it is called the *anterior circulation*) and the vertebrobasilar arterial system supplies the posterior third of the brain (hence it is called the *posterior circulation*).

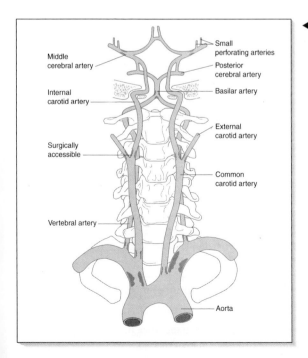

◀ **Fig 4.1** The anatomy of the arterial blood supply to the brain. Sites that are most often affected by atherosclerosis are shown as dark indentations in the arterial lumen. Adapted with permission from Hankey & Warlow 1994.[1]

Labels on figure:
Middle cerebral artery
Internal carotid artery
Surgically accessible
Vertebral artery
Small perforating arteries
Posterior cerebral artery
Basilar artery
External carotid artery
Common carotid artery
Aorta

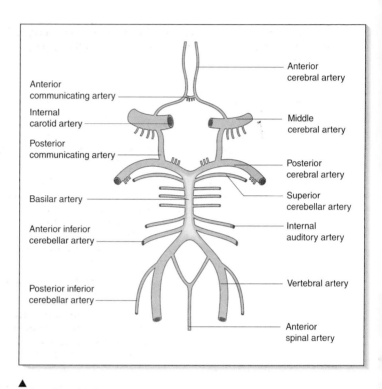

Fig 4.2 Diagrammatic representation of the circle of Willis at the base of the brain, as seen from below in relation to the optic chiasm. Adapted with permission from Hankey & Warlow 1994.[1]

4.2 What clinical syndromes may be caused by ischaemia in the region supplied by the carotid artery?

Complete internal carotid artery occlusion, if symptomatic, usually produces symptoms of ischaemia in the middle cerebral artery territory, but the ophthalmic and anterior cerebral artery territories can also be involved, alone or in combination with the middle cerebral artery, depending on collateral supply (*Table 4.1*).

4.3 What symptoms indicate definite carotid territory ischaemia?

Definite carotid symptoms include:

■ Monocular visual loss in all or part of the visual field (amaurosis fugax)
■ Language disturbance (dominant hemisphere).

TABLE 4.1 Branches of the internal carotid artery and typical clinical syndromes caused by ischaemia of the brain or eye in the region supplied by them

Branches	Region supplied	Syndrome caused by ischaemia
Ophthalmic artery	Retina and optic nerve	Monocular blindness or altitudinal field defect
Anterior choroidal artery	Globus pallidus Internal capsule Choroid plexus	Contralateral hemiparesis, hemisensory loss and homonymous hemianopia
Middle cerebral artery	Frontal lobe Parietal lobe Superior temporal lobe	Contralateral facial weakness, hemiparesis and hemisensory loss (arm > leg), homonymous hemianopia, and global aphasia (dominant hemisphere) or visual–spatial–perceptual dysfunction (non-dominant hemisphere)
Medial lenticulostriate artery	Internal capsule	Contralateral pure motor hemiparesis
Lateral lenticulostriate artery	Putamen Globus pallidus Caudate nucleus Internal capsule Corona radiata	Contralateral hemiparesis, dysphasia (dominant hemisphere) or visual–spatial–perceptual dysfunction (non-dominant hemisphere)
Superior division of middle cerebral artery Prerolandic branch Rolandic branch Anterior parietal branch	Frontal and anterior parietal lobes	Contralateral central facial weakness, hemiparesis and hemisensory loss, ipsilateral deviation of head and eyes, and global or motor aphasia (dominant hemisphere) Contralateral face and arm weakness, and motor aphasia (dominant hemisphere) Contralateral central facial weakness, hemiparesis and hemisensory loss, and dysarthria (resembling lacunar syndrome) Conduction aphasia and bilateral ideomotor apraxia

TABLE 4.1 (*Cont'd*)

Branches	Region supplied	Syndrome caused by ischaemia

Inferior division of middle cerebral artery
  Posterior parietal branch
  Angular branch
  Posterior temporal branch
  Anterior temporal branch
  Temporal polar branch
	Inferior parietal and lateral temporal lobes	Homonymous hemianopia, Wernicke's aphasia or agitated confusional state (dominant hemisphere), left visual neglect (right-sided lesion)

Anterior cerebral artery	Anterior and superior medial frontal lobe	Contralateral foot and leg weakness or hemiparesis (leg > arm), abulia, incontinence, grasp reflexes

4.4 What clinical syndromes may be caused by ischaemia in the region supplied by the vertebrobasilar artery system?

Occlusion of the vertebral or basilar artery may also cause ischaemia in the territory of supply of one or both posterior cerebral arteries (which are branches of the basilar artery; *Table 4.2*). Incomplete syndromes are common, and the symptoms of infarction and haemorrhage are similar.

4.5 What symptoms indicate definite vertebrobasilar territory ischaemia?

Definite vertebrobasilar events include combinations of:

■ Tetraparesis
■ Diplopia
■ Vertigo
■ Cortical blindness
■ Cerebellar ataxia.

4.6 What symptoms may be due to either carotid or vertebrobasilar ischaemia?

More often than not, it is difficult to be certain which arterial territory is involved in an ischaemic event of the brain, particularly if the symptoms and signs have resolved and it is not possible to elicit any associated co-lateralising signs. This is because certain pathways (e.g. corticospinal tract, ascending sensory pathways, optic radiation, etc.) receive their blood supply

TABLE 4.2 Branches of the vertebral arteries and basilar artery and typical clinical syndromes caused by ischaemia of the brain in the region supplied by them

Branches	Region supplied	Syndrome caused by ischaemia
Vertebral and basilar artery	Brainstem and cerebellum	Various syndromes including: diplopia, ophthalmoplegia or gaze palsies; vertigo, nausea and nystagmus; dysarthria, dysphagia and bulbar weakness; ipsilateral facial sensory loss and weakness (nuclear or infranuclear); hiccups and respiratory failure; contralateral hemiparesis or tetraparesis; contralateral or bilateral sensory loss; coma
Basilar artery Top of basilar artery	Rostral midbrain Part of thalamus Inferior temporal occipital lobes	Variable pupillary abnormalities Ptosis or lid retraction Supranuclear vertical gaze paresis Somnolence Hemiballismus Amnesia Cortical blindness
Superior cerebellar artery	Midbrain (dorsolateral) Superior cerebellar peduncle Superior cerebellum	Ipsilateral Horner's syndrome Ipsilateral limb ataxia and tremor Contralateral spinothalamic sensory loss Contralateral central facial weakness Sometimes contralateral IVth nerve palsy
Anterior inferior cerebellar artery	Base of pons Rostral medulla Inferior cerebellum Cochlea Vestibule	Ipsilateral Horner's syndrome Ipsilateral facial sensory loss (pain, temperature) Ipsilateral nuclear facial and abducens palsy Ipsilateral deafness and tinnitus Vertigo, nausea, vomiting and nystagmus Ipsilateral ataxia of limbs and dysarthria

TABLE 4.2 (*Cont'd*)

Branches	Region supplied	Syndrome caused by ischaemia
Posterior inferior cerebellar artery	Lateral medulla Inferior cerebellum	Ipsilateral Horner's syndrome Ipsilateral facial sensory loss (pain, temp) Vertigo, nausea, vomiting and nystagmus Ipsilateral paralysis of palate (dysphagia) Ipsilateral paralysis of larynx (dysphonia) Ipsilateral ataxia of limbs Contralateral hemisensory loss below neck
Paramedian branches	Paramedian pons	Any of the lacunar syndromes: Pure motor hemiparesis Pure hemisensory loss Hemiparesis-hemisensory loss Ataxic hemiparesis Internuclear ophthalmoplegia Locked-in syndrome, if bilateral
Thalamic-subthalamic (thalamoperforating)	Posteromedial thalamus inferiorly	Hemisensory loss, amnesia
Paramedian mesencephalic arteries	Rostral medial midbrain	Hemisensory-motor loss
Posterior cerebral artery	Occipital lobe Inferior temporal lobe	Contralateral homonymous hemianopia Cortical blindness if bilateral Amnesia (especially if bilateral)
Thalamogeniculate	Ventrolateral thalamus	Pure hemisensory loss
Posterior choroidal arteries	Anterior and posterior thalamus	Hemisensory loss, amnesia
Posterior communicating artery Polar arteries (tuberothalamic)	Anterior lateral thalamus	Hemisensory loss, amnesia

from both the carotid and vertebrobasilar arteries at different levels. Symptoms and signs that can occur with carotid or vertebrobasilar ischaemia (*Table 4.3*) include:

- Hemiparesis
- Hemisensory deficit
- Dysarthria.

TABLE 4.3 Which vascular territory is involved?

Symptom	Carotid	Either	Vertebrobasilar
Dysphasia	+		
Monocular visual loss	+		
Unilateral weakness*		+	
Unilateral sensory disturbance*		+	
Dysarthria[†]		+	
Homonymous hemianopia		+	
Unsteadiness/ataxia[†]		+	
Dysphagia[†]		+	
Diplopia[†]			+
Vertigo			+
Bilateral simultaneous visual loss			+
Bilteral simultaneous weakness			+
Bilateral simultaneous sensory disturbance			+
Crossed sensory/motor loss			+

* Usually regarded as carotid distribution.
[†] NOT necessarily a TIA/stroke if an isolated symptom, only if associated with more than one other symptom on the list.

4.7 Why distinguish between carotid and vertebrobasilar territory ischaemic events?

It is important to distinguish between carotid and vertebrobasilar territory symptoms if carotid endarterectomy is to be considered.

The risk of stroke (and thus the benefit of carotid endarterectomy) is considerably greater for symptomatic than for asymptomatic carotid stenosis (*see Q. 7.16*). Therefore, the benefits of carotid endarterectomy are greater in patients with symptoms of carotid territory ischaemia who have a severe carotid stenosis on the symptomatic side (i.e. the side of the ischaemic brain or eye) than in patients without neurological symptoms or with neurological symptoms stemming from another vascular territory (asymptomatic carotid stenosis).

However, about 10–15% of the population have a normal cerebrovascular anatomy variant whereby the carotid artery on one side gives rise not only to the anterior and middle cerebral arteries but also to the posterior cerebral artery. Occasionally, therefore, a posterior cerebral artery ischaemic stroke involving the medial temporal lobe, thalamus and occipital lobe can be due to a *symptomatic* carotid stenosis. This variant can only be identified, however, by cerebral angiography (magnetic resonance angiography, catheter cerebral angiography and possibly computerised tomographic angiography).

4.8 How reliable is the clinical distinction between carotid and vertebrobasilar territory TIAs?

The clinical distinction between carotid and vertebrobasilar territory TIAs is not very reliable, even among experienced neurologists. Kraaijeveld et al[2] investigated the interobserver agreement for the diagnosis of carotid and vertebrobasilar territory TIA among eight senior neurologists from the same department who interviewed 36 TIA patients in alternating pairs. Both neurologists agreed that 16 patients had a carotid TIA and 8 had not, but they disagreed about 12 patients (κ = 0.31; for perfect agreement κ = 1.0; *Table 4.4*).

TABLE 4.4 Interobserver variation in the diagnosis of carotid or vertebrobasilar territory TIA

| | Neurologist 1 | | |
	Carotid	Vertebrobasilar	Total
Neurologist 2			
Carotid	16	4	20
Vertebrobasilar	8	8	16
Total	24	12	36

Agreement over and above chance (κ statistic): 31% (0.31)
Eight neurologists; 36 patients with TIA.

STROKE SYNDROMES

4.9 What are the common clinical syndromes of stroke and TIA?

Common clinical stroke syndromes

- Total anterior circulation syndrome (TACS) – about 20% of cases
- Partial anterior circulation syndrome (PACS) – about 30% of cases
- Lacunar syndrome (LACS) – about 25% of cases
- Posterior circulation syndrome (POCS) – about 25% of cases
- About 1% of stroke patients do not fit one of these syndromes.

These syndromes are based on clinical features but can be further refined, if necessary, by CT imaging.[3,4] They provide valuable information about the anatomical and vascular location, aetiology, and prognosis of the stroke (*Table 4.5*).

4.10 What is a total anterior circulation syndrome (TACS)?

A total anterior circulation syndrome (TACS) is the combination of *all* the following:

■ Hemiparesis, with or without a sensory deficit, involving the whole of at least two of the three body areas (face, arm, leg)
  and
■ Homonymous visual field defect
  and
■ Higher cerebral (or 'cortical') dysfunction – dysphasia if the dominant cerebral hemisphere for language is affected (usually left hemisphere) or neglect and other visual–spatial–perceptual problems if the nondominant cerebral hemisphere is involved – all of which must be *new*.

These patients are not infrequently drowsy and so any cognitive or visual field defects sometimes have to be assumed. Deviation of the eyes towards the affected hemisphere is common but generally recovers in a few days.

This is the typical 'big stroke' we are all taught about in medical school.

4.11 What are the causes of a TACS?

The causes of TACS include a large infarct involving the cerebral cortex, basal ganglia and internal capsule (a total anterior circulation infarct –TACI) in the middle cerebral or middle and anterior cerebral artery territories (about 70–80% of cases), or a large haematoma involving the lobes of one cerebral hemisphere or a smaller deep haematoma in the basal ganglia region (about 20–30% of cases; *see Chapter 5*).

A large haematoma may cause midline shift, transtentorial herniation and coma within 24 hours, whereas these changes usually take 2–3 days to evolve with large infarcts, as it takes some time (i.e. hours to days) for cerebral oedema to develop.

4.12 What are the causes of total anterior circulation infarction (TACI)?

Total anterior circulation infarcts (TACIs) are usually caused by an acute occlusion of the internal carotid artery (e.g. embolism from the heart, atherothrombosis, dissection), or embolic occlusion of the proximal middle cerebral artery from a cardiac or proximal arterial source (*Fig. 4.3*; *see Chapter 6*).

TABLE 4.5 Common clinical stroke syndromes

	Total anterior circulation syndrome (TACS)	Partial anterior circulation syndrome (PACS)	Lacunar syndrome (LACS)	Posterior circulation syndrome (POCS)
Clinical features	1) Hemiparesis and hemisensory loss and 2) Homonymous hemianopia and 3) Cortical dysfunction (dysphasia or visual–spatial–perceptual dysfunction)	Any two of preceding three in TACS [(1) and (2), or (2) and (3) or (1) and (3)] or (3) alone.	Hemiparesis or Hemisensory loss or Hemisensorimotor loss or Ataxic hemiparesis No hemianopia or cortical dysfunction	Brainstem symptoms and signs (e.g. diplopia, vertigo, dysphagia, ataxia, bilateral limb deficits, hemianopia or cortical blindness)
Anatomy	Fronto-temporal-parietal lobes or Thalamus/internal capsule/occipital lobe	Lobar	Small deep lesion in either corona radiata, internal capsule, thalamus or ventral pons	Brainstem and/or cerebellum
Pathology	Infarction (85%) or Haemorrhage (15%)	Infarction (85%) or Haemorrhage (15%)	Infarction (95–98%) or Haemorrhage (2–5%)	Infarction (85%) or Haemorrhage (15%)
Aetiology	*Infarction:* occlusion of ipsilateral ICA or MCA, and occasionally PCA, by embolism from heart, aortic arch or carotid or vertebrobasilar arteries; or in-situ thrombosis. *Haemorrhage:* any of possible causes	*Infarction:* occlusion of branch of MCA or PCA by embolism from heart, aortic arch or carotid or vertebrobasilar arteries *Haemorrhage:* any of possible causes.	*Infarction:* usually perforating artery microatheroma/lipophyalinosis; rarely arteritis or embolism *Haemorrhage:* any, but usually hypertensive small-vessel disease	*Infarction:* occlusion of VBA or PCA, or branches by in-situ thrombosis or embolism from heart, aortic arch or VBA *Haemorrhage:* any of possible causes

TABLE 4.5 *(Cont'd)*

	Total anterior circulation syndrome (TACS)	Partial anterior circulation syndrome (PACS)	Lacunar syndrome (LACS)	Posterior circulation syndrome (POCS)
Recurrence rates	Low	High in first 3 months	Low but steady over 12 months	High first 2 months then steady over 12 months
Prognosis at 1 year (%)	Poor	Fair	Fair	Fair
Dead	60	15	10	20
Dependent	35	30	30	20
Independent	5	55	60	60

ICA, internal carotid artery; MCA, middle cerebral artery; PCA, posterior cerebral artery; VBA, vertebrobasilar artery

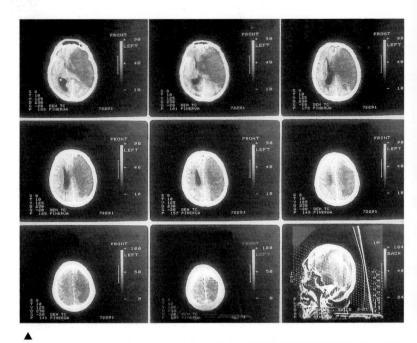

▲

Fig 4.3 Plain cranial CT scan, eight slices in the axial plane, showing a large area of low density, due to infarction, in the territory of supply of the left middle cerebral artery, causing a total left anterior circulation syndrome.

4.13 What is a partial anterior circulation syndrome (PACS)?

A partial anterior circulation syndrome (PACS) is a more restricted clinical syndrome consisting of:

■ Only two of the three components of the total anterior circulation syndrome (*see Q. 4.10*)
or

■ Isolated higher cortical dysfunction such as dysphasia
or

■ A predominantly proprioceptive deficit in one limb
or

■ A motor/sensory deficit restricted to one body area or part of one body area (out of the face, upper limb, and lower limb) (i.e. a monoparesis)..

If the 'cortical' signs are rather subtle and are not detected (e.g. dressing apraxia, neglect, dysphasia mistaken for dysarthria, etc.), the patient may be misclassified as having a 'lacunar' syndrome (*see Q. 4.16*)

4.14 What are the causes of a PACS?

These include a cortical/subcortical infarct (about 80% of cases of PACS) or a lobar haemorrhage (about 20% of cases). (*See Figs 3.9, 3.11, 3.14, 3.15 & 3.16 and Chapter 5*)

4.15 What are the causes of partial anterior circulation infarction (PACI)?

Partial anterior circulation – or cortical – infarcts (PACIs) are commonly caused by occlusion of a branch of the middle cerebral artery, or rarely the trunk of the anterior cerebral artery, usually as a consequence of embolism from the heart or proximal large arteries (aortic arch, extracranial carotid arteries). The causes are therefore the same as for TACIs (*see Q. 4.12 and Chapter 6*)

Sometimes a PACI is caused by a more proximal occlusion of the main stem of the middle cerebral artery in patients who have a good pial collateral circulation or rapid recanalisation of the occluded artery, so that the overlying cerebral cortex is relatively spared and infarction is largely subcortical in the distribution of several lenticulostriate arteries; this causes a characteristic area of 'striatocapsular infarction' on computed tomography (CT; *Fig. 4.4*). This clinical syndrome often comprises a hemiparesis and cognitive deficit, without a homonymous hemianopia.[5]

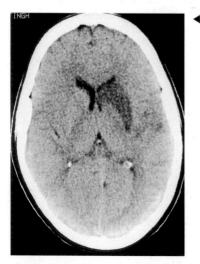

Fig 4.4 Plain cranial CT scan showing a comma-shaped area of low density, due to infarction, in the left putamen, internal capsule (anterior limb) and caudate nucleus. This is called a striatocapsular infarct.

A PACI may also be caused by occlusion of an anterior cerebral artery, which causes contralateral weakness predominantly of the lower limb, perhaps with some cortical sensory loss, and aphasia if in the dominant hemisphere (*see Table 4.1*). Left, and rarely right, anterior cerebral infarcts can cause a curious dyspraxia of the left upper limb due to infarction of the corpus callosum disconnecting the right motor centres from the left language centres. Bilateral leg and even additional bilateral arm weakness has been described when both anterior cerebral arteries are supplied from one stenosed internal carotid artery, or both anterior cerebral arteries are occluded by embolism, so mimicking a brainstem or spinal cord syndrome.

Some anterior circulation syndromes, usually classified as PACS, are caused by boundary zone infarcts (*see Q. 4.26 and Fig. 4.6*). Anterior choroidal artery distribution infarcts (*see Table 4.1*), which can be defined only by the CT/MR pattern, are rare, are probably due to microvascular disease as well as embolism and can cause a PACS or lacunar syndrome.

4.16 What is a lacunar syndrome (LACS)?

There are four main lacunar syndromes (LACS).

- *Pure motor hemiparesis* (about 50% of lacunar cases) – unilateral motor weakness involving two or three areas (face, upper limb, lower limb), including the whole of each area affected. There are often sensory symptoms but no sensory signs. The muscle weakness is in a pyramidal/corticospinal tract distribution (i.e. mainly of the antigravity muscles – shoulder abduction and external rotation, elbow extension, supination, wrist extension, finger extension, hip flexion and abduction, knee flexion, and ankle and toe dorsiflexion). There may be a flurry of immediately preceding TIAs, the so-called 'capsular warning syndrome'.

- *Pure hemisensory loss* (about 5% of cases) – symptoms of sensory loss, with or without sensory signs affecting all modalities equally (light touch, pain, temperature, joint position sense – proprioception), or sparing proprioception, in all of the face and arm, arm and leg, or face, arm and leg (i.e. the same distribution as the weakness in a pure motor hemiparesis).

- *Hemisensorimotor loss* (about 35% of cases) – the combination of weakness and sensory loss in all of the face and arm, arm and leg, or face, arm and leg, without any other abnormalities.

- *Ataxic hemiparesis* (about 10% of cases) – the combination of corticospinal/pyramidal distribution weakness and cerebellar ataxia affecting the arm and/or leg on one side of the body. This entity includes the syndrome in which there is dysarthria and clumsiness of one hand.

With each of these four lacunar syndromes, there is:
- No visual field defect
- No new cortical defect (such as dysphasia, visuospatial disturbance or predominantly proprioceptive sensory loss)
- No impairment of consciousness
- Nothing to suggest a brainstem syndrome (such as diplopia, crossed motor and sensory deficit, etc.).

4.17 Where in the brain are the lesions that cause LACS?

- *Pure motor hemiparesis* – the lesion is where the motor pathways are closely packed together, separate from other pathways: usually in the internal capsule or pons, sometimes the corona radiata or cerebral peduncle, rarely the medullary pyramid.
- *Pure hemisensory loss* – the lesion is usually in the thalamus but can be in the brainstem.
- *Hemisensorimotor loss* – the lesion is usually in the thalamus or internal capsule but can be in the corona radiata or pons. Compared with other LACS, sensorimotor stroke is more often due to larger cortical and subcortical infarcts.
- *Ataxic hemiparesis* – the lesion is usually in the pons, internal capsule or cerebral peduncle. Dysarthria, with or without upper motor neurone facial weakness, may also be a lacunar syndrome with similar lesion localisation as ataxic hemiparesis, but there are other localising possibilities as well.

4.18 What are the causes of a LACS?

The most common pathology is a small deep infarct (about 98% of cases) affecting the motor and/or sensory pathways in the corona radiata, internal capsule, thalamus, cerebral peduncle or pons (*Fig. 4.5*), but occasionally the pathology is a small deep haemorrhage in one of these regions[6,7] (*see Figs 3.6 & 3.8 and Chapter 5*).

4.19 What are the causes of lacunar infarction (LACI)?

Lacunar infarcts (LACI) are caused by presumed occlusion of a small perforating artery affected by degenerative intracranial small vessel disease (lipohyalinosis/microatheroma; *see Chapter 6*).[6]

4.20 What is a posterior circulation syndrome (POCS)?

A posterior circulation syndrome (POCS) comprises symptoms and signs of dysfunction of the brainstem, cerebellum, thalamus or occipital lobe (which are supplied by the vertebrobasilar (posterior) circulation), usually in some

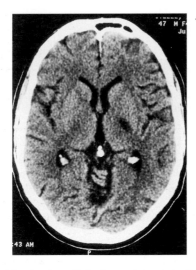

◀ **Fig 4.5** Plain cranial CT scan showing a small, deep infarct in the posterior limb of the left internal capsule in a patient with a lacunar syndrome (pure right hemisensorimotor loss).

combination (e.g. diplopia, vertigo, ataxia, facial sensory loss, Horner's syndrome and bilateral limb weakness and sensory loss; (*see Q. 4.5*).

Various syndromes have been described, such as the 'top of the basilar' syndrome, other midbrain syndromes, the locked-in syndrome, pontine syndromes and the lateral and medial medullary syndromes (*see Table 4.2*).[8] Recognising these syndromes is more important for passing medical exams than managing patients, except for being able to accurately identify a cerebellar stroke (which may require life-saving surgical treatment) and distinguishing it from a thalamic stroke, which can cause diagnostic confusion.

4.21 What are the two most important POCS to identify?

The two most important POCS to identify are cerebellar and thalamic strokes.

4.22 Why is it important to identify cerebellar strokes?

Importance of identifying cerebellar strokes

■ Although uncommon, cerebellar strokes have a wide clinical spectrum and can be rapidly fatal if unrecognised and inappropriately managed.

■ Mild syndromes, limited to sudden vertigo, nausea, imbalance and horizontal nystagmus that soon pass, are frequently misdiagnosed as 'labyrinthitis'.[9]

■ Larger lesions cause additional ipsilateral limb and truncal ataxia, as well as dysarthria.

- Even more extensive cerebellar strokes cause occipital headache, vomiting and sometimes only depressed consciousness, which can make it impossible to detect limb or truncal ataxia.[10] Usually, there are additional brainstem signs (e.g. ipsilateral facial weakness and sensory loss, a gaze palsy to the side of the lesion, ipsilateral deafness and tinnitus, and bilateral extensor plantar responses) because of pressure from a large oedematous infarct or haematoma, or because an occluded artery supplying the cerebellum so often supplies parts of the brainstem as well. Mass effect can obstruct flow of cerebrospinal fluid (CSF) from the fourth ventricle to cause acute or subacute hydrocephalus with subsequent coma and meningism, which is very easily confused with subarachnoid haemorrhage, particularly if there is no obvious weakness or sensory loss in the limbs, which is usually the case. CT scan will reveal a haematoma but the signs of an infarct are more subtle, with disappearance or shift of the fourth ventricle due to mass effect before the low density of the lesion itself appears. Magnetic resonance imaging (MRI) is more sensitive and provides detail of any additional brainstem involvement.
- Patients who become acutely or subacutely comatose have a very poor prognosis. However, if there is little evidence of primary brainstem infarction, then drainage of any hydrocephalus and/or decompression of the posterior fossa may sometimes be followed by relatively good-quality survival.[11]

4.23   Why is it important to identify thalamic strokes?

Importance of identifying thalamic strokes

- Thalamic strokes are like cerebellar strokes in that they are uncommon but have a wide clinical spectrum and can be rapidly fatal if unrecognised and inappropriately managed.
- If the thalamic lesion is small, it may cause only a pure hemisensory stroke or hemisensorimotor stroke (i.e. a lacunar syndrome). The affected limbs may also manifest cerebellar ataxia (involvement of the dentato (dentate nucleus in cerebellum)–rubro (red nucleus in midbrain)–thalamic tract). However, thalamic lesions that involve thalamocortical projections may also cause aphasia and impairment of verbal memory (dominant side), visuospatial dysfunction (non-dominant side) and visual hallucinations.
- Larger thalamic lesions, which compress the adjacent midbrain, cause various additional deficits such as paralysis of upward gaze, small pupils, apathy, depressed consciousness, hypersomnolence and apathy. Furthermore, severe retrograde and anterograde amnesia can be a manifestation of *bilateral* paramedian thalamic infarction caused by occlusion of a *single* small branch of the proximal posterior cerebral artery.
- Therefore, thalamic stroke may present in many ways, sometimes only with somnolence, confusion or amnesia, but the sudden onset is a clue.

4.24 What are the causes of a POCS?

Most commonly, a POCS is caused by infarction in the distribution of the vertebrobasilar (i.e. posterior) circulation and less commonly by a localised haemorrhage in the brainstem, cerebellum, thalamus or occipital lobe[12,13] (*see Chapter 5*).

4.25 What are the causes of posterior circulation infarction (POCI)?

The causes of infarction in the vertebrobasilar territory are rather heterogeneous and, in individual patients, difficult to work out, particularly because vertebral angiography is seldom carried out (because it can be risky), non-invasive arterial imaging (i.e. ultrasound and magnetic resonance angiography) is often difficult to interpret, and pathological studies are uncommon for many reasons, one of which is that fatality is relatively low.

A combination of brainstem and occipital lobe signs is highly suggestive of infarction due to thromboembolism within the regions supplied by the basilar and posterior cerebral arteries (*see Chapter 6*). However, occasionally occlusion of the proximal posterior cerebral artery causes sufficient temporal, thalamic and internal capsule or midbrain compression/infarction to result in a TACS, with some contralateral hemiparesis and sensory loss and a marked cognitive deficit such as aphasia, as well as the expected homonymous hemianopia. The condition can therefore be confused with occlusion of the middle cerebral artery or one of its branches.[14] This has been called the 'walking TACS' because, although it fulfils the definition of a TACS, the motor loss is slight.

Some lacunar syndromes are caused by small brainstem or thalamic infarcts as a consequence of small vessel occlusion (perhaps intracranial small-vessel disease, or perhaps atheroma at the mouth of small perforating arteries). However, both small and large infarcts can be due to:

■ Embolism from the heart and atherothrombosis or dissection affecting the vertebral arteries
■ Thrombotic occlusion complicating atheroma of the basilar artery or its major branches
■ Low flow distal to vertebral and other arterial occlusions.

BOUNDARY ZONE INFARCTIONS

4.26 What is a boundary zone infarct?

Boundary zone (or border zone) infarcts are infarcts in the border zones between arterial territories.

4.27   What are the major border zones between arterial territories?

There are three major boundary zones, which lie between:

■ the superficial territories of the middle cerebral artery and anterior cerebral artery in the frontoparasagittal region (anterior boundary zone; *Fig. 4.6*)

■ the superficial territories of the middle cerebral artery and posterior cerebral artery in the parieto-occipital region (posterior boundary zone)

■ the superficial medullary penetrators and deep lenticulostriate territories of the middle cerebral artery in the paraventricular white matter of the corona radiata (subcortical boundary zone).

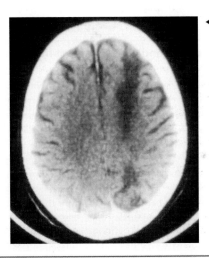

◀ **Fig 4.6** Plain cranial CT scan showing a linear region of low attenuation, consistent with infarction, in the border zone between the arterial territory of supply of the left middle and anterior cerebral arteries.

4.28   How common are boundary zone infarcts?

Boundary zone infarcts are uncommon, accounting for only a small percentage of strokes.

4.29   What causes boundary zone infarcts?

Boundary zone infarcts are usually caused by low flow to the brain.[15] This usually occurs under two main sets of circumstances:

■ *Sudden, profound systemic hypotension*, as during cardiac arrest, which can cause bilateral infarcts usually in the posterior boundary zones, presumably where blood flow is at its most precarious. Clinical features include cortical blindness, visual disorientation and agnosia, and amnesia.

■ *Internal carotid occlusion*, or extreme stenosis, may predispose to unilateral boundary zone infarction when there is a relatively small drop in systemic blood pressure, or perhaps just because collateral blood flow is so poor and perfusion reserve is exhausted. Anterior boundary zone and subcortical boundary zone infarcts are the most common, and cause contralateral weakness of the leg more than the arm, with sparing of the face, some impaired sensation in the same areas and aphasia if in the dominant hemisphere. Unilateral posterior boundary zone infarcts are less common and cause contralateral hemianopia and cortical sensory loss, along with aphasia if in the dominant hemisphere.

Occasionally, microemboli obstructing the circulation (platelets, cholesterol, tumour), rather than low flow, cause infarction in boundary zones.

4.30 How is the diagnosis of a boundary zone infarct made?

The diagnosis is frequently difficult and uncertain. Although it is not that difficult to determine where the lesion is, from the clinical features and brain imaging, nor the state of the cerebral circulation, from arterial imaging, it can be quite difficult to be certain of exactly why the stroke has occurred. The site of the infarct is not a reliable guide to a particular boundary zone because of the variability of the territorial supply of the cerebral arteries (*see Chapter 3*). Therefore, the diagnosis of 'low flow' rather than embolic occlusion depends more on the preceding and precipitating circumstances. For instance, it may have been likely that there was a drop in systemic blood pressure at or just before stroke onset, or the internal carotid artery may have been clamped during endarterectomy. Internal carotid artery occlusion or severe stenosis is a clue in unilateral cases but, even so, there are many cases of doubt and embolic infarction is still possible, even within a so-called border zone area.[16] Sometimes these 'low-flow' infarcts seem to develop and progress gradually over days or weeks.

4.31 Can the clinical classification of stroke, based on the clinical syndrome, be modified by the findings on CT?

The clinical syndrome attributed to an ischaemic stroke patient following clinical assessment may need to be modified if subsequent brain imaging shows a recent, relevant infarct in a different area to that expected clinically (*see Chapter 7*). This is quite common in patients who present with a TACS (thought to be due to an internal carotid or middle cerebral artery occlusion) but in whom the CT scan shows extensive infarction in the territory of the posterior cerebral artery (i.e. a posterior circulation syndrome). Another common misclassification is a patient who appears to have a pure motor hemiparesis on the left (LACS) but in whom the CT scan shows a large right frontoparietal infarct (due to occlusion of a branch of the middle cerebral artery) and the assessment by the occupational therapist reveals evidence of visual–spatial–perceptual dysfunction that was not detected by the doctor at the bedside.

Pathological diagnosis (what is the nature of the lesion?)

5.1 What pathologies cause stroke and how common are they?

In white people, about 80–85% of strokes are due to cerebral infarction, 10–15% to primary intracerebral haemorrhage and 5% to subarachnoid haemorrhage.[1] In Asians and blacks, the proportion of haemorrhagic stroke is reported to be higher, about 30–40%.

5.2 Why distinguish between an ischaemic and a haemorrhagic stroke?

It is important to accurately distinguish between an ischaemic and a haemorrhagic stroke because the respective causes, prognoses and acute and prophylactic treatments for ischaemic and haemorrhagic stroke are different.

5.3 How is a recent ischaemic stroke differentiated from a recent haemorrhagic stroke?

> **Differentiating ischaemic from haemorrhagic stroke**
> The only reliable method of differentiating ischaemic stroke from primary intracerebral haemorrhage or subarachnoid haemorrhage is early brain imaging by plain CT scan within the first week after onset of stroke (*Fig. 5.1*).

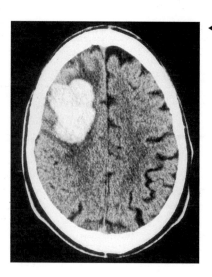

Fig 5.1 Plain cranial CT scan showing a right frontal lobe haemorrhage (as a focal area of high density in the right frontal lobe cortex and subcortex) due to a ruptured arteriovenous malformation.

5.4 Why does CT imaging need to be carried out within the first few days of stroke?

Haemorrhage in the brain is visible immediately on CT (i.e. it doesn't take a few hours to develop its characteristic white appearance) but the distinct appearance of the fresh haemorrhage changes with time, disappearing slowly in the subsequent days to weeks, depending on the size of the haemorrhage. Thereafter the haemorrhage appears as a region of low density on CT scan, which can be mistaken for an old infarct (*see Q. 3.27 & Fig. 3.8*).

5.5 How reliable is early CT imaging in differentiating ischaemic from haemorrhagic stroke?

Early CT imaging is 100% reliable in diagnosing primary intracerebral haemorrhage (PICH), but it is 'only' positive in 95–97% of patients with subarachnoid haemorrhage (SAH). Consequently, there are a small number of patients with SAH in whom brain imaging is equivocal (about 3%) and in whom examination of the cerebrospinal fluid (CSF) by lumbar puncture between 12 hours and 2 weeks after onset is required to confirm or exclude SAH (*see Q. 3.49 & Q. 3.50*).

5.6 Does lumbar puncture have any other role in distinguishing ischaemic from haemorrhagic stroke?

No. Besides its role in the diagnosis of CT-negative SAH, examination of the cerebrospinal fluid by lumbar puncture has no place in differentiating cerebral infarction from primary intracerebral haemorrhage; it is useless and potentially hazardous.

5.7 How useful are clinical features in differentiating ischaemic from haemorrhagic stroke?

The clinical features of the stroke are not specific enough to differentiate ischaemic from haemorrhagic stroke.

Before the days of CT brain imaging, the clinical features considered typical of haemorrhagic stroke (e.g. drowsiness and severe headache) were derived from clinicopathological correlation of severe cases of intraparenchymal and intraventricular haemorrhage that were examined at autopsy. When CT imaging became available, it was soon clear that many smaller, non-fatal PICHs were not associated with these 'typical' features. A number of clinical scoring systems were then devised specifically to differentiate PICH from infarction, for use when CT imaging was not available: the Allen score,[2,3] the Siriraj score[4] and a method suggested by Besson et al.[5] Although these systems do increase clinical diagnostic accuracy, prospective studies have shown that, even in patients with a low probability of cerebral haemorrhage on the basis of these scores, at least 7% (with the Allen score) and 5% (with the Siriraj score) of patients do actually have an intracerebral haemorrhage visible on CT.[6,7]

Indeed, none of the clinical scoring systems devised to help differentiate between infarction and haemorrhage is sufficiently accurate to guide investigation, treatment and prognosis in any individual patient.

5.8 How is an old ischaemic stroke differentiated from an old haemorrhagic stroke?

If CT imaging is delayed for more than a few weeks after stroke, it is not possible to reliably distinguish ischaemic from haemorrhagic stroke because the CT appearances of haemorrhage (i.e. a white hyperdense area) will have changed to resemble the CT scan appearances of an infarct (i.e. a black hypodense area).

However, appropriate magnetic resonance imaging (MRI) sequences can help diagnose intracerebral haemorrhage months or even years after the event when the CT shows only a hypodense area indistinguishable from an infarct (*Fig. 5.2*). This is because the characteristic signal changes of parenchymal haemorrhage due to haemosiderin formation persist indefinitely. The only drawback is that not all haematomas form haemosiderin during their resolution and therefore not all haematomas are discernible as such on MRI performed late after the stroke.

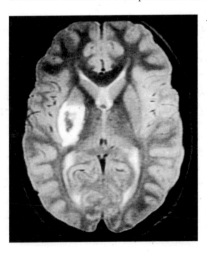

Fig 5.2 MRI T2-weighted brain scan, axial plane, within 48 hours of onset of stroke, showing a haematoma in the right posterior putamen and globus pallidus (basal ganglia) as an area of low density in the centre of the haemorrhage (caused by deoxyhaemoglobin in hypoxic red cells) surrounded by a rim of high intensity (caused presumably by oedema).

5.9 What are the distinguishing features of arterial haemorrhagic transformation of the infarct?

Haemorrhagic transformation (HTI) occurs in a substantial minority of cerebral infarcts, particularly in large infarcts and patients with high blood pressure. It tends to occur early, within the first few days, but can happen up to weeks after cerebral infarction. However, the clinical relevance of HTI is frequently uncertain.[8]

Although early brain CT will reliably identify intracerebral haemorrhage, the distinction between a PICH and HTI is unreliable and difficult (*see Q. 3.35 & Fig. 3.14*). The CT appearances of HTI range from small petechial haemorrhages (small white spots in an area of low density) to frank haematomas (a large white blob), which may or may not have been symptomatic (i.e. accompanied by clinical deterioration). The only definitive way of diagnosing HTI is to have identified a definite infarct, or at least to have excluded PICH, on an earlier scan and then to see haemorrhage in the same region on a follow-up scan. This is another reason for recommending CT brain scan as soon as possible after suspected stroke, ideally at the time of initial assessment.

5.10 Should all patients with suspected stroke have a CT brain scan?

Yes, all patients with suspected stroke should have a CT scan to:

- Help confirm the clinical diagnosis of stroke
- Distinguish ischaemic from haemorrhagic stroke
- Obtain important clues as to the likely cause of the cerebral infarction, primary intracerebral haemorrhage or subarachnoid haemorrhage (all of which aid clinical decisions about further investigation, treatment and secondary prevention strategies).

If these issues are not relevant to patient management (e.g. in a patient with terminal malignancy undergoing palliative care) then CT brain imaging is not necessary.

Computed tomography is likely to remain the principal imaging technique for stroke patients for the foreseeable future, not only because it excludes several non-stroke pathologies and reliably distinguishes haemorrhage from infarction but because it is far more widely available, less expensive and easier and safer to use in acutely ill stroke patients. However, where available, MRI and its specific sequences, such as diffusion-weighted imaging, perfusion-weighted imaging and MR angiography, can add substantially to the understanding of the mechanisms of stroke.

PATIENT QUESTIONS

5.11 What types of stroke are there?

Ischaemic stroke

About 85% of all strokes are caused by a blockage in an artery (blood vessel), which prevents blood getting to part of the brain. The artery may be blocked by a blood clot or it may be affected by a disease that makes the artery too narrow for blood to get through. The reduced blood flow to the brain cells in the area supplied by the artery causes them initially to stop functioning. The part of the brain which is deprived of blood (and oxygen and glucose) supply is said to be *ischaemic*. If the lack of blood supply (ischaemia) is not restored, and persists for several hours, then that part of the brain dies because of lack of oxygen and glucose. This is called *infarction* of the brain.

Haemorrhagic stroke

About 15% of all strokes are caused by rupture/bursting of an artery (not blockage of an artery), which leads to bleeding (haemorrhage) into the brain or over the surface of it. This is called a haemorrhagic stroke.

Bleeding into the brain is called *intracerebral haemorrhage* and bleeding over the surface of the brain is called *subarachnoid haemorrhage*.

ESTABLISHING THE CAUSE OF BRAIN HAEMORRHAGE

PQ PATIENT QUESTIONS

ESTABLISHING THE CAUSE OF STROKE

6.1 Is stroke a single disease entity or a syndrome with many underlying diseases?

Stroke and transient ischaemic attacks (TIAs) are merely symptoms and signs of one of a number of possible underlying disease processes, which need to be identified in order to minimise brain damage and prevent recurrence. There are many potential diseases that can cause a stroke or TIA, and these generally differ for ischaemic and haemorrhagic stroke, although some conditions, such as hypertension, can cause both.

6.2 How is the cause of stroke determined?

The clinical syndrome, derived by the history and examination, and the stroke pathology, derived from an early CT brain scan, often provide several clues to the underlying cause, but the results of special investigations are frequently required to ascertain the underlying cause of the cerebral infarct or haemorrhage.

6.3 Is it possible to establish the cause of stroke in all cases?

Even after extensive investigation, the underlying cause cannot be definitely established in up to 40% of patients with ischaemic stroke. Furthermore, many patients have several concurrent conditions that may be causes (e.g. carotid stenosis and atrial fibrillation (AF) in a patient with an embolic ischaemic carotid territory stroke). Thus, in practice, the precise cause of the stroke is often uncertain. This must be accepted when interpreting the data in this chapter.

6.4 What are the common causes of stroke?

Common underlying causes of stroke

- Embolism of thrombus via or from the heart (20%)
- Large artery atherothrombosis or thromboembolism (45–50%)
- Small artery microatheroma/lipohyalinosis (25%)
- Other arteriopathies such as dissection and arteritis (5%)
- Haematological disorders causing a prothrombotic state (< 5%).[1]

Among the 80% of all strokes that are ischaemic (i.e. caused by cerebral infarction), the mechanism is usually sudden thrombotic or embolic occlusion of a cerebral artery or, less often, low flow distal to an already occluded or highly stenosed artery. The common underlying causes are listed in the box.

Various rare but sometimes treatable conditions (e.g. arteritis, infective endocarditis) are more common in young stroke patients, in whom 'degenerative' arterial disease is unusual, but may still be the cause of stroke in the elderly. The common causes of intracerebral and subarachnoid haemorrhage are also listed in *Table 6.1*.

TABLE 6.1 Causes of stroke

Cause	%
Cerebral infarction	75–80
Large artery atherothromboembolism	(50)
Extracranial (aorta, carotid, vertebral arteries)	[40–45]
Intracranial (interior/middle/anterior/posterior carotid, vertebral, basilar arteries)	[5–10]
Small artery microatheroma/lipohyalinosis (lacunar syndromes)	(20–25)
Embolism from the heart	(20)
Non-atheromatous arterial disease (e.g. dissection, arteritis)	(5)
Blood disease (thrombophilia)	(< 5)
Intracerebral haemorrhage	10–15
Hypertensive lipophyalinosis and microaneurysms	(40)
Bleeding diatheses (e.g. antithrombotic drugs, thrombocytopenia)	(10)
Arteriovenous malformation	(10)
Amyloid angiopathy	(10)
Haemorrhagic transformation of cerebral infarct	(10)
Aneurysm	(5)
Intracerebral tumour	(5)
Arteritis	(< 5)
Drugs: sympathomimetics (e.g. amphetamines, cocaine)	(< 5)
Arterial dissection	(< 5)
Intracranial venous thrombosis	(< 5)
Subarachnoid haemorrhage	5
Aneurysm	
Arteriovenous malformation	
Undetermined	5

This chapter will concentrate on large-artery atherothromboembolism, intracranial small-artery disease and embolism from the heart, the 'big three' causes of ischaemic stroke.

ATHEROSCLEROSIS AS A CAUSE OF ISCHAEMIC STROKE

6.5 What is arteriosclerosis?

Arteriosclerosis is a generic term embracing all varieties of structural changes that result in hardening (and thickening) of the wall of large and small, and elastic and muscular arteries, and arterioles ('arteriolosclerosis').

6.6 What is atherosclerosis?

Atherosclerosis is one form of arteriosclerosis, characterised by an intimal pool of necrotic, proteinaceous and fatty substances in the hardened arterial wall (Greek *athere*, 'porridge' or 'gruel').

6.7 What are the common arterial sites of atherosclerosis?

> Atherosclerosis (or atheroma) mainly affects large (e.g. aortic arch) and medium-sized arteries at places of arterial branching (e.g. carotid bifurcation), tortuosity (e.g. carotid siphon) and confluence (e.g. basilar artery) (*Fig. 4.1*). These are sites of haemodynamic shear stress, turbulent blood flow, boundary layer separation, stagnation of blood, and endothelial trauma.
>
> Curiously, some parts of the arterial tree are free of atheroma, such as the region of the internal carotid artery (ICA) between the origin and siphon, and the main cerebral arteries distal to the circle of Willis.

However, in any given individual, atheroma in one site tends to be accompanied by atheroma in other segments of the same artery and atheroma in other arteries to the brain and other organs (e.g. the heart, kidneys and limbs). Precisely where atheroma occurs is probably determined by the anatomy of the arteries, although it is curious how, in an individual, one arterial site can be affected severely while its counterpart on the other side of the body is normal. Perhaps this is because of subtle asymmetries. Presumably who gets atheroma is determined by individual genetic susceptibility (to develop atheroma in response to exposure to causal risk factors such as hypertension) as well as the degree and duration of exposure to causal vascular risk factors (see below).

6.8 What causes atherosclerosis?

> Although atheroma seems to be an almost inevitable accompaniment of ageing, at least in developed countries, it is not a 'degenerative' disease. Indeed, atheroma is a dynamic condition that begins in childhood, probably in response to endothelial injury. The nature of the endothelial injury is uncertain but is possibly inflammatory; inflammation in the vessel wall seems to play an essential part in the initiation of atheroma (as well as in the progression and erosion and rupture of atherosclerotic plaque).[2]

> Genetically predisposed individuals (strong family history of atherosclerotic disease due to presumed polygenic inheritance) are likely to develop atheroma prematurely or to have particularly extensive or severe atheroma when exposed to causal risk factors for atheroma (e.g. cigarette smoking, raised blood pressure, raised serum cholesterol and diabetes mellitus; *see Chapter 7*).

6.9 How does atherosclerosis evolve?

Atheroma begins as intimal fatty streaks. Over many years, circulating monocyte-derived macrophages adhere to and invade the arterial wall. Intracellular (and later extracellular) cholesterol and other lipids are deposited, particularly in macrophages, which are then described as foam cells. An inflammatory response is evoked, with cytokine production and T-lymphocyte activation. Smooth muscle cells proliferate and fibrosis occurs, forming fibrolipid plaques. These atheromatous plaques invade the media and gradually spread around and along the arterial wall. The arterial lumen narrows and, at times, the vessel dilates. The plaques may become 'active' or 'unstable' from time to time and complicated by erosion or fissuring of thin parts of the fibrous cap, haemorrhage into the plaque or rupture of the plaque, with subsequent platelet adhesion, activation, aggregation and thrombus formation (see below).

Otherwise, advanced plaques may become calcified or necrotic. Heavily calcified and fibrotic plaques make the whole artery rigid, elongated, tortuous and sometimes ectatic. Ectasia and aneurysmal bulging, particularly of the basilar artery, may compress adjacent structures such as the lower cranial nerves and brainstem (as well as cause thromboembolism). However, arterial rupture is exceptional.

6.10 What causes an atherosclerotic plaque to become unstable?

It remains uncertain exactly what triggers a 'dormant' atherosclerotic plaque to become unstable and then rupture. In contrast to a stable atherosclerotic plaque, which has a small lipid core and a strong, fibrous cap, ruptured plaques contain a large core of eccentrically located lipid-laden macrophages (foam cells) engorged with oxidised low density lipoprotein (LDL) cholesterol, and a thin friable overlying fibrous cap devoid of smooth muscle cells.

It appears that the oxidised LDL within the lipid core stimulates plaque inflammation, which undermines the structural integrity of the plaque and activates the endothelium to a proinflammatory and procoagulant state. The oxidised LDL and other inflammatory stimuli initiate recruitment of inflammatory cells into the lesion, and serve as a second messenger to enhance the synthesis of other vascular inflammatory products such as adhesion molecules and cytokines. Cytokines and metalloproteinases weaken the fibrous cap. The plaque is believed to rupture because the large lipid core redistributes the shear stress on the thin fibrous cap and very high loads are imparted upon localised areas of the weakened cap.[3]

6.11 What triggers an unstable atherosclerotic plaque to rupture?

Plaque inflammation and rupture may be triggered by an endogenous systemic factor or exposure (acute or chronic) to an exogenous antigen, such as a microorganism. There is a consistent significant relationship between symptomatic coronary artery disease and moderately elevated markers of inflammation that are unrelated to chronic infection (e.g. fibrinogen, C-reactive protein, albumin, serum amyloid A and leukocyte count), particularly C-reactive protein. Some studies have identified a higher than expected incidence of chronic infections of the teeth, gums and lungs, and with *Chlamydia pneumoniae*, *Helicobacter pylori* and cytomegalovirus. Although there is emerging evidence that these associations with chronic infections may be coincidental rather than causal, a similar, yet less robust, body of evidence is also mounting for the role of a systemic, low-grade, inflammatory response being an integral part of the pathogenesis of acute ischaemic stroke due to atherosclerosis.[4,5]

6.12 How does thrombus form on a ruptured atherosclerotic plaque?

PLATELET-MEDIATED THROMBOSIS

Following plaque rupture or erosion of the vascular endothelium, blood is exposed to the endothelial basement membrane and extracellular matrix. Von Willebrand factor (vWF), which is a large, multimeric protein synthesised by the endothelium and secreted into the subendothelium, binds to extracellular collagen. Platelets adhere to the subendothelial collagen, vWF and fibronectin by means of platelet-membrane glycoprotein receptors, which are receptors for adhesive proteins.[6] The largest glycoprotein (Gp) is designated I, the smallest IX. Letters a and b were added when better techniques allowed resolution of single protein bands on electrophoresis into two separate bands (e.g. glycoprotein I became Ia and Ib). The most abundant platelet-membrane glycoprotein receptor is the integrin family, which are heterodimeric molecules composed of α and β subunits.

Under conditions of low shear stress, platelets adhere to subendothelial collagen and fibronectin through the binding of platelet glycoprotein Ia–IIa receptors. Under conditions of high shear stress, platelets adhere to subendothelial vWF by means of platelet glycoprotein Ib–V–IX (Ib/IX).

Platelets become activated when specific platelet receptors bind to various agonists such as collagen (in the vessel wall), thrombin, thromboxane A_2, adenosine diphosphate (ADP), adrenaline (epinephrine) and arachidonic acid. A series of intracellular reactions takes place. The final common pathway of platelet activation is the assembly of the glycoprotein IIb/IIIa receptor on the surface of activated platelets.[7] Under resting conditions, the surface of a platelet contains 50 000–80 000 copies of the GpIIb–IIIa ($\alpha_{IIb}\beta_3$) receptor. Upon platelet activation, the platelet GpIIb–IIIa receptor undergoes a conformational change, enabling it to bind both vWF and fibrinogen, resulting in irreversible platelet adhesion and aggregation, respectively. The dimeric nature of the fibrinogen molecule allows it to bind to GpIIb–IIIa receptors on two separate platelets, resulting in interplatelet bridging, platelet aggregation and growth of the primary platelet clot.

Adherent, activated platelets recruit additional platelets into the growing thrombus by releasing ADP and arachidonic acid, the latter of which is metabolised by platelet cyclooxygenase thromboxane A_2. Activated platelets also promote the assembly of clotting factors on the platelet surface (V, X, VIII), thereby amplifying thrombin generation. Thrombin is central to platelet aggregation.

COAGULATION

Coagulation is initiated by exposure of blood to tissue factors (TFs) located in the necrotic core of ruptured atherosclerotic plaques, in the subendothelium of injured vessels and on the surface of activated leukocytes attracted to the damaged vessel.[8]

The original cascade/waterfall hypothesis of blood coagulation is that there are two activating pathways:

- The TF or extrinsic pathway
- The contact or intrinsic pathway.

A revised hypothesis of blood coagulation maintains that there is a single coagulation pathway, triggered by vessel injury and TF.[9] TF binds factor VIIa and the resulting factor VIIa/TF complex activates both factors IX and X (i.e. the intrinsic and extrinsic pathways are integrated in vivo). Factor IXa assembles on the surface of activated platelets as part of the intrinsic tenase complex, which comprises factor IXa, factor VIIIa and calcium. Factor Xa, generated through the extrinsic (factor VIIa/TF) and the intrinsic tenase complex, assembles on the surface of activated platelets as part of the prothrombin-activating (prothrombinase) complex, which consists of factor Xa, factor Va and calcium. When assembled in this way, the prothrombinase complex generates a burst of thrombin activity. Thrombin (IIa) activates platelets and factors V and VIII and also converts fibrinogen to fibrin; thrombin then binds to fibrin, where it remains active.

As blood clot forms at the site of vessel injury, plasminogen, an inert circulating protein closely bound to the deposited fibrin, is slowly activated (by tissue plasminogen activator, which has been activated by kallikrein) to form plasmin, which digests the fibrin clot to give fibrin degradation products. The net result is that platelets and later fibrin accumulate at, and are limited to, the site of vascular injury. The rest of the vasculature remains free of platelet and fibrin deposits because, in circulating blood, the tendency of the coagulation mechanism to be activated is counterbalanced by inhibitory factors in the blood such as antithrombin III (which inactivates factors IX, X, XI and XII). However, at the point of vessel injury, the activation of the coagulation mechanism is so powerful that the inhibitors are overwhelmed.

The three major inhibitory systems that modulate the coagulation pathway are:

- The protein C anticoagulant pathway
- The TF pathway inhibitor (TFPI)
- Antithrombin.

Protein C is activated by the thrombin/thrombomodulin complex on the endothelial cell surface. When thrombin binds to thrombomodulin (an endothelial membrane protein) it undergoes a conformational change at its active site that converts it from a procoagulant enzyme to a potent activator of protein C. Activated protein C acts as an anticoagulant in the presence of protein S by proteolytic degradation and inactivation of factors Va and VIIIa (*see Q. 6.55*). TFPI binds and inactivates factor Xa and the TFPI/factor Xa complex, and then inactivates factor VIIa within the factor VIIa/TF complex. Antithrombin inactivates free thrombin and factor Xa, but these clotting enzymes are protected from inactivation by antithrombin when they are bound to fibrin and activated platelets, respectively (*see Q. 6.54*).

6.13 What happens to thrombus on an atherosclerotic plaque?

Thrombus on an atherosclerotic plaque may:

- Become incorporated into the atheromatous plaque with subsequent re-endothelialisation ('healing') of the plaque
- Grow to obstruct the arterial lumen and then propagate proximally or distally in the stagnant column of blood as far as the next branching point or beyond
- Be lysed by natural fibrinolytic mechanisms in the vessel wall
- Embolise in whole or in part to occlude a distal artery, usually at a branching point. Such artery-to-artery emboli vary in size and shape, and usually consist not only of platelet aggregates but also of some combination of cholesterol debris (from the atheromatous plaque) and

fibrin, which may be newly formed and relatively friable or old and well organised. Depending on local blood flow and on the size, composition and consistency of the impacted emboli, they may be lysed, fragment and vanish into the microcirculation, or remain to occlude the artery and promote local thrombosis.

6.14 Why is atherothrombosis regarded as a dynamic, acute-on-chronic disease?

Atherothrombotic plaques are dynamic lesions, progressing and regressing in various parts of the arterial tree at different rates and at different times, usually showing layers of thrombus of different ages. At any one time a plaque may be static and quiescent with a thick fibrous cap, slowly growing but asymptomatic, or active with ongoing thrombosis and embolisation which may or may not be symptomatic depending on the degree and duration of the consequent ischaemia. It is now possible to monitor the release of emboli from carotid plaques, and elsewhere, into the cerebral circulation with transcranial Doppler ultrasound of the middle cerebral artery, which is a further indication of plaque 'instability'. Not surprisingly, high-intensity embolic signals are more common distal to symptomatic rather than asymptomatic stenoses.

This concept may explain the tendencies for TIAs to cluster, for stroke to occur early after a TIA and to affect the same arterial territory, for presumed artery-to-artery embolic strokes to recur early, and for the risk of stroke to decline with time even distal to a severe symptomatic stenosis (*see Chapter 9*).

6.15 What is an atherosclerotic TIA or ischaemic stroke?

Atherosclerotic TIA and ischaemic stroke are cerebral ischaemia and infarction caused by insufficient blood flow to a part of the brain as a result of the complications of atherosclerosis in the feeding artery:

- Acute in-situ thrombotic arterial occlusion
- Low flow distal to a severely narrowed or occluded artery
- Embolism of atherosclerotic plaque or thrombus from a proximal artery (such as the carotid bifurcation) to occlude a smaller intracranial artery (such as the mainstem or branch of the middle cerebral artery – MCA).

Occasionally, emboli may reach the brain via the collateral circulation, e.g. from a stenosed internal carotid artery (ICA) across the circle of Willis into the MCA distal to an occluded contralateral ICA, or from thrombus in the blind proximal stump of an occluded contralateral ICA, a stenosed proximal external carotid artery (ECA) or more proximal sites of atheroma, but all via the ECA and through the ophthalmic circulation to the carotid siphon and beyond. Also, emboli may arise from the distal end of a thrombus occluding the ICA. Furthermore, focal ischaemia may occur between arterial territories (i.e. in boundary zones), usually because of low flow distal to an occluded artery (*see Q. 4.26*).

6.16 How is atherosclerotic TIA or ischaemic stroke diagnosed?

There are no 'hard and fast' diagnostic criteria for atherosclerotic TIA and ischaemic stroke. Extracranial large artery atherothromboembolism is *more likely* to be the cause of ischaemic stroke or TIA in the case of:

- An elderly patient – more than 60 years of age
- Total or partial anterior circulation infarction/ischaemia (clinical syndrome plus computed tomography/magnetic resonance imaging – CT/MRI – evidence; *see Chapter 4 & Fig. 4.3; Fig. 6.1*)
- Posterior cerebral artery territory infarction/ischaemia
- Boundary zone infarction/ischaemia (clinical syndrome plus CT/MRI evidence)
- Cerebellar infarction/ischaemia
- Carotid, subclavian or vertebral bruit; absent carotid pulses; unequal radial pulses
- Ultrasound or angiographic evidence of more than 50% stenosis of the symptomatic artery
- Other clinical complications of atherothrombosis – angina, past myocardial infarction, claudication, femoral bruits, absent foot pulses.

Extracranial large-artery atherothromboembolism is *less likely* to be the cause of ischaemic stroke or TIA in the case of:

- A young patient – less than 40 years of age
- Lacunar infarct/TIA (clinical syndrome plus CT/MRI evidence; *Fig. 6.2*)
- Definite cardiac embolic source (see below)
- Clear evidence of an alternative mechanism (e.g. migrainous stroke, high erythrocyte sedimentation rate and giant-cell arteritis, arterial dissection, etc.)
- No vascular bruits, normal pulses
- No arterial stenosis on Duplex sonography or angiography
- No evidence of atherothrombosis elsewhere.

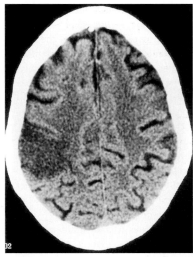

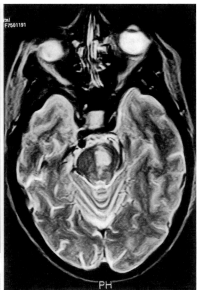

Fig 6.1 Plain cranial CT scan showing a wedge-shaped area of low attenuation, consistent with infarction, in the right parietal lobe, due to embolic occlusion of a branch of the upper division of the middle cerebral artery from a more proximal source in the heart or large arteries and causing a partial anterior circulation syndrome (left hemiparesis – mild – and visual–spatial–perceptual dysfunction). This patient later experienced haemorrhagic transformation of the infarct, as shown in *Fig. 3.14*.

Fig 6.2 MRI brain scan showing a small area of low attenuation in the ventral and paramedian part of the pons on the left side. This is a small pontine infarct caused by occlusion of a small paramedian penetrating branch of the basilar artery and causing a lacunar syndrome characterised by a contralateral (i.e. right-sided) pure motor hemiparesis.

6.17 Why are the diagnostic criteria for atherosclerotic TIA and ischaemic stroke unreliable?

It is rarely possible to attribute an ischaemic stroke or TIA confidently to atherosclerosis because in any individual patient with acute focal ischaemia or infarction (the latter confirmed by CT imaging) it is difficult to visualise the arterial occlusion and the underlying arterial disease and even more difficult to determine exactly how the occlusion has occurred. One reason for this is that angiography is seldom performed early, if at all, and in any case angiography only images the lumen of the artery and not the wall. Ultrasound can non-invasively image the wall and lumen of extracranial arteries but not of the intracranial circulation.

To add to these limitations, even when angiography or ultrasound of the extra- and intracranial circulation is done early, the study is not infrequently normal because many occluded arteries, particularly the mainstem of the MCA, have already spontaneously recanalised (i.e. within the first few hours to days). And if the angiogram or ultrasound does reveal an occluded artery, it is not possible to be sure of the underlying disease and the mechanism of arterial occlusion, unless the appearance is characteristic. Furthermore, it is not possible to be sure that the occlusion was recent, that it was embolic rather than due to in situ thrombosis, that any embolism arose from the parent artery rather than via collaterals or from the distal end of the occluded thrombus – or whether the ischaemia was due to low flow distal to an old occlusion.

However, although it is generally not possible to be certain of the exact cause of the arterial occlusion, it is reasonable to assume that atherothromboembolism has occurred at some stage (and is likely to occur again) if angiography or ultrasound demonstrates arterial pathology, consistent with atheroma, in the relevant cerebral circulation, as well as in other common sites such as the aorta, neck arteries, basilar artery and circle of Willis. If little or no arterial pathology is demonstrated by vascular imaging, or macroscopically at post-mortem, then focal ischaemia is most probably due to embolism from the heart or to intracranial small-vessel disease (see below).

INTRACRANIAL SMALL-VESSEL DISEASE AS A CAUSE OF STROKE

6.18 What is intracranial small vessel disease?

The intracranial small vessels are the small penetrating arteries of the brain (less than about 500 μm in diameter), i.e. the lenticulostriate branches of the MCA, the thalamoperforating branches of the proximal posterior cerebral artery, and the perforating arteries to the brainstem.

There are four major types of intracranial small vessel disease:

- *Arteriolosclerosis* (hyaline arteriolosclerosis, 'simple' small-vessel disease) – a uniform, concentric/circumferential, hyaline thickening and mineralisation/calcification of the arteriolar wall that is frequently seen at post-mortem in elderly, hypertensive, diabetic patients and is associated with cognitive decline (e.g. vascular dementia) but is not a proven cause of lacunar infarction.
- *Atherosclerosis* (microatheroma) – affects larger perforating arteries (> 300 μm in diameter) and the circle of Willis. It is almost like larger-artery atheroma that has been 'driven down the vascular tree' by hypertension and causes about one-third of cases of lacunar infarction.

It is uncertain whether plaque instability plays a role, as in larger artery atherosclerosis.

■ *Lipohyalinosis* ('complex' small-vessel disease) – circumferential subintimal collections of foamy macrophages (intimal xanthoma) that may ultimately occlude the lumen of the smaller, distal perforating arteries (40–300 μm in diameter). The appearance is similar to that of fatty streaks seen in early childhood atheroma in larger arteries. It is usually asymptomatic. However, acute symptomatic lesions, which cause about two-thirds of cases of lacunar infarction, are characterised by a destructive lesion characterised by fibrinoid necrosis. This lesion is also the cause of intracranial haemorrhages in the areas supplied by small perforating arteries (e.g. pons, thalamus, putamen).

■ *Rarities* – arteritis, platelet emboli.

6.19 How does intracranial small-vessel disease cause TIA and stroke?

Because the small perforating arteries are not supported by a good collateral circulation, occlusion usually causes infarction, albeit in a small restricted area of brain. Such 'lacunar' infarcts comprise about one-quarter of first ischaemic strokes and TIAs, and usually cause a lacunar syndrome (*see* Q. 4.16). Because the case fatality is so low (about 1%), there are few pathological data, but it does seem that these small arteries are much less likely to be occluded by emboli, either from the heart or from extracranial sites of atherothrombosis, than the trunk or cortical branches of the MCA. Furthermore, ischaemic lacunar strokes are less often associated with MCA emboli detected with transcranial Doppler ultrasound.

Diseased intracranial small vessels can also rupture and cause small, deep haemorrhages (as well as lacunar infarcts); indeed, both types of stroke have been described in the same patients.

6.20 What causes intracranial small-vessel disease?

Although hypertension, cigarette smoking, diabetes and advanced age are common in patients with lacunar infarction, they cannot explain every case and in any event the risk factors, including hypertension, seem to be rather similar to those of ischaemic stroke patients with presumed atherothrombotic arterial disease. Perhaps the same individuals are susceptible to both atherothrombosis of large and medium-sized arteries *and* small-vessel disease, but one becomes symptomatic before the other. Or perhaps the concept of a distinct small-vessel disease causing lacunar infarction is incorrect. Certainly, at least some small infarcts in the brainstem and internal capsule are caused by atheroma at the mouth of the small penetrating vessels spreading from atheroma of the larger parent artery.

6.21 How is TIA or ischaemic stroke due to intracranial small-vessel disease diagnosed?

There are no reliable diagnostic criteria. Intracranial small vessel disease is *more likely* to be the cause of ischaemic stroke or TIA:

- In the case of lacunar syndrome (clinically defined)
- Where CT/MRI shows a small, deep and relevant infarct in the internal capsule/basal ganglia area, cerebral peduncle or pons (*see Figs 4.5 & 6.2*), or is normal
- If there is no clinical (cervical bruit) or ultrasonographic/angiographic evidence of more than 50% stenosis, or occlusion, of the symptomatic artery in the neck
- If there is no evidence of a cardiac embolic source
- When vascular risk factors are present, particularly hypertension, smoking and diabetes.

EMBOLISM FROM THE HEART AS A CAUSE OF ISCHAEMIC STROKE

6.22 What are the cardiac sources of embolism to the brain?

The cardiac sources of embolism that may travel to the brain are listed in *Box 6.1.*

BOX 6.1 Cardiac sources of embolism (in anatomical sequence)

Right to left shunt (paradoxical emboli from the venous system) via:
- Patent foramen ovale
- Atrial septal defect
- Ventricular septal defect
- Pulmonary arteriovenous malformation

Left atrium
- Thrombus:
  - Atrial fibrillation*
  - Sinoatrial disease (sick sinus syndrome)
  - Atrial septal aneurysm
- Myxoma and other tumours*

Mitral valve
- Rheumatic endocarditis (stenosis* or regurgitation)
- Infective endocarditis*

BOX 6.1 (Cont'd)

■ Mitral annulus calcification
■ Mitral valve prolapse
■ Non-bacterial thrombotic (marantic) endocarditis
■ Libman–Sacks endocarditis
■ Antiphospholipid-protein antibody syndrome
■ Prosthetic heart valve*
■ Papillary fibroelastoma

Left ventricle
■ Mural thrombus:
  – Acute myocardial infarction (within previous few weeks)*
  – Left ventricular aneurysm or akinetic segment
  – Dilated cardiomyopathy*
  – Mechanical 'artificial' heart*
  – Blunt chest injury (myocardial contusion)
■ Myxoma and other tumours*
■ Hydatid cyst
■ Primary oxalosis

Aortic valve
■ Rheumatic endocarditis (stenosis or regurgitation)
■ Infective endocarditis*
■ Syphilis
■ Non-infective thrombotic (marantic) endocarditis
■ Libman–Sacks endocarditis
■ Antiphospholipid antibody syndrome
■ Prosthetic heart valve*
■ Calcific stenosis/sclerosis/calcification

Congenital heart disease (particularly with right to left shunt)
**Cardiac manipulation/surgery/catheterisation/valvuloplasty/
angioplasty**

* Substantial risk of embolism

6.23 **What are the common cardiac sources of embolism to the brain?**

The most common source of embolism from the heart is a dilated, fibrillating left atrium (non-rheumatic AF) causing stasis of blood in the left atrial appendage.

Other major sources are:

■ Thrombus in a dilated left atrium caused by rheumatic AF

TABLE 6.2 Prevalence of potential cardiac sources of embolism in patients with first-ever ischaemic stroke[10]

Source	%
Any atrial fibrillation	13
Without rheumatic heart disease	12
With rheumatic heart disease	1
Mitral regurgitation	6
Recent (< 6 weeks) myocardial infarction	5
Prosthetic valve	1
Mitral stenosis	1
Paradoxical embolism	1
Any of the above	*20*
Other sources of uncertain significance (aortic stenosis/sclerosis; mitral annulus calcification, mitral valve prolapse, etc.)	11

■ Valvular heart disease due to prosthetic heart valves, rheumatic mitral stenosis or infective endocarditis

■ Thrombus overlying an akinetic or dyskinetic left ventricle due to recent myocardial infarction or a dilated cardiomyopathy

■ Intracardiac tumour.

The prevalence of such sources of embolism are listed in *Table 6.2*.

6.24 What are the high risk cardiac sources of embolism?

Relative risk of cardiac sources of embolism

High risk of embolism
■ Atrial fibrillation (rheumatic or non-rheumatic)
■ Infective endocarditis
■ Prosthetic heart valve
■ Recent myocardial infarction,
■ Dilated cardiomyopathy
■ Intracardiac tumour
■ Rheumatic mitral stenosis

Low risk of embolism
■ Mitral valve prolapse (uncomplicated)
■ Mitral annulus calcification
■ Patent foramen ovale with no evidence of deep venous thrombosis
■ Atrial septal aneurysm
■ Aortic sclerosis

6.25   What is the composition of emboli from the heart to the brain?

Emboli from the heart vary in their composition from mostly fibrin (AF) to mostly platelets (mitral leaflet prolapse), calcium (mitral annulus calcification), tumour (myxoma) or infected vegetations (infective endocarditis).

6.26   What is the size of emboli from the heart to the brain?

Emboli from the heart also vary in size, so they may impact in a medium-sized artery to cause a substantial infarct (e.g. MCA origin, basilar artery) or in a smaller artery to cause merely a restricted defect (e.g. branch of the central retinal artery, cortical branch of MCA). Like other causes of cerebral ischaemia, some emboli, perhaps even most, may be completely asymptomatic.

6.27   How does AF cause embolism from the heart to the brain?

Atrial fibrillation predisposes to stasis of blood in the left atrium and left atrial appendage, which may clot. This may soon embolise to the brain as a fresh clot, or later as an organised thrombus.

However, AF is not always the direct cause of stroke because:

- Other possible causes of stroke, which may also be the cause of the AF, such as ischaemic heart disease and hypertension (e.g. carotid atheroma, intracerebral haemorrhage), are present in about 20% of fibrillating stroke patients
- Some patients with AF have lacunar (presumed non-embolic) syndromes due to intracranial small-vessel disease
- 'Only' about 13% of non-rheumatic fibrillating patients have detectable (by transoesophageal echocardiography) thrombus in the left atrium (although some thrombi may have embolised or be too small to be detected) and it is unknown whether or not these patients have a higher stroke risk than those without detectable thrombi
- In a few cases the AF is caused by the stroke.

Atrial fibrillation may also be associated with stroke due to infective endocarditis and haemorrhagic stroke due to excessive anticoagulation.

6.28   What is the risk of stroke associated with AF?

The average absolute risk of stroke in unanticoagulated non-rheumatic AF patients is about 5% per annum (six times greater than in those in sinus rhythm) and about 12% per annum in unanticoagulated fibrillating TIA/stroke patients.[11]

6.29 What is the risk of stroke associated with prosthetic heart valves?

- The risk of embolism is about 2% per annum for all prosthetic valves, provided patients with mechanical valves are on anticoagulants.
- Mechanical valves have a higher risk of embolism than tissue valves, but there is no difference in stroke risk between the different types of mechanical valve.
- Some Bjork–Shiley tilting disc valves have disintegrated and embolised pieces to the brain.
- Prosthetic mitral valves are more prone to thrombosis than aortic valves.
- Infective endocarditis is a potential risk for any type of prosthetic valve.

6.30 Does mitral valve prolapse cause embolism from the heart to the brain?

No, unless it is associated with, or complicated by, another heart disease such as severe mitral incompetence, AF or infective endocarditis.[12–14]

Mitral-valve prolapse is now understood to be not a single entity but a spectrum of abnormalities with varied clinical, echocardiographic and pathological features. At one end of the spectrum (the severe end) are patients with leaflet redundancy as a result of marked myxomatous proliferation of the spongiosa and elongation of the chordal apparatus. At the other end (the mild end) are those with morphologically normal-appearing leaflets that bulge into the left atrium. Only those with abnormal valve morphology appear to be at risk of complications, and those patients can be identified by echocardiography.

The prevalence of mitral-valve prolapse is also now understood to be as low as 2.4% in the community and is no more common among young patients with unexplained cerebral ischaemia than among control subjects. The majority of patients with a diagnosis of mitral-valve prolapse have 'normal variants', with mild bowing and normal-appearing leaflets, and are not at high risk of stroke, but there is a subgroup with abnormalities on echocardiography who may develop severe mitral regurgitation or infective endocarditis. A single echocardiographic examination is therefore warranted for patients with a midsystolic click or characteristic murmur.

6.31 Does non-rheumatic sclerosis/calcification of the aortic and mitral valves cause embolism from the heart to the brain?

Non-rheumatic sclerosis/calcification of the aortic and mitral valves may be a source of embolism in some patients but unless calcific emboli are seen in the retina (*Fig. 6.3*) or on CT it is difficult to confidently attribute the TIA

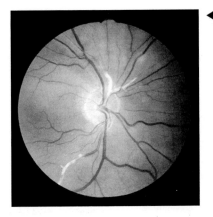

◀ **Fig 6.3** The fundus of a patient with mitral annulus calcification who presented with an ischaemic stroke and in whom ophthalmoscopy revealed calcific emboli in the retinal arterioles.

or ischaemic stroke to this condition, which is very common in normal elderly people.

6.32 Does sinoatrial disease cause embolism from the heart to the brain?

Sinoatrial disease (sick sinus syndrome) may be associated with intracardiac thrombus and embolism, particularly if bradycardia alternates with tachycardia or the patient is in AF.

6.33 Is a patent foramen ovale a common cause of embolism through the heart to the brain?

No, a patent foramen ovale (PFO) is uncommonly the cause of embolism from the venous system or right atrium to the brain. Although a PFO is probably the cause in some of the 30% of patients with stroke in whom the cause is otherwise undetermined (cryptogenic stroke), particularly in younger patients, it is probably more often a coincidental finding.[15]

In 19–36% of people, the foramen ovale fails to close completely after birth, and echocardiographic studies show that about 25% of the general population have an incidental PFO. The size of the defect varies from 1–19 mm (mean 4.9 mm) and is much like a flap valve, sealed closed by the higher pressure in the left atrium. However, at times of elevated right atrial pressure, blood may pass from the right into the left atrium and thence into the systemic arterial circulation.

This paradoxical route for venous embolic material to reach the systemic arterial circulation has been recognised through rare autopsy findings of thrombus straddling a PFO in the setting of fatal stroke. Paradoxical embolism in the context of PFO has also been documented, with stroke during pulmonary embolus, cerebral lesions from gas embolism in divers and cerebral infarction from fat embolism following orthopaedic trauma. However, these clinical settings are often associated with increased pressure in the right heart and therefore predispose to paradoxical embolism. Nevertheless, right-to-left shunting may occur with normal right heart pressures during normal respiration or be precipitated by the Valsalva manoeuvre.

The possible predictors of a causative PFO are: larger size, greater shunting, association with an interseptal aneurysm, evidence of a venous embolic source and clinical features supporting paradoxical embolism. However, these parameters are yet to be confirmed.

6.34 What factors predispose to infective endocarditis?

HEART ABNORMALITIES
- Rheumatic heart disease (especially mitral valve defects)
- Congenital heart disease (especially bicuspid aortic valve in the elderly)
- Mitral valve prolapse – eightfold excess risk
- Degenerative heart disease:
  - Calcified mitral valve annulus
  - Postinfarct mural thrombosis.

IATROGENIC AND LIFESTYLE-ASSOCIATED FACTORS
- Pre-existing dental caries
- Intravenous drug misuse
- Prosthetic heart valves.

PROCEDURES INVOLVING MUCOSAL SURFACES ASSOCIATED WITH BACTERAEMIA
- Upper airway – oral/dental procedures (15–40%)
- Gastrointestinal (10%)
- Urological (10–30%)
- Obstetric (< 10%).

PAEDIATRIC RISK FACTORS
- Previous cardiac surgery
- Congenital heart defects, particularly those involving the septum
- Intravascular catheterisation.

6.35 Which organisms cause infective endocarditis?

- Streptococci – 60–80% of cases
- Staphylococci – < 30%
- Gram-negative bacteria (*Salmonella*, other Enterobacteriaceae, *Pseudomonas* spp.) – < 10%

- Fungi (*Candida albicans, Aspergillus*) – < 4%
- *Coxiella burnetii* (Q fever)
- *Chlamydia* spp.
- *Mycoplasma* spp.
- Non toxigenic *Corynebacterium diphtheriae* biovar. *gravis*.

6.36 Can infective endocarditis be difficult to diagnose?

Yes. The diagnosis of infective endocarditis is often made after pursuing a high index of suspicion in patients with an unexplained stroke, particularly if a cardiac murmur is present (and changes). Sometimes echocardiography fails to image any valvular vegetations, and sometimes the blood cultures are negative.

6.37 How is embolism from the heart to the brain or eye diagnosed?

Diagnosis of embolism from the heart

There are no reliable, valid and standardised diagnostic criteria for TIA or ischaemic stroke due to embolism from the heart (as for other causes of ischaemic stroke).

The diagnosis of embolism from the heart is *more likely* to be the cause of ischaemic stroke or TIA in the case of:

- An identified cardiac source of embolism, particularly one with a substantial embolic risk (*see Q. 6.24*)
- Ischaemic events in more than one arterial territory, particularly if more than one organ is involved
- No evidence clinically (bruits, palpation), on ultrasound or by angiography, of arterial disease (> 50% stenosis) in the neck
- Calcific emboli in the retina (very rare)
- Calcific emboli on brain CT (even rarer)
- No vascular risk factors
- Age less than 50
- No other explanation for the stroke.

Embolism from the heart is *less likely* in the case of:

- Lacunar syndrome (clinical syndrome plus CT/MRI evidence)
- Low flow infarction/ischaemia (clinical syndrome plus possibly CT/MRI evidence).

Embolism from the heart is *uncertain* in the case of:

- Haemorrhagic transformation of the infarct
- Past TIA.

RARER CAUSES OF ISCHAEMIC STROKE

6.38 What are the important less common causes of TIA and ischaemic stroke?

> ### Important less common causes of TIA and ischaemic stroke
>
> *Arterial diseases*
> - Dissection (*see* Q. 6.39–Q. 6.44)
> - Inflammatory and infectious vascular diseases (non-septic and septic arteritis) (*see* Q. 6.45 & Q. 6.46)
> - Cholesterol embolisation syndrome (*see* Q. 6.47)
> - Trauma
> - Fibromuscular dysplasia
> - Congenital arterial anomalies
> - Moyamoya syndrome
> - Embolism from arterial aneurysms
> - Leukoaraiosis
> - Irradiation
>
> *Cardiac sources of embolism (see Box 6.1 & Table 6.3)*
> *Haematological diseases (see Q. 6.48–Q. 6.58).*

6.39 What is arterial dissection and how does it cause a stroke?

Arterial dissection is a tear in the intima or media of the artery. Dissection of a cerebral artery, such as the carotid or vertebral artery, leads to bleeding within the arterial wall, which tracks or dissects longitudinally and circumferentially between the intima and media, or media and adventitia, of the arterial wall. This may cause an ischaemic stroke or TIA if the dissected artery becomes occluded by the false lumen or superimposed thrombus, or if thrombus forms on the intimal flap or in the wall and then embolises distally to occlude intracranial artery.

6.40 Which arteries are prone to dissection?

Most dissections occur at the origin of the internal carotid artery, just above the bifurcation of the common carotid artery into the internal and external carotid arteries. Common carotid artery and intracranial carotid and MCA dissections are less common.

Dissection of the vertebrobasilar arterial system is also not uncommon. When it does occur it happens at the C2 level in more than 80% of cases, possibly reflecting increased susceptibility to mechanical torsion and stretch at this location.

6.41   What causes arterial dissection?

Carotid and vertebral arteries may dissect spontaneously or as a result of local trauma. Predisposing factors are listed in *Box 6.2.*

BOX 6.2   Factors predisposing to arterial dissection

Spontaneous dissection
- Genetic disorders of collagen (family history of arterial dissection in 5% of cases)
- Point mutation in one allele of the *COL1A1* gene, which encodes the proα1(I) chains of type I procollagen, resulting in substitution of alanine for glycine (G13A) in about half of the α1(I) chains of type I collagen
- Marfan's syndrome
- Ehlers–Danlos syndrome types IV and VI
- Cystic medial necrosis
- Osteogenesis imperfecta
- Pseudoxanthoma elasticum
- Polycystic kidney disease
- Fibromuscular dysplasia
- Reticular fibre deficiency
- Accumulation of mucopolysaccharides
- Possibly atheromatous risk factors (hypertension, diabetes, smoking, high cholesterol, hyperhomocystinaemia)

Traumatic dissection
- Sports
- Whiplash injury
- Neck manipulation
- Reversing the car
- Painting the ceiling
- Iatrogenic: cerebral angiography

6.42   What are the characteristic clinical features of carotid artery dissection?

The clinical features of carotid artery dissection are listed in *Box. 6.3.*

6.43   What are the characteristic clinical features of vertebral artery dissection?

The clinical features of vertebral artery dissection are listed in *Box. 6.3.*

BOX 6.3 Characteristic clinical features of carotid artery and vertebral artery dissection

Carotid artery dissection

■ Pain around the eye or frontal region, sometimes in the neck, and sometimes generalised and non-specific, is common and may be the only feature

■ Acute or delayed focal monocular or carotid territory ischaemic symptoms:
  – Ipsilateral visual loss
  – Contralateral hemisensorimotor deficit
  – Difficulty speaking

■ The onset of ischaemic symptoms is usually within a few days of dissection but can be as long as several weeks and even a few months

■ Pulsatile tinnitus may occur

■ Dysgeusia (altered taste)

■ Horner's syndrome ipsilaterally (involvement of the cervical sympathetic chain, ascending in the wall of the carotid artery)

■ Cranial nerve palsy (single or multiple) – III, IV, V, VI, VII, IX, X, XI, XII, in at least 10% of patients with extracranial internal carotid artery (ICA) dissection. The lower cranial nerves, IX–XII, lie close to the ICA below the jugular foramen in the retrostyloid and posterior retroparotid space and may be compressed or stretched by the dissected ICA if it is expanded or aneurysmal because of the extra blood in its wall. Alternatively, the blood supply to the cranial nerves may be compromised by the dissection; the nutrient vessels to the cranial nerves are small (200–300 μm in diameter) branches of the ICA

■ Neck bruit.

Vertebral artery dissection

■ Pain in the neck and back of the head

■ Focal vertebrobasilar ischaemic symptoms: occipital/temporal lobe, brainstem, cerebellum; most commonly features of a lateral medullary or cerebellar infarct

■ Upper limb peripheral motor deficits: bilateral distal upper limb amyotrophy.

6.44 How is the diagnosis of TIA or ischaemic stroke due to arterial dissection made?

Diagnosis of stroke due to artery dissection

■ The clinical features are consistent with the diagnosis (*see Q. 6.42 & Q. 6.43*)

■ *CT (or MRI) brain scan* shows an ischaemic stroke in the territory of supply of a major cerebral artery

■ *Doppler/duplex ultrasound* demonstrates very poor flow in the artery, giving a 'to and fro' high-resistance signal. Occasionally, the line of the dissection and a double lumen can be imaged. Vertebrobasilar ultrasound is more difficult technically and not as reliable

■ *MRI of brain and neck* – T1 images through the narrowed segment of the artery may show a narrowed arterial lumen (as a narrower flow void) with a rim of high signal, which is the thrombus in the arterial wall. Intramural haemorrhage is almost pathognomonic of dissection and differentiates dissection from vasospasm in patients with subarachnoid haemorrhage

■ *Magnetic resonance angiography (MRA)* – may show a stenosed or occluded internal or common carotid artery, or tapering of the lumen at the dissection

■ *Contrast intra-arterial angiography* is the gold standard for diagnosis but is often not required if duplex and MR scanning are available. Angiography of a carotid dissection shows a smoothly stenosed internal or common carotid artery with a double lumen or intimal flap, or a smooth tapering occlusion. The 'string sign' is due to haematoma in the wall of the artery compressing the normal lumen to a 'fine thread'. Sometimes the artery is completely occluded but the occlusive stump often has a tapered shape, suggestive of dissection. Other angiographic findings include intraluminal clot, intimal flaps, pseudoaneurysm formation (usually at the base of the skull) and evidence of distal emboli obstructing smaller intracranial arteries.

6.45 When should CNS vasculitis be suspected?

■ Vasculitis of the central nervous system (CNS) is variable in onset, nature and duration.

■ The clinical features are determined partly by the size and location of the involved vessel(s).

■ It most commonly presents as an acute or subacute, focal or diffuse, encephalopathy or meningoencephalopathy with headache, altered mentation, seizures and cognitive and behavioural abnormalities, with multifocal neurological signs.

■ Less commonly, patients present with a multiple-sclerosis-like picture (i.e. relapsing and spontaneously remitting focal neurological dysfunction), features of a rapidly progressive space-occupying lesion,

multiple cranial neuropathies (e.g. Wegener's granulomatosis) and, rarely, a spinal cord syndrome, extrapyramidal syndrome or stroke syndrome.
■ Systemic symptoms and signs may be present such as fever, headache, malaise, weight loss, joint aches and pains, facial rash, livido reticularis.

6.46 When should giant cell arteritis be suspected?

The common symptoms and signs of giant cell arteritis are listed in *Box 6.4.*

BOX 6.4 Common symptoms and signs of giant cell arteritis

Symptoms
■ Systemic upset (fever, malaise, fatigue, anorexia, weight loss, night sweats, depression and arthralgias)
■ Myalgia (pain and stiffness in the neck, shoulders and buttocks)
■ Headache (temporal, occipital or generalised; severe and persistent)
■ Pain, swelling, redness and tenderness over the affected arteries (e.g. superficial temporal arteries may stand out and be tender on brushing the hair)
■ Pain on chewing (jaw and tongue claudication due to maxillary and lingual artery occlusion)
■ Ischaemic symptoms of the eye (usually sudden, painless deterioration of vision in one eye) or brain.

Signs
■ Thickening, tenderness and nodularity of the temporal arteries, sometimes with reduced or absent pulsation
■ Visual acuity varies from 6/6 to no light perception
■ Visual field defects: particularly altitudinal visual field defects (loss of either the upper or more commonly the lower half of the field in one eye)
■ Ophthalmoscopic findings of distended veins, a swollen optic disc (may be segmental) and, occasionally, cotton-wool spots and splinter- or flame-shaped haemorrhages at or near the disc margin.

The criteria for the diagnosis of temporal arteritis are at least three of the following:

■ Age at disease onset > 50 years
■ New onset of localised headache
■ Abnormal temporal artery clinically – tenderness or decreased pulse
■ Elevated erythrocyte sedimentation rate (> 50 mm/h)
■ Abnormal temporal artery biopsy.

The triad of temporal headache, blindness, and jaw claudication (aching of the jaw on repeated chewing caused by involvement of the branches of the external carotid artery), if present in an elderly person, is almost pathognomonic for the diagnosis of temporal arteritis.[16]

6.47 What is the cholesterol embolisation syndrome?

The cholesterol embolisation syndrome is a rare clinical syndrome, very similar to that seen in systemic vasculitis and infective endocarditis, characterised by the subacute onset of malaise, fever, abdominal pain, proteinuria and renal failure, stroke-like episodes, drowsiness, confusion, skin petechiae, splinter haemorrhages, livedo reticularis, cyanosis of fingers and toes, raised erythrocyte sedimentation rate, neutrophil leukocytosis and eosinophilia. Patients are usually elderly with widespread atherosclerotic disease, and may have undergone instrumentation or surgery within the preceding few hours or days.

The cause is thought to be rupture of atheromatous plaques, either spontaneously or, probably more often, as a complication of instrumentation or surgery of large atheromatous arteries such as the aorta, and possibly of anticoagulation or therapeutic thrombolysis. Cholesterol debris is released and embolises to the microcirculation of many organs throughout the body, including the brain and spinal cord.

The diagnosis is made by finding cholesterol debris in the microcirculation of biopsy material, usually from the kidney but sometimes from skin or muscle.

6.48 What are the thrombophilias?

The thrombophilias are disorders of the blood that predispose to recurrent venous and possibly arterial thrombosis (i.e. they predispose to a procoagulant state)

These include:

- The antiphospholipid syndrome
- Hereditary deficiency of natural coagulation inhibitors:
  - Antithrombin III
  - Protein C
  - Protein S
- Single point mutations in coagulation molecules:
  - Factor V Leiden (1691G/A): activated protein C resistance
  - The 3' untranslated region of the prothrombin gene (factor II; 20210 G/A)
- Hereditary abnormalities of fibrinolysis:
  - Plasminogen deficiency and/or abnormality
- Polycythaemia rubra vera

- Essential thrombocythaemia
- Sickle-cell disease
- Paraproteinaemias
- Thrombotic thrombocytopenic purpura
- Heparin-induced thrombocytopenia
- Cancer
- Nephrotic syndrome
- Pregnancy and the puerperium.

6.49 What is the antiphospholipid syndrome?

The antiphospholipid syndrome is a heterogeneous disorder, both in terms of its clinical manifestations and range of autoantibodies, which is characterised by thrombosis (venous or arterial), recurrent miscarriage or both, in association with persistent positive laboratory tests for antiphospholipid protein antibody (APA) – lupus anticoagulant (LA), anticardiolipin antibody (ACA) or both – on repeated studies. Thrombocytopenia is an occasional feature.

6.50 What are antiphospholipid antibodies?

Antiphospholipid-protein antibodies are a family of antibodies that are specific for several plasma proteins, such as human prothrombin and $\beta2$ glycoprotein ($\beta2$ GpI), which may bind to phospholipid surfaces.[17]

6.51 What are lupus anticoagulants and anticardiolipin antibodies?

Lupus anticoagulants and anticardiolipin antibodies are different antiphospholipid antibodies but occur together in about 60% of patients with the phospholipid antibody syndrome; in the remaining 40%, only one is present.

Lupus anticoagulants are immunoglobulins (IgG, IgM, IgA or mixtures) that interfere with one or more of the in vitro phospholipid-dependent tests of coagulation – e.g. activated partial thromboplastin time (APTT), dilute Russell viper venom time (dRVVT), dilute prothrombin time (dPT) and kaolin clotting time (KCT). They slow the rate of thrombin generation and therefore clot formation in vitro.

Anticardiolipin antibodies are detected by immunoassay, most commonly enzyme-linked immunosorbent assay, in which the anionic phospholipid cardiolipin is used to coat wells on plastic microtitre plates.

6.52 What is the cause of the antiphospholipid syndrome?

In the primary antiphospholipid syndrome there is no evidence of other underlying disease.

The secondary antiphospholipid syndrome is associated with:

■ Rheumatic and connective tissue disorders:
  – Systemic lupus erythematosus (SLE): about 30–40% of patients
    with SLE have lupus anticoagulants
  – Rheumatoid arthritis
  – Systemic sclerosis
  – Temporal arteritis
  – Sjögren's syndrome
  – Psoriatic arthropathy
  – Behçet's syndrome
  – Others
■ Infections
  – Viral (e.g. HIV1, varicella, hepatitis C)
  – Bacterial (e.g. syphilis)
  – Parasitic (e.g. malaria)
■ Drug exposure
  – Chlorpromazine
  – Hydralazine
  – Quinidine
  – Quinine
  – Antibiotics
  – Phenytoin
  – Valproate
  – Procainamide
■ Lymphoproliferative diseases
  – Malignant lymphoma
  – Paraproteinaemia
■ Miscellaneous conditions
  – Autoimmune thrombocytopenia
  – Autoimmune haemolytic anaemia
  – Sickle-cell disease
  – Intravenous drug abuse
  – Livedo reticularis
  – Guillain–Barré syndrome.

6.53 What are the clinical features of the antiphospholipid syndrome?

Any vascular site can be affected so there is a wide range of clinical
manifestations (*Box 6.5*). Venous thromboembolic events account for about
70% of cases and arterial events for the remaining 30%. The most common
site for arterial thrombi is the cerebral circulation.

BOX 6.5 Clinical features of the antiphospholipid syndrome

Neurologic
- TIA, stroke or multifocal encephalopathy due to arterial or venous thrombosis in any size of vessel
- Migraine-like headaches

Dermatologic
- Sneddon's syndrome – livedo reticularis, stroke-like episodes and hypertension
- Non-healing ulceration of the ankles and skin necrosis

Obstetric
- Recurrent spontaneous miscarriage/fetal loss due to intrauterine death in the latter part of the first trimester or early second trimester
- Intrauterine fetal growth retardation
- Early-onset pre-eclampsia
- Prematurity

Paediatric
- Postinfectious (e.g. varicella) thromboembolic events.

6.54 How may antithrombin III deficiency predispose to TIA and ischaemic stroke?

Antithrombin III is a plasma glycoprotein produced primarily in the liver as well as the endothelium. It binds to and inactivates thrombin (factor IIa) and activated factors X, IX, XI and XII (but not VII). It exerts its greatest antithrombotic effect through inhibition of thrombin and factor Xa (*see Q. 6.12*).

It is an important mediator of the anticoagulant effect of heparin; heparin increases the activity of antithrombin III 100-fold. Indeed, heparin resistance is a clue to low antithrombin III activity.

Antithrombin III deficiency may be inherited as an autosomal dominant trait with variable penetrance in about one in every 2000–5000 people, or acquired as a result of severe liver disease (reduced synthesis), intravascular thrombosis (consumption), the nephrotic syndrome (renal loss) or the use of medications such as L-asparaginase or the oral contraceptive pill.

Inherited antithrombin III deficiency carries a high risk of venous thrombosis, and it has been linked to odd case reports and series of ischaemic stroke, but a causal association with ischaemic stroke has not been established.

6.55 How may protein C deficiency predispose to TIA and ischaemic stroke?

Protein C is a vitamin-K-dependent plasma glycoprotein produced in the liver as a zymogen (serine protease precursor). When activated by thrombin in the presence of calcium and the endothelial protein, thrombomodulin, activated protein C inhibits thrombosis by inactivating factors Va and factor VIIIa, and promotes fibrinolysis by inactivating plasminogen activator inhibitor 1, with the assistance of protein S as a cofactor (*see Q. 6.12*).

Protein C deficiency may be inherited as an autosomal dominant trait, or acquired as a result of warfarin therapy or severe liver disease (reduced synthesis), disseminated intravascular coagulation and acute thrombosis.

Children with the homozygous forms of protein C deficiency do not survive infancy. The heterozygous forms of protein C deficiency lead to a hypercoagulable state in adults, with an increased risk of deep vein thrombosis (DVT) that may account for up to 10% of cases of venous thrombosis. Any association with ischaemic stroke has been limited to anecdotal case reports and series.

6.56 How may protein S deficiency predispose to TIA and ischaemic stroke?

Protein S is a vitamin-K-dependent plasma glycoprotein produced primarily in the liver and also in endothelial cells and platelets. About 40% is free in the plasma and about 60% is bound to C4b-binding protein.

The free form of protein S acts as an anticoagulant by serving as a cofactor for protein-C-induced inhibition of factors Va and VIIIa. Free protein S increases the affinity of protein C for phospholipid and enhances the inactivation of factors Va and VIIIa by activated protein C.

Protein S deficiency may be inherited as an autosomal dominant trait or acquired as a result of warfarin therapy, severe liver disease (reduced synthesis) and the nephrotic syndrome.

When there is a deficiency of protein S, protein C is not activated and there is an increased risk of thrombosis. The heterozygous form of protein S deficiency is associated with an increased risk of DVT that may account for up to 5% of cases. Any association with ischaemic stroke has been limited to anecdotal case reports and series.

6.57 What is activated protein C resistance?

Inherited resistance to activated protein C (APCR) was first reported in 1993 by a Swedish team, which identified a family with a tendency to thrombosis (thrombophilia) who had a poor anticoagulant response to protein C.[18]

In 1994; Bertina and colleagues from Leiden in the Netherlands demonstrated that APCR can occur as a result of a mutation in the factor V gene (substitution of glutamine for arginine-506) that is inherited in an autosomal dominant fashion. They named this inherited defect the Leiden factor V mutation (FV Leiden).[19] In patients with FV Leiden, one of the factor Va sites normally cleaved by activated protein C is eliminated and unmodulated factor V results in the occurrence of inappropriate thrombosis.

Inherited resistance to activated protein C due to FV Leiden is now recognised as the most common inherited cause of venous thrombosis. It is present in 0.45–7.8% of the general population (depending on different studies, countries and ethnic groups) and 15–64% of patients with a history of venous thrombosis but less than 5% of patients with arterial thrombosis such as ischaemic stroke (i.e. no more common than the general population). Therefore, in contrast to its established causal role in cerebral venous thrombosis, its causal role in cerebral arterial occlusion is uncertain.

6.58 How is ischaemic stroke due to a procoagulant state diagnosed?

It can be very difficult to confidently attribute the cause of the ischaemic stroke to the haematological disorder (i.e. thrombophilia) if the patient has other disease that could have caused the stroke. More often than not, the haematological disorder is one of several factors predisposing to thrombus formation, such as activated protein C resistance with coexistent atherothrombosis, trauma or dehydration.[20] Irrespective of this, the haematological disorder frequently needs treating in its own right (e.g. ?antiplatelet therapy, ?oral anticoagulant therapy).

ESTABLISHING THE CAUSE OF BRAIN HAEMORRAGE

6.59 What are the common causes of intracerebral haemorrhage?

Common causes of intracerebral haemorrhage

Most haemorrhagic strokes are thought to be due to intracranial small vessel disease (lipohyalinosis – fibrinoid necrosis), which is often associated with hypertension (*Box 6.6*). These haemorrhages are usually deep in the brain, in the areas supplied by small penetrating arteries, such as the thalamus, putamen, pons and cerebellum.

The most common cause of lobar haemorrhages is amyloid angiopathy in older individuals and vascular abnormalities such as arteriovenous malformations and aneurysms in younger individuals. However, the use of illicit drugs such as cocaine and amphetamines increasingly underlies intracerebral haemorrhage in younger people, and anticoagulant drugs with poorly controlled anticoagulation (i.e. international normalised ratios above 4) continue to be an important cause of intracerebral haemorrhage in older individuals.

The age of the patient is the biggest clue to the cause of a primary intracerebral haemorrhage: arteriovenous malformations are the most common cause in the young, 'degenerative' small-vessel disease in middle and early old age, and amyloid angiopathy in old age.

BOX 6.6 Causes of primary intracerebral haemorrhage

Arterial disease

- Lipohyalinosis (fibrinoid necrosis) in small penetrating vessels
  - Most common cause in middle and old age
  - Haemorrhages often deep in putamen (40%), caudate nucleus (8%), thalamus (15%), cerebral hemispheres (lobar) (20%), cerebellum (8%) and brainstem (8%).
- Amyloid (congophilic) angiopathy*
  - Most common cause in old age
  - May be associated with dementia
- Vascular malformations (arteriovenous and cavernous angiomas)
  - Dural or brain
  - Most common cause in young normotensive people
  - Seizures and headaches commonly antedate haemorrhage
  - Cavernous angiomas tend to be multiple and familial
- Caroticocavernous fistula
- Hereditary haemorrhagic telangiectasia
- Saccular aneurysms – cause one in 13 intracerebral haemorrhages (two in 13 < 65 years old), usually in conjunction with subarachnoid haemorrhage
- Atheromatous aneurysm
- Septic arteritis and mycotic aneurysms
- Necrotising angiitis of the CNS*
- Arterial dissection
- Intracerebral tumours
  - Primary (glioblastoma, oligodendroglioma, medulloblastoma, haemangioblastoma)
  - Metastases (melanoma, bronchial/renal/endometrial carcinoma, choriocarcinoma)
- Intracranial venous thrombosis*
- Moyamoya syndrome
- Occult head injury*
- Trauma
- Haemorrhagic brain infarction

Raised blood pressure

- Acute arterial hypertension
  - Alcohol (also antiplatelet action and coexistent liver disease)
  - Amphetamines (may also cause a vasculitis)
  - Cocaine and other sympathomimetic drugs
  - Monoamine oxidase A inhibitors
  - Exposure to extreme cold
  - Trigeminal nerve stimulation

BOX 6.6 (Cont'd)

- Post carotid endarterectomy
- Post heart transplantation
- Post correction of congenital heart lesions
■ Chronic arterial hypertension, causing lipohyalinosis and microaneurysms (see below)

Bleeding diathesis*

■ Anticoagulants
- Risk of intracranial haemorrhage is about 1% per year
- Increased risk if elderly, previous stroke, hypertensive and if INR > 4.0
■ Antiplatelet drugs – probably a relatively minor contributory factor
■ Thrombolytic treatment – 0.75% of patients with myocardial infarction: > 2% risk if elderly (> 65 years), low body weight (< 70 kg), hypertensive and given alteplase as opposed to streptokinase; 0.3% risk if none of these
■ Thrombocytopenia
■ Haemophilia
■ Hereditary factor V deficiency – usually autosomal recessive
■ Leukaemia
■ Diffuse intravascular coagulation
■ Occult head injury.

* Causes of multiple haemorrhages in the brain parenchyma

6.60 What features of the clinical history are suggestive of a primary intracerebral haemorrhage and its causes?

PRECEDING CIRCUMSTANCES

■ Neck trauma (arterial dissection)
■ Physical activity– heavy exertion, defaecation, lifting, sexual intercourse
■ Administration of recreational drugs (e.g. amphetamines)
■ Ischaemic stroke (haemorrhagic transformation of an infarct)
■ Puerperium (choriocarcinoma, intracranial venous thrombosis).

ONSET

■ Sudden, with symptoms and signs gradually increasing over seconds or minutes, or rarely hours
■ During physical activity.

SYMPTOMS
- Altered consciousness and/or a focal neurological deficit reflecting a loss of function of the site of bleeding in the brain
- Headache – localised (but may be generalised) at first, often in occipital area, and may later become generalised and spread down back of neck
- Seizures are common in patients with cortical/subcortical haematomas.

PAST HISTORY
- Haemophilia
- Haemorrhage in other sites of the body (haemostatic disorder)
- Hypertension (lipohyalinosis or microaneurysms) – past history of hypertension in about 50% of patients with spontaneous intracranial haemorrhage
- Cancer (particularly melanoma, bronchial or renal carcinoma)
- Epileptic seizures (cortical arteriovenous malformation – AVM, tumour, amyloid angiopathy)
- Headache (AVM)
- Valvular heart disease (septic embolism).

MEDICATIONS/DRUGS
- Oral anticoagulant drugs
- Recreational drugs such as cocaine and amphetamines.

FAMILY HISTORY
- Intracranial haemorrhage:
  - Haemophilia and other inherited coagulation and platelet disorders
  - Sickle-cell disease/trait
  - Vascular malformations sometimes
  - Saccular aneurysm sometimes
  - Hereditary haemorrhagic telangiectasia
  - Amyloid (congophilic) angiopathy – autosomal dominant inheritance (Iceland and Netherlands)
  - Von Hippel–Lindau syndrome
  - Ehlers–Danlos syndrome
  - Pseudoxanthoma elasticum.
- Dementia:
  - Alzheimer's disease
  - Vascular dementia – amyloid angiopathy.

6.61 What features of the clinical examination are suggestive of a primary intracerebral haemorrhage and its causes?

GENERAL

- Petechiae or bruising (generalised haemostatic disorder)
- Signs of malignant disease (clubbing, cutaneous melanoma, hepatosplenomegaly, lung collapse)
- Needle marks (drug addict)
- Hypertension and hypertensive end-organ disease (retinopathy, cardiomegaly)
- Subhyaloid (pre-retinal) haemorrhages
- Heart murmur (infective endocarditis).

NEUROLOGICAL

- Focal neurological deficits: determined by site and size of haematoma – if the intracranial haemorrhage becomes large, with raised intracranial pressure, headache, vomiting and decreased level of consciousness occur
- Depressed consciousness level – about one-third of patients; determined by site and size of haematoma
- Dementia.

6.62 What are the causes of subarachnoid haemorrhage?

Causes of subarachnoid haemorrhage

Saccular aneurysms (85% of cases)
Conditions associated with saccular aneurysms:
- Disorders of connective tissue
  - Marfan's syndrome
  - Ehlers–Danlos syndrome type IV
  - Pseudoxanthoma elasticum
  - α_1-antitrypsin deficiency
  - Neurofibromatosis
- Disorders of angiogenesis
  - Hereditary haemorrhagic telangiectasia
- Associated hypertension
  - Coarctation of the aorta
  - Polycystic kidney disease – hypertension and developmental factors contribute to the development of intracranial aneurysms
- Haemodynamic stress
  - Anomalies of the circle of Willis
  - Arteriovenous malformations
  - Moyamoya syndrome

> *Non-aneurysmal perimesencephalic haemorrhage (10% of cases)*
> *Arterial dissection*
> *Rare conditions*
> ■ Cerebral arteriovenous malformation
> ■ Dural arteriovenous fistula
> ■ Spinal arteriovenous malformation
> ■ Saccular aneurysm of a spinal artery
> ■ Head trauma
> ■ Mycotic aneurysms
> ■ Metastasis of cardiac myxoma
> ■ Cocaine abuse
> ■ Sickle-cell disease
> ■ Coagulation disorders
> ■ Pituitary apoplexy
> ■ Spinal meningioma
> ■ Rupture of circumferential artery of the brainstem.

6.63 What features of the clinical history are suggestive of subarachnoid haemorrhage and its causes?

■ Sudden loss of consciousness (one-half of patients, *see Q. 3.47*)
■ Headache (two-thirds of patients)
  – May be the only symptom
  – *Onset* – sudden, in a split second, like a 'blow' or 'explosion' on/in the head; gradual over minutes rather than seconds in about 10–15%
  – Maximal in seconds
  – *Location* – diffuse and poorly localised but may be occipital or retro-orbital
  – *Severity* – unusually severe, 'the worst headache in my life'
  – *Precipitants* (uncommon) – weight-lifting, sexual activity
  – *Duration* – hours (possibly minutes, we don't know) to weeks; may be biphasic in SAH because of vertebral artery dissection.

It is not clear how frequently patients with aneurysmal subarachnoid haemorrhage have had preceding and unrecognised 'warning leaks'.

■ Epileptic seizures – about 10% of patients
■ Confusion/delirium – less than 5% of patients
■ Nausea
■ Vomiting
■ Neck stiffness – takes about 3–12 (usually 6–12) hours after onset to develop, in response to blood in the subarachnoid space, which acts as a meningeal irritant

■ Pain and stiffness in the back and legs, hours to days after onset – blood irritating lumbosacral nerve roots
■ Photophobia
■ Family history of subarachnoid haemorrhage (6–9% of patients) – in first-degree relatives of patients with SAH, the risk is three to seven times higher than in second-degree relatives or in the general population.

6.64 What features of the examination are suggestive of subarachnoid haemorrhage and its causes?

■ None (very often)
■ Meningism (but absence of neck stiffness does not exclude SAH)
■ Focal neurological signs:
 – *IIIrd nerve palsy* – aneurysm of the terminal internal carotid artery, or at the origin of posterior communicating artery; rarely aneurysm of basilar artery or superior cerebellar artery
 – *VIth nerve palsy* – false localising sign of a non-specific rise in cerebrospinal fluid pressure
 – *IX–XIIth nerve palsy* – compression by subadventitial vertebral artery dissection
 – *Hemiparesis* – large subarachnoid haematoma in Sylvian fissure (middle cerebral artery aneurysm)
 – *Paraparesis* – Aneurysm of anterior communicating artery
 – *Cerebellar ataxia, Wallenberg's syndrome or both* – vertebral artery dissection.

NB. Intraparenchymal haematomas may give rise to other deficits, depending on their site.

■ Subhyaloid haemorrhages in optic fundi (20%)
■ Fever (if due to blood in subarachnoid space, the heart rate is normal; if due to infection, the heart rate is increased)
■ Raised blood pressure
■ Kernig's sign – passive extension of the knee with the hip flexed elicits pain in the back and leg and resistance to hamstring stretch
■ Brudzinski's sign – forward flexion of the neck elicits flexion at the hip and knee
■ Altered consciousness.

PATIENT QUESTIONS

6.65 What causes strokes?

Ischaemic stroke

About 80% of strokes and TIAs are caused by a lack of blood supply to the brain or eye (ischaemic stroke or transient ischaemic attacks of the brain and eye). The most common cause of narrowing of the arteries to the brain is hardening of the arteries (atherosclerosis), which occurs in everyone to a greater or lesser degree as they get older. This process is similar that which affects the water pipes in our houses; they gradually become 'furred up' and narrowed on the inside as they get older. Atherosclerosis (hardening of the arteries) also affects arteries (blood vessels) to other organs of the body – a heart attack (myocardial infarction) is caused by hardening of the arteries supplying blood to a part of the heart muscle. As atherosclerosis tends to affect the arteries to the brain as well as the heart (and legs), it is therefore not surprising that people who suffer a heart attack are also at increased risk of suffering a stroke, and vice-versa. Indeed, among survivors of stroke, the most common cause of death is a heart attack (not another stroke).

Less commonly, ischaemic stroke and TIA are caused by blood clots in the heart, which break away and are carried in the blood stream until they lodge in a smaller blood vessel (artery) in the brain and block the blood flow there. The heart diseases that predispose most to the formation of blood clots in the heart (and thus stroke) are previous heart attacks, diseases of the heart valves and a disturbance of the regular rhythm of the heart beat called atrial fibrillation.

Haemorrhagic stroke

About 20% of strokes are caused by a ruptured artery (blood vessel) in the brain, which causes bleeding (haemorrhage) into the brain (intracerebral haemorrhage) or over the surface of the brain (subarachnoid haemorrhage).

The most common cause of intracerebral haemorrhage is high blood pressure (hypertension), which damages the small arteries in the brain and makes them prone to rupture. Other common causes include malformations of blood vessels (arteriovenous malformations), degenerative changes in blood vessels (e.g. amyloid angiopathy), and disorders of blood clotting (e.g. haemophilia and excessive anticoagulation with medication).

The most common cause of subarachnoid haemorrhage is a ruptured aneurysm (blister) on one of the arteries on the surface of the brain. High blood pressure is an important modifiable risk factor for aneurysm formation and subarachnoid haemorrhage.

GENERAL RISK FACTORS

7.1 What is a risk factor for stroke?

Risk factors for stroke are characteristics of an individual, or of a population, that are associated with an increased risk of stroke compared with an individual, or a population, without those characteristics (*Table 7.1*).

TABLE 7.1 Risk factors for cerebral infarction		
Risk factor	**Relative risk**	**Estimated-age-standardised prevalence of exposure in population (%)**
Definite		
Increasing age		
Male gender		
Increasing blood pressure	2–4	30
Cigarette smoking	2–4	25
Diabetes mellitus	2	3
Atrial fibrillation	6	1
Ischaemic heart disease (IHD)	1–3	20
Carotid bruit/stenosis	3–15	4
Transient ischaemic attack or previous stroke	7	2
Peripheral vascular disease (intermittent claudication)	1–4	3
Increasing plasma fibrinogen		
Possible		
Hyperlipidaemia* (definite for IHD)	1–2	5
Hyperhomocystinaemia		
Activation of the renin–angiotensin–aldosterone system		
High plasma factor VII coagulant activity		
Low blood fibrinolytic activity		
Raised haematocrit		
Raise von Willebrand factor antigen		
Raised tissue plasminogen activity antigen		
Plasma viscosity (largely determined by plasma fibrinogen)		
Physical inactivity		
Obesity		
Snoring and sleep apnoea		
Recent infection		
Family history of stroke		
Diet (salt, fat)		

TABLE 7.1 (*Cont'd*)		
Risk factor	**Relative risk**	**Estimated-age-standardised prevalence of exposure in population (%)**
Alcohol (none, or heavy drinking)	1–4	5
Race		
Social deprivation		
Stress		
* Probable weak (or under-researched) positive association with ischaemic stroke, and possible weak inverse/negative association with haemorrhagic stroke		

The strength of any association between a risk factor and the occurrence of stroke is expressed by a ratio (relative risk or relative odds), which describes the number of times greater the frequency of stroke is in a group of individuals with the risk factor compared to those without it. However, the presence of an association does not necessarily imply causality.

7.2 What distinguishes a causal association between a risk factor and the occurrence of stroke from a coincidental association?

A causal association between a risk factor and stroke is inferred by:

- The strength of the association (high relative risk or relative odds)
- The consistency of the association in different studies and populations
- The presence of a dose–response relationship (the more of the risk factor, the higher the frequency of the disease)
- Independence from confounding factors
- A temporal sequence in which the risk factor is followed by the disease, remembering that stroke may occur years after the onset of the underlying pathology (e.g. atheroma, aneurysm)
- Biological and epidemiological plausibility
- The effect on the incidence of stroke of experimental removal of the risk factor in randomised trials.

7.3 What determines the importance of a risk factor for stroke?

The importance and relevance of the association of a risk factor with incidence of stroke is determined by causality and the absolute risk difference between those with and those without the causal risk factor.

Even if the relative risk is high, the relevance will be small if the risk factor is rarely present in the population. For example, although the relative risk of stroke for patients with rheumatic atrial fibrillation is very high, the fact that rheumatic heart disease is now so rare in developed countries means that it is still a very rare cause of stroke, i.e. it 'explains' only a small proportion of strokes and so has a low attributable risk. On the other hand, a risk factor that is common (e.g. mild hypertension) will 'explain' a much higher proportion of strokes, even though it does not carry a particularly high relative risk (compared with severe hypertension, which is rare). Indeed, about three-quarters of stroke deaths attributed to hypertension arise in people whose diastolic blood pressure is less than 110 mmHg. Also, if the background risk of stroke in a particular population group is very low (as it is in young women), exposure to quite a high relative risk (by taking oral contraceptives) does not make the absolute risk of stroke high.

The effect of risk factors on subsequent stroke incidence is usually additive or multiplicative, so that the presence of several risk factors puts an individual at particularly high risk. Consequently, general practitioners are now encouraged to stratify individuals into categories of stroke risk on the basis of their risk factor profile.[1,2]

7.4 What is the most important and relevant causal risk factor for stroke?

High blood pressure (hypertension) is the most important causal risk factor for stroke because:

- The strength of the association between blood pressure and risk of stroke is so strong
- It is consistent throughout many studies
- It is biologically plausible
- Treating hypertension reduces stroke risk
- Hypertension, particularly mild to moderate hypertension, is so prevalent in the general population (*Tables 7.2 & 7.3*).[3,4]

Therefore, the population-attributable risk for mild-moderate hypertension is greater than for severe hypertension, and greater than for any other risk factor.

Observational studies of healthy cohorts of both sexes, followed-up over many years, show that increasing blood pressure is strongly associated with subsequent increasing risk of all types of stroke, even after allowing for the increased risk of stroke associated with increasing age. The results are similar however blood pressure is measured; i.e. for diastolic blood pressure, systolic blood pressure and probably even 'isolated' systolic hypertension.

TABLE 7.2 Prevalence of vascular risk factors in 244 patients with a first-ever-in-a-lifetime ischaemic stroke in the Oxfordshire Community Stroke Project[5]

Risk factor	n	(%)
Hypertension (BP > 160/90 mmHg × 2 pre-stroke)	126	(52)
Angina and/or myocardial infarction	92	(38)
Current smoker*	66	(27)
Claudication and/or absent foot pulses	60	(25)
Major cardiac embolic source	50	(20)
Transient ischaemic attack	35	(14)
Cervical arterial bruit	33	(14)
Diabetes mellitus	24	(10)
Any of the above	196	(80)

TABLE 7.3 Population-attributable mortality from stroke in males arising at different levels of blood pressure: the Whitehall Study[6]

Diastolic blood pressure (mmHg)	Cumulative % of excess deaths attributable to hypertension
< 80	0
< 90	14
< 100	25
< 110	73

Throughout the range of diastolic blood pressure of 70–110 mmHg, the relationship with stroke is 'log-linear'. The risk of stroke doubles with each 7.5 mmHg increase in usual diastolic blood pressure in Western populations, and with each 5.0 mmHg increase in Japanese and Chinese populations.[7,8] There is no evidence of a threshold below which the risk becomes stable, even in patients who have already had cerebrovascular symptoms (*Fig. 7.1*). Studies that have shown a J-shaped curve, with increasing risk of stroke at the lowest blood pressures, have probably been subject to publication bias and almost certainly included patients with prior vascular disease or treated hypertension that might have led to higher risks at low blood pressures.

The association between increasing blood pressure and stroke is not as strong in the elderly as in middle age,[9] and it is not clear if hypertension is a risk factor for stroke in the *very* elderly, where stroke may be also associated with low pressures, perhaps because low pressures are a reflection of pre-existing cardiovascular and other disease.[4]

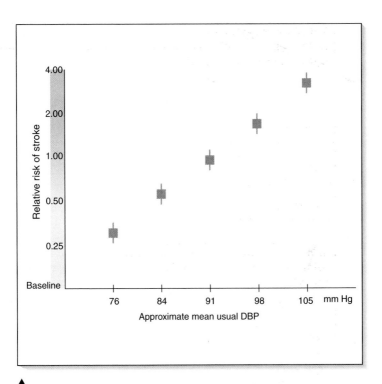

Fig 7.1 The relationship between blood pressure and stroke in Western populations, drawn from the data from seven prospective observational studies including a total of 843 events. Throughout the range of diastolic blood pressure (DBP) of 70–110 mmHg, the risk of stroke doubles with each increase of 7.5 mmHg. There is no evidence of a threshold level of diastolic blood pressure in this range below which there is a change in the log-linear relationship. Adapted with permission from MacMahon et al.[7]

The association between hypertension and stroke risk is biologically plausible because hypertension accelerates the formation, and increases the extent and severity, of atheroma in large and medium sized arteries[10] and small vessel disease in the perforating arteries within the brain.

7.5   What is the strongest risk factor for stroke?

Age is the strongest risk factor for ischaemic stroke, primary intracerebral haemorrhage and subarachnoid haemorrhage[11] and almost certainly for the subtypes of ischaemic stroke as well (e.g. lacunar infarction). For example, stroke in people aged 75–84 is about 25 times more common than in people aged 45–54.

7.6   Is gender a risk factor for stroke?

Men have a slightly greater risk of stroke, particularly in middle to old age. However, this excess risk among men is not present in the very elderly or the young. It is curious how the male predominance is so much less than in the other two main clinical manifestations of atheroma, myocardial infarction (MI) and peripheral vascular disease. Perhaps this reflects the pathological and aetiological heterogeneity of stroke but, even so, most strokes are due to infarction and most infarcts are due to atherothromboembolism.

7.7   Is cigarette smoking a strong and causal risk factor for stroke?

Cigarette smoking and stroke

- Up to one-quarter of all strokes are directly attributable to cigarette smoking, which independently increases the relative risk of stroke by about threefold[11]
- The risk is increased, dose-dependent and consistent for all pathological subtypes of stroke, and is strongest for subarachnoid haemorrhage and cortical ischaemic stroke due to arterial atherothromboembolism[12]
- The relative risk of stroke is equally high among male and female smokers, and is maximal (compared with non-smokers) in middle age, declining with advancing years
- Evidence is accumulating to implicate pipe and cigar smoking also as risk factors for stroke, and passive exposure to environmental smoke as a risk factor for atherogenesis
- The mechanisms by which smoking causes stroke are uncertain but are probably multifactorial (increased fibrinogen concentration, increased haematocrit, increased platelet aggregability, reduced fibrinolytic activity, vasoconstriction) and primarily atherogenic. Smoking has been related to the extent of carotid disease in patients selected for angiography, by ultrasound, and in identical twins discordant for smoking.

7.8   Does quitting smoking reduce the risk of stroke?

Yes. The risk of stroke declines considerably within 5 years after quitting smoking, so supporting a causal relationship, even though it has proved impossible to conduct a satisfactory randomised controlled trial of smoking cessation.

7.9   Is diabetes mellitus a risk factor for stroke?

Diabetes mellitus has long been recognised as a risk factor for atherosclerotic vascular disease of the brain, heart and limbs. Diabetics have double the risk of stroke compared with non-diabetics, probably independently of any association with other risk factors such as hypertension.[14] However, care must be taken when interpreting any relationship between diabetes and mortality since strokes in diabetics are more likely to be fatal.[15]

CARDIOVASCULAR RISK FACTORS

7.10 Is atrial fibrillation a risk factor for stroke?

Yes. Atrial fibrillation (AF) is associated with an increased risk of systemic thromboembolism and stroke (*Q. 6.27 & Q. 6.28*). The risk of stroke averages about 5% per year among all individuals in AF, which is about five to six times greater than for people of the same age who are in sinus rhythm.[16]

The association between AF and stroke is certainly plausible, because AF induces blood stasis and blood clot formation in the left atrium and its appendage. However, some of the association between AF and stroke is coincidental rather than causal: AF is commonly caused by coronary and hypertensive heart disease, both of which may also cause stroke, and stroke is commonly caused by mechanisms other than embolism from the fibrillating left atrium. These include embolism from an akinetic left ventricle or a carotid atherosclerotic plaque, or hypertensive intracranial small-vessel disease causing lacunar infarction, or primary intracerebral haemorrhage. Also, AF may even be caused by the stroke (i.e. be a consequence rather than a cause). So, AF may be coincidental to the underlying cause. Furthermore, the fact that anticoagulation markedly reduces the risk of first or recurrent stroke among AF patients (*see Chapter 14*) is not sufficient evidence to confirm causality because, although it is unlikely, this treatment may be working in other ways, such as by inhibiting artery-to-artery embolism. However, for most patients with AF and stroke, the association is probably causal.

The proportion of strokes that can be attributed to AF is highest in the very elderly because the prevalence of AF increases with age, from about 2% in the general population to 5% in people older than 65 years and 10% in people older than 75 years.[16] However, the population-attributable risk cannot be greater than 20%. AF is present in fewer than 20% of all ischaemic stroke patients and, as stated above, some have other, equally likely causes for their stroke, such as embolism from the left ventricle, carotid stenosis or intracranial small-vessel disease.

Atrial fibrillation may occur as a single episode, a series of recurrent episodes ('paroxysmal' AF), or continuously ('permanent' or 'chronic' AF) but the epidemiological and clinical evidence is insufficient to link either the onset or the chronicity of AF with the development of embolic stroke, nor is it clear whether paroxysmal AF is particularly likely or unlikely to cause stroke. However, it would seem intuitive (if our understanding is correct) that frequent and prolonged paroxysms of AF are more likely to predispose to left atrial thrombus and embolism than infrequent, brief paroxysms.

7.11 Which individuals with AF are at particularly low and high risk of stroke?

The risk of stroke varies substantially among individuals in AF. Some are at quite low risk (< 1% per year) such as those with 'lone' AF (i.e. no other heart disease). On the other hand, there are others who are at particularly high risk of stroke (e.g. > 6% per year). These include the elderly (> 75 years of age), those with hypertension or diabetes, those who have had a previous embolic event in the brain (transient ischaemic attack – TIA – or ischaemic stroke) or elsewhere, and those with echocardiographic evidence of left ventricular dysfunction, an enlarged left atrium and left atrial spontaneous echo densities/contrast ('smoke'), which is possibly indicative of stasis of blood.[17]

These risk factors are cumulative. For people younger than 65 years with no risk factors the untreated annual risk of stroke is about 1%, whereas with one or more risk factors it is about 5%. For people aged 65–75 years with no risk factors the annual risk of stroke is about 4%, and with one or more risk factors it is about 6% per year. For people older than 75 years with no risk factors, risk of stroke is about 3–4%, whereas with one or more risk factors it is about 8% (*Box 7.1*).

BOX 7.1 Risk stratification in atrial fibrillation

High risk (6–12% per year risk of stroke)
- Age > 65 years and hypertension or diabetes
- Previous transient ischaemic attack (TIA) or stroke
- Valvular heart disease
- Heart failure
- Recent myocardial infarction
- Impaired left ventricular function on echocardiography
- Thyroid disease
- Left atrial thrombus or left atrial spontaneous echo contrast (transoesophageal echocardiography done on basis of clinical suspicion)

BOX 7.1 (*Cont'd*)

Moderate risk (3–5% per year risk of stroke)
- Age < 65 years and hypertension or diabetes
- Age > 65 years and not in high risk group

Low risk (< 1% per year risk of stroke)
- Age < 65 and no hypertension, diabetes, TIA, stroke or other clinical risk factor

---

7.12 Are transient ischaemic attacks a risk factor for stroke?

Yes. TIAs of the brain and eye are risk factors for stroke. Among all individuals in the community who experience a TIA, the risk of stroke in the first year after the TIA is about 10%. Thereafter the risk falls to at about 5% per annum and remains like that, at least for the next 5 years or so. This risk is about seven times the expected risk in the background population of the same age and gender.[18] The risk of stroke among TIA patients referred to hospital is lower, probably because the patients are younger with fewer vascular risk factors.[19]

Patients with TIAs of the eye have half the risk of stroke and other serious vascular events than patients with TIAs of the brain.[18]

7.13 When is the risk of stroke highest after a TIA?

The risk of stroke is greatest early, within the first few days and weeks after a TIA, particularly in patients with symptomatic carotid stenosis and those with a partial anterior circulation rather than a lacunar TIA syndrome (*see Q. 9.8–Q. 9.11*).

7.14 Which TIA patients have a high risk of stroke soon after TIA and why?

The higher rate of stroke soon after the TIA (*Q. 9.11*) is probably in those patients whose TIA was caused by embolism of thrombus from a ruptured atherosclerotic plaque (e.g. those with markers of a heavy burden of atheroma – such as older patients, those with ischaemic heart disease and peripheral arterial disease, and those with carotid stenosis). Also, patients with TIAs of the brain have twice the risk of stroke and other serious vascular events than patients with TIAs of the eye. The reason for this remains uncertain.

> The risk for TIA patients of a recurrent thromboembolic event to the brain so soon after the initial TIA is probably high because either the plaque hasn't had time to heal (by repair of the endothelium) or collateral channels have not had time to develop to restore a reasonable blood supply beyond a stenotic lesion.
>
> Whatever the explanation, preventive treatments (e.g. carotid endarterectomy, antiplatelet therapy) should be started as soon as possible after a TIA to avoid a major, if not fatal, recurrence.

7.15 Are TIAs also a risk factor for coronary events?

Yes. The risk of a serious cardiac event (e.g. fatal or non-fatal myocardial infarction, sudden presumed cardiac death) after a TIA is substantial (about 3–5% per annum), presumably because of the association of atheroma in one artery with atheroma in another artery in the same susceptible individual (see Q. 9.10). However, there is no early high-risk period, presumably because the coronary arterial lesion is in a different place and may not be 'unstable' at the same time as the recently symptomatic cerebral arterial lesion.

It is therefore appropriate to consider the patient as a whole, and likewise the risk of all serious vascular events together (i.e. stroke, MI and other vascular death). They are almost all caused by the same underlying pathology (atheroma) and are all potentially preventable by the control of vascular risk factors, antithrombotic drugs and appropriate revascularisation procedures. Furthermore, in the long-term, death from cardiovascular disease is more frequent than death from stroke and as time goes by non-vascular deaths, such as cancer, become relatively more frequent.

The risk of the composite outcome of stroke, MI or vascular death among TIA patients in the community is about 9% per year.

7.16 Is carotid stenosis a risk factor for stroke?

Yes, increasing degrees of carotid stenosis are a strong causal risk factor for stroke but the risk is modified by other factors, such as whether or not the carotid stenosis has recently become unstable and active, causing focal neurological symptoms of a TIA or ischaemic stroke.

For patients with neurologically asymptomatic severe carotid stenosis (i.e. at least 70% stenosis of the arterial lumen), the risk of any stroke is about 3% per year, and the risk of ipsilateral ischaemic stroke (which is what may be caused by the carotid stenosis) is about 2%. With extreme stenosis (> 90%), there is some evidence that the risk of ipsilateral ischaemic stroke is greater, but this information is derived from very small numbers of patients and about one-third of the strokes are not due to the carotid stenosis but are due to intracranial small vessel disease (lacunar) or embolism from the heart.[20]

For patients with neurologically symptomatic severe carotid stenosis (i.e. at least 70% of the lumen of the artery), the risk of any stroke is about 12–15% per year, and the annual risk of ipsilateral ischaemic stroke (which is what may be caused by the carotid stenosis) is about 10–14%. With extreme stenosis (> 90%), the annual risk of ipsilateral ischaemic stroke is even higher (18–20%) than for patients with 80–89% stenosis (11–15%) and patients with 70–79% stenosis (6–10%).[21,22] Again, up to one-third of these strokes are due to intracranial small-vessel disease (lacunar) or embolism from the heart, and so are unlikely to be prevented by carotid endarterectomy. Furthermore, the risk of stroke in patients with severe symptomatic carotid stenosis, if not operated upon by carotid endarterectomy, falls rapidly in the first 2 years after the initial symptomatic event (TIA or ischaemic stroke) and within 3 years it is the same as in patients with mild carotid stenosis (less than 5% per year; *see Q. 14.45–Q. 14.53*).

7.17 Is a neck bruit a risk factor for stroke?

Carotid and supraclavicular arterial (i.e. cervical) bruits are neither sufficiently specific nor sufficiently sensitive to diagnose stenosis of the underlying arteries. Their absence does not exclude a tight carotid stenosis and their presence does not mean that the patient has tight common or internal carotid artery stenosis. A carotid bruit can be:

- A normal finding in young adults
- Due to external carotid stenosis (which is usually irrelevant to the patient's symptoms)
- Transmitted from the heart and great vessels in patients with aortic or mitral valve disease, patent ductus arteriosus or coarctation of the aorta
- Part of a diffuse neck bruit in patients with thyrotoxicosis or a hyperdynamic circulation associated with pregnancy, anaemia, fever and haemodialysis.

Nevertheless, there is a reasonable correlation between neck bruits and severity of carotid stenosis and so, not surprisingly, neck bruits, like carotid stenosis, are risk factors for subsequent stroke. However, the stroke may not necessarily be in the same arterial territory because the disease (usually atherothrombotic) in one carotid artery is likely to be associated with disease in other arteries in the same (predisposed) individual.

Both neck bruits and carotid stenosis become more prevalent with age and about 5% of the normal elderly have severe carotid stenosis.[23]

7.18 Are ischaemic heart disease and cardiac failure risk factors for stroke?

Ischaemic heart disease (a past history of MI, coronary artery bypass surgery or current angina) is present in about 20% of patients with TIA and ischaemic stroke.

Stroke may occur in up to 5% of patients with recent acute MI, due to:

■ Embolism of left ventricular mural thrombus
■ Systemic hypotension
■ Intracerebral haemorrhage secondary to thrombolysis, anticoagulants or aspirin
■ Embolism of catheter thrombus during coronary angioplasty/stenting
■ Concurrent non-cardiac cause of stroke; i.e. atherosclerotic TIA and ischaemic stroke (ischaemic heart disease is a marker of carotid and vertebral artery atherosclerotic disease).

After the acute period of myocardial ischaemia, the risk of stroke is much lower – about 1% in the first year, perhaps higher if there is persisting left ventricular thrombus.

Chronic left ventricular aneurysm after MI often contains thrombus but embolisation is uncommon.

Besides ischaemic heart disease (i.e. angina or MI), heart failure and electrocardiographic abnormalities reflecting hypertension (e.g. left ventricular hypertrophy) or ischaemic heart disease are, not surprisingly, also associated with stroke.

7.19 Is peripheral vascular disease a risk factor for stroke?

Yes. Like ischaemic heart disease, peripheral arterial disease is a strong marker of multifocal atherosclerotic disease. Individuals with intermittent claudication and asymptomatic peripheral vascular disease (as defined by an abnormal low ankle-brachial systolic pressure index) are at excess risk of stroke and MI, presumably reflecting the association of atheromatous disease in different parts of the circulation in the same (predisposed) individuals.[24]

METABOLIC RISK FACTORS

7.20 Is hyperlipidaemia a risk factor for stroke?

Observational cohort studies of about 500 000 people who were followed up over many years and among whom about 13 500 subsequent stroke events were recorded do not suggest that raised plasma cholesterol is a risk factor for all stroke.[8,9] The studies identified no clear relation between plasma cholesterol and total (fatal and non-fatal) stroke.

However the studies did reveal that increasing plasma concentration of cholesterol is a weak risk factor for ischaemic stroke and that decreasing plasma concentration may be a weak risk factor for haemorrhagic stroke,[9] although more recent evidence suggests that low total serum cholesterol may not be a risk factor for haemorrhagic stroke.[25]

Clinical trials ($n = 16$) have shown that lowering plasma concentrations of cholesterol in about 39 000 patients at fairly low risk of stroke (e.g. patients with a history of coronary heart disease) reduces the odds of stroke by about 25% (95% confidence interval, CI 14–41%) and the absolute annual risk of stroke by about 0.17% (i.e. 1.7 strokes per 1000 patient-years of treatment).[26,27] However, there is uncertainty about the effects of statins on haemorrhagic stroke and fatal stroke, so the results are awaited of ongoing clinical trials using them to lower plasma concentrations of cholesterol in TIA and stroke patients. It is hoped that cholesterol lowering will prevent recurrent ischaemic stroke (as well as ischaemic coronary events) and not increase the risk of haemorrhagic stroke (*see Q. 14.11*).

Of course, the relationship between lipids and stroke is quantitatively at least (and perhaps qualitatively) quite different from the relationship between lipids and coronary heart disease. There is unequivocal evidence that increasing concentrations of total plasma cholesterol and low-density-lipoprotein cholesterol, and to a lesser extent decreasing concentrations of high-density-lipoprotein cholesterol, are strong causal risk factors for coronary heart disease.[28] Long-term lowering of plasma cholesterol by 0.6 mmol/L reduces the risk of coronary events by about 25% (more so in the young than in the elderly). The relationship between blood triglyceride levels and coronary heart disease is less clear.[29]

It is not clear why there is such a contrast between the effects of increasing plasma cholesterol levels on cardiovascular and cerebrovascular disease. The most popular hypothesis is that the presumed negative association between cholesterol and intracranial haemorrhage minimises, and possibly even obscures, the presumed positive association with ischaemic stroke in studies of 'all strokes' and particularly studies of fatal strokes (which include a greater proportion of haemorrhagic strokes). Other possible reasons include less influence of high plasma lipid levels on vascular events in older people (in whom more strokes occur) than in younger people (in whom more coronary events occur), and methodological limitations of the studies completed, such as confounding in case-control and cohort studies, data from only a relatively narrow range of blood cholesterol concentrations, and lack of statistical power in cohort studies and randomised trials, which have usually focused on coronary events rather than on the smaller number of strokes, especially pathological and aetiological subtypes of stroke.

7.21 Is activation of the renin–angiotensin–aldosterone system a risk factor for stroke?

The results of the recently published large multicentre Heart Outcomes Prevention Evaluation (HOPE) trial suggest that activation of the renin–angiotensin system is an independent risk factor for recurrent stroke and other serious vascular events among patients with a history of ischaemic stroke due to atherothromboembolism.[30] A total of 9297 patients with a history of symptomatic atherothrombosis of the cerebral, coronary or peripheral arteries, or diabetes with one other vascular risk factor, were randomised to receive either ramipril 10 mg daily or placebo, in addition to otherwise best medical therapy. There was a significant reduction in the rate of subsequent stroke, MI or death from vascular causes in the patients allocated ramipril (13.9%) compared with those given placebo (17.5%). This represents a relative risk reduction of 22% (95% confidence interval, CI 14–30%) and an absolute risk reduction of 3.6% over about 5 years of follow-up.

The reduction in vascular events was about 60% greater than might have been expected from the size of the reductions in blood pressure (3 mmHg systolic, 1 mm Hg diastolic). This supports the hypothesis that inhibition of angiotensin-converting enzyme is effective not only by reducing blood pressure but also by other mechanisms, perhaps acting on the vessel wall (e.g. anti-atherogenic).

7.22 Is plasma fibrinogen a risk factor for stroke?

Increasing plasma concentrations of fibrinogen are associated with an increased risk of stroke. The association is understandable because raised plasma fibrinogen could cause stroke by increasing plasma viscosity or by promoting thrombosis. Indeed, as stated above (*see Q. 7.7*) it is possible that the adverse vascular effect of cigarette smoking is mediated, at least in part, by increasing fibrinogen levels and thus accelerating thrombosis. However, the strength of the association between fibrinogen and stroke is attenuated by adjusting for cigarette smoking and other confounding variables such as infections and even social class.[31] Furthermore, it is difficult to lower plasma fibrinogen consistently and no randomised trials have been carried out.

7.23 What other haematostatic variables may be risk factors for stroke?

Haematocrit has a strong effect on cerebral blood flow but any association between increasing haematocrit and risk of stroke, or type of stroke, is weak and confounded by cigarette smoking, blood pressure and plasma fibrinogen.

Raised plasma factor VII coagulant activity, raised tissue plasminogen activator antigen, low blood fibrinolytic activity and raised von Willebrand factor are risk factors for coronary heart disease and may also be risk factors for stroke.[32] Although other platelet, coagulation and fibrinolytic parameters have been associated with vascular disease, the associations have been limited by the lack of large cohort studies, the failure to eliminate the effect of the stroke itself on the plasma concentrations of these factors (are they the cause of the stroke or caused by the stroke?) and inconsistency among studies.

7.24 Is inherited thrombophilia a risk factor for stroke?

No, or very rarely, perhaps for certain subtypes of stroke such as cardioembolic ischaemic stroke (*see Q. 6.48–Q. 6.58*).

In recent years, an increasing number of largely inherited abnormalities of blood coagulation have been commonly associated with venous thromboembolism and sometimes arterial thrombosis. These conditions, the thrombophilias, include deficiencies of the natural anticoagulants – such as antithrombin III, protein S and protein C – and single point mutations in coagulation molecules such as factor V Leiden (1691G/A) or in the 3' untranslated region of the prothrombin gene (factor II; 20210 G/A).

There is little doubt that inherited thrombophilias can cause venous thrombosis but most individuals with a single genetic risk factor do not experience a thrombotic event in the absence of circumstantial risk factors such as immobility or the oral contraceptive pill.

One in seven patients with first-ever acute ischaemic stroke or TIA tests positive for one of the inherited thrombophilias but in almost all cases the relationship is coincidental rather than causal, irrespective of the aetiological subtype of the ischaemic stroke. Therefore, routine testing for thrombophilia in most patients with acute ischaemic stroke and TIA is probably unnecessary. Whether the thrombophilias are important in younger patients presenting with ischaemic stroke or in predicting complications (e.g. venous thrombosis) and stroke outcome remains uncertain.

7.25 Is hyperhomocysteinaemia a risk factor for stroke?

Possibly. Systematic reviews of observational studies reveal an independent relationship between higher mean plasma concentrations of total homocysteine (tHcy – either fasting or after methionine load), a greater frequency of elevated tHcy, or both, in individuals with cerebral, coronary and peripheral arterial disease compared with those without vascular disease.[33] Furthermore, high tHcy has been associated with specific aetiological subtypes of ischaemic stroke caused by large-artery disease, and less strongly with small-artery disease, but not with cardioembolic or other non-atherosclerotic causes of stroke.[34] The association between elevated tHcy and atherosclerotic disease is also dose-related (i.e. the risk is greater with higher tHcy concentrations), strong, independent and biologically plausible: experimental studies suggest that supraphysiological concentrations of non-physiological forms of homocysteine are both atherogenic and thrombogenic.[35]

However, the results obtained by different epidemiological methods are inconsistent. Stronger associations have been found in studies using less robust designs, and smaller associations or no association have been reported from most prospective cohort studies.[36] In addition, the temporal relationship between the onset of elevated tHcy and the onset of stroke is unclear. The finding of a stronger association in case-control studies than in cohort studies suggests that elevated tHcy may be an acute-phase reactant that rises or falls after the stroke or other vascular event in response to tissue damage or tissue repair. Furthermore, there is no clear relationship between a polymorphism in methylenetetrahydrofolate reductase (C677T), which is associated with high tHcy in the plasma, and increased cardiovascular risk.

It therefore remains uncertain whether the epidemiological and statistical association between plasma tHcy and arterial disease is causal or confounded. Proof of a causal relationship requires large randomised controlled trials to show reliably that lowering the level of plasma tHcy is followed by a reduction in the incidence of major vascular events.

It is possible to lower plasma tHcy by about 25% (95% CI 23–28%) with folic acid 0.5–5 mg daily, and by a further 7% (95% CI 3–10%) with vitamin B_{12} 0.02–1 mg daily.[37] The addition of vitamin B_6 to folic acid may also lower plasma tHcy.

Randomised controlled trials have shown that lowering tHcy, by means of folic acid and/or vitamins B_6 and B_{12}, improves surrogate markers of cardiovascular disease but it is still not known whether lowering homocysteine prevents 'hard' clinical vascular events. A number of trials investigating the effect of lowering tHcy by means of multivitamin therapy on stroke, MI and vascular death in patients at high risk of vascular disease are now in progress. Two trials are studying patients with TIA and stroke: the Vitamins in Stroke Prevention (VISP) Trial (Bowman Gray School of Medicine, USA) and the VITAmins TO Prevent Stroke (VITATOPS) Study (Royal Perth Hospital, University of Western Australia).

HORMONAL RISK FACTORS

7.26 Is oestrogen a risk factor for stroke?

There is some indirect evidence that oestrogen is a risk factor for stroke.

■ Men with coronary heart disease have higher rather than lower levels of female sex hormones

- Exogenous high-dose oestrogen given to elderly men with prostatic cancer increases their risk of vascular death[38]
- Oral contraceptives increase the risk of ischaemic stroke, and less so, haemorrhagic strokes.

Hence, it is unlikely that the lower incidence of stroke (and other ischaemic vascular events) in women compared with men is due to 'protection' by their endogenous female sex hormones.

7.27 By how much does the oral contraceptive pill increase the risk of stroke?

Current users of the 'modern' oral contraceptive pill, which is a progestagen-only or low oestrogen pill, increase their risk of ischaemic stroke by up to about threefold (relative risk 2.75, 95% CI 2.24–3.38). Smaller oestrogen doses are associated with a lower relative risk, but the relative risk is significantly elevated for all dosages (relative risk 1.93, 95% CI 1.35–2.74). However, the absolute risk is so low that even a tripling of stroke risk is not sufficient reason to withhold it.[39] Non-smoking, normotensive women using low-oestrogen oral contraceptives are at risk of an additional 4.1 ischaemic strokes per 100 000 per year, or one additional ischaemic stroke per year per 24 000 of them. Contrary to what was previously believed, the summary results from a meta-analysis of all studies indicated that the relative risk of stroke due to oral contraceptive use is not different in women who smoke, have migraines or have hypertension.[40] Nevertheless, because a woman taking the oral contraceptive pill who is hypertensive, a cigarette smoker and over the age of about 30 has a relatively high absolute risk of stroke, it is probably advisable, although not evidence-based, to advise other means of contraception (or better still, for her to stop smoking and lower her blood pressure by lifestyle modification).

Of course, women taking the oral contraceptive pill who are carriers of mutations causing thrombophilias (e.g. factor V Leiden) are at particular risk of intracranial venous thrombosis already and should also be advised to consider other means of contraception.[41]

7.28 Does previous use of the oral contraceptive pill increase the risk of stroke?

No, ex-users of the oral contraceptive pill have no excess risk of stroke.

7.29 What proportion of strokes in young women are attributable to the oral contraceptive pill?

Only up to about 10% of strokes in young women are likely to be due to oral contraceptives, even assuming that the association is causal.[39]

7.30 Is post-menopausal oestrogen replacement therapy a risk factor for stroke?

Data from observation studies suggest that postmenopausal oestrogen replacement is not associated with any increased risk of stroke or coronary events and may even be associated with a lower risk. Indeed, cardiovascular mortality is higher in women who have had an early menopause, and bilateral oophorectomy without oestrogen replacement about doubles the risk. The effect of added progestagen is not known.

However, the results of two recent clinical trials of oestrogen-replacement therapy suggest that oestrogen does not reduce mortality or recurrent stroke in postmenopausal women with previous recent ischaemic stroke or TIA[42], or coronary artery disease.[43] The ongoing Women's Health Initiative, a randomised trial, should help clarify the role of oestrogen in the primary prevention of stroke and other vascular diseases (if any – particularly given the small increase in risk of breast and uterine cancer, and venous thromboembolism[44] associated with postmenopausal oestrogen replacement).

7.31 Is pregnancy and the puerperium a risk factor for stroke?

The relative risk of stroke in the pregnant woman is about 13 times the risk in the non-pregnant woman of the same age but the absolute risk of stroke in the last trimester of pregnancy and the puerperium is no more than 30 per 100 000 deliveries (i.e. about one in every 3000 deliveries)

About three-quarters of ischaemic strokes are due to arterial occlusion and one-quarter to venous occlusion. Causes of stroke during pregnancy and the puerperium are listed in *Box. 7.2.*

BOX 7.2 Causes of stroke during pregnancy and the puerperium

Common
- Paradoxical embolism from the venous system of the pelvis or legs
- Valvular heart disease
- Cardiomyopathy of pregnancy
- Arterial dissection during labour
- Haematological disorders

Less common
- Amniotic fluid embolism
- Air or fat embolism
- Metastatic choriocarcinoma.

LIFESTYLE RISK FACTORS

7.32 Is alcohol a risk factor for stroke?

Studies that have attempted to correlate alcohol consumption and stroke have been plagued by several methodological limitations such as:

■ Difficulty in selecting appropriate controls and excluding ex-heavy-drinkers, who may be at high risk

■ Difficulty in measuring alcohol consumption accurately, particularly over prolonged periods of time

■ Confounding by the association of alcohol consumption with other risk factors for stroke, such as cigarette smoking (positive association with alcohol), physical exercise (negative association) and socioeconomic status

■ Other biases inherent in case-control studies

■ Difficulty in distinguishing ischaemic and haemorrhagic strokes, which may be affected differently by alcohol consumption

■ Difficulty in determining whether different patterns of drinking behaviour have different effects on stroke risk

■ Difficulty in unravelling whether any effect on stroke is due to alcohol per se or to the type of alcoholic beverage

■ Difficulty in determining the mechanism by which alcohol consumption might cause stroke – alcohol is known to raise blood pressure, alter blood lipids, induce atrial fibrillation and cause cardiomyopathy

■ Difficulty in excluding the effects of chance, as many studies are small.

Alcohol and stroke

Despite these limitations, there is a large body of evidence suggesting that heavy consumption of alcohol (including binge drinking) is an independent and causal risk factor for stroke, particularly for haemorrhagic stroke. However, modest consumption is probably protective for ischaemic stroke.[45] The mechanism for this apparent protective effect in modest drinkers compared with heavy drinkers and non-drinkers remains unclear.

7.33 Is diet a risk factor for stroke?

> ### Dietary risk factors for stroke
>
> ■ Salt increases blood pressure and probably increases the risk of stroke by this mechanism, despite the claims of the food industry.[46]
> ■ Dietary deficiency of the following may be associated with an increased risk of stroke and coronary heart disease:
>   – Potassium
>   – Calcium
>   – Fresh fruit and vegetables
>   – Fish (high in long-chain, omega-3 polyunsaturated fatty acids and low in saturated fatty acids)
>   – Antioxidants such as vitamin C, vitamin E, beta-carotene and flavonols.
>   However, randomised trials of dietary interventions to supplement some of these factors have been disappointing.
> ■ A systematic review of randomised controlled trials of modified dietary fat intake in healthy adult participants over at least 6 months does show that modification or reduction of dietary fat intake results in a small but potentially important reduction (16%) in cardiovascular risk (95% CI 1–28%), but only in trials of at least 2 years duration. There is little effect on total mortality. There is still only limited and inconclusive evidence of the effects of modification of total, saturated, monounsaturated or polyunsaturated fats on cardiovascular morbidity and mortality.[47]
> ■ There is no association between coffee consumption and stroke or other vascular disease, despite the fact that coffee may have a small hyperlipidaemic effect.

Of course, studies relating various dietary constituents to the risk of stroke and other vascular diseases are fraught with methodological problems, because not only are dietary questionnaires difficult to construct but diets change with time, geography (i.e. where people live), occurrence of disease, and even believing oneself to be at risk of disease. Furthermore, a particular dietary constituent is often associated with another (e.g. coffee and milk) so it is almost impossible to tease out which is the relevant factor (if any). Moreover, individuals who eat so-called healthy diets often have an inherently healthy lifestyle, which confounds any association that might be observed between a healthy diet and reduced risk of stroke. Finally, even 'negative' clinical trials of dietary interventions can be misleading because it is conceivable that an intervention is too late to influence the underlying vascular disease, which is the cause of stroke.

7.34 Is obesity a risk factor for stroke?

Stroke and overall mortality are more common in obese individuals but the relationship between obesity and stroke is likely to be confounded by the positive association of obesity with hypertension, diabetes, physical inactivity and hypercholesterolaemia, and the negative association with smoking (non-smokers are heavier than smokers) and concurrent illness.

However, there is little doubt that the risk of coronary events, in men and women, is greater in the obese, particularly if the weight has been gained in middle age or has fluctuated substantially.

The measurement of obesity is also variable. A raised waist-to-hip ratio as a measure of central obesity, and perhaps change in body weight, may be stronger risk factors than the traditional measure of weight for a given height.[48]

7.35 Is physical inactivity a risk factor for stroke?

Physical inactivity is indeed associated with an increased risk of stroke and coronary heart disease.[49,50] A causal association is plausible because physical activity (i.e. exercise) reduces body weight, blood pressure, plasma cholesterol and fibrinogen, and the risk of non-insulin-dependent diabetes mellitus. However, physical activity is also associated with less cigarette smoking, which may be a confounding factor.

To date there is insufficient evidence from randomised trials to be certain that deliberately increasing exercise levels reduces the risk of stroke and other vascular events, but a lack of proof of effect doesn't mean proof of a lack of effect.

7.36 Is infection a risk factor for stroke?

Despite increasing interest in the notion that chronic and acute infection may contribute to the development, progression and instability of atheromatous plaques, there is little supportive evidence from studies of infections in general, specific infections (e.g. chronic dental infection) or infections with specific organisms such as *Helicobacter pylori*, *Chlamydia pneumoniae* and cytomegalovirus. There is definite evidence of chlamydial infection in atherosclerotic plaques but, of course, reverse causality is possible (i.e. atheroma is prone to become infected, rather than infection promoting atheroma).

7.37 Is social deprivation a risk factor for stroke?

Social deprivation, low socioeconomic class and unemployment are all associated with an increased risk of stroke. This is partly because deprived populations have a higher prevalence of vascular risk factors (smoking, physical inactivity), stress and adverse health behaviours (poor diet).

7.38 Is 'stress' a risk factor for stroke?

There is some evidence that severely life-threatening events, anxiety and depression, higher levels of anger expression,[51] and psychological stress may trigger the onset of stroke, perhaps in individuals already at risk of stroke.

GENETIC RISK FACTORS

7.39 Is race a risk factor for stroke?

From the limited data available, it seems that stroke incidence is greater in blacks than in whites living in Western countries, probably in part because blacks have a higher prevalence of hypertension, diabetes, sickle-cell trait and social deprivation. Similarly, Maori and Pacific people living in New Zealand have a higher stroke risk than white New Zealanders, and South Asian populations in the UK have a higher stroke mortality than white populations, by virtue of higher serum lipoprotein (a) concentrations and a higher prevalence of central obesity, insulin resistance, diabetes mellitus and coronary heart disease.

7.40 Which genetic disorders are risk factors for stroke?

A few strokes clearly have an underlying cause that is 'familial' with a simple mendelian pattern of inheritance (*Box 7.3*).[52]

There is also evidence that parental history of stroke is a risk factor for stroke.[53] However, stroke has several causes, many of which are probably polygenic disorders, characterised by complex gene-gene and gene-environment interactions.

Indeed, many of the classic vascular risk factors are genetically determined in part (e.g. hypertension and hyperlipidaemia) but environmental influences modify them (e.g. salt and saturated fat consumption, respectively).

Disentangling the interactions, identifying the gene(s) involved and working out the pathway from genotype to disease and stroke phenotype are major challenges for the future.[54,55]

BOX 7.3   Some causes of stroke that can be 'familial' (including intracranial venous thrombosis and intracranial haemorrhage)

Vascular anomalies	Intracranial vascular malformation
	Saccular aneurysm
	Hereditary haemorrhagic telangiectasia
Connective tissue anomalies	Ehlers–Danlos syndrome
	Pseudoxanthoma elasticum
	Marfan's syndrome
	Fibromuscular dysplasia
	Polycystic kidney disease
	Mitral leaflet prolapse
Haematological diseases	Haemophilia and other coagulation factor deficiencies
	Sickle-cell disease/trait
	Antithrombin III deficiency
	Protein C deficiency
	Activated protein C resistance
	Protein S deficiency
	Plasminogen abnormality/deficiency
	Dysfibrinogenaemia
Others	Familial hypercholesterolaemia
	Cerebral amyloid angiopathy (Icelandic and Dutch forms)
	Neurofibromatosis
	Tuberous sclerosis
	Homocysteinaemia
	Fabry's disease
	Migraine
	Cardiac myxoma
	Cardiomyopathy
	Von Hippel–Lindau disease
	Mitochondrial cytopathy
	Cerebral autosomal dominant arteriopathy with subcortical infarcts and leucoencephalopathy (CADASIL).

PATIENT QUESTIONS

7.41 What causes hardening of the arteries (atherosclerosis)?

Atherosclerosis occurs in us all as we get older, but the process is accelerated substantially if we are exposed over a long period of time to high blood pressure, cigarette smoking, high blood cholesterol and the disease diabetes mellitus. Other indirect causes are physical inactivity and obesity, because they lead both to high blood pressure and high blood cholesterol. These conditions (high blood pressure, smoking, high cholesterol, diabetes, physical inactivity, obesity), because they increase the risk of us having the blood vessel disease called atherosclerosis, are therefore called vascular risk factors (or risk factors for vascular disease).

Our genetic make-up (the genes we have inherited from our parents; 'the way we are made') is also important in determining how we respond to exposure to the vascular risk factors just mentioned. The odd person is 'blessed' with 'good genes' and can harbour many risk factors for many years without experiencing a stroke or heart attack, but the vast majority of us will suffer these major adverse health outcomes much earlier if we are exposed to the risk factors for any length of time.

7.42 Does stroke run in families?

Because strokes and TIAs occur quite commonly it is not unusual for more than one person in a family to have a stroke or TIA through chance alone. However, some families have a greater tendency to experience strokes (and heart attacks). Sometimes this is because they have inherited a genetic predisposition to have high concentrations of cholesterol (fat) in the blood and/or high blood pressure, but it can also be because members of family indulge in the same adverse behaviours (e.g. they all smoke or all eat fatty foods).

Aetiological diagnosis 3 (what investigations are needed?)

8.1 What investigations should be performed in all, or nearly all, patients?

The decision to investigate, and choice of investigations, is based on: the patient's symptoms, age, pre- and poststroke condition; the patient's willingness to accept any risks, costs or inconvenience; and the purpose and cost-effectiveness of the investigations. However, all patients with transient ischaemic attack (TIA) or stroke in whom active management is being considered should undergo at least the following first-line investigations, even if the clinical assessment strongly suggests a common cause.[1]

Investigations for all stroke and TIA patients

- Full blood count
- Erythrocyte sedimentation rate (ESR)
- Plasma glucose
- Plasma urea and electrolytes
- Random plasma cholesterol
- Urinalysis
- 12-lead electrocardiogram (ECG; *Fig. 8.1*)
- Urgent plain brain computed tomography (CT) scan:
  - To exclude non-vascular causes of the suspected TIA or stroke (e.g. tumour)
  - To distinguish intracranial haemorrhage from cerebral infarction (CT must be done within about a week of stroke onset)
  - To ascertain the likely cause of the ischaemic or haemorrhagic stroke
- Duplex carotid ultrasound if the patient has a non-disabling carotid ischaemic event (i.e. carotid TIA or mild ischaemic stroke) and is fit and willing for carotid angiography and endarterectomy (or stent) should severe symptomatic carotid stenosis be identified.

These investigations may reveal important modifiable vascular risk factors and suggest rare, unanticipated causes of stroke (e.g. polycythaemia, thrombocythaemia, giant cell arteritis, infective endocarditis; *Table 8.1*).

More specialised investigations are reserved for patients in whom the cause of stroke remains uncertain or in whom the results of the clinical assessment or simple investigations suggest an abnormality.

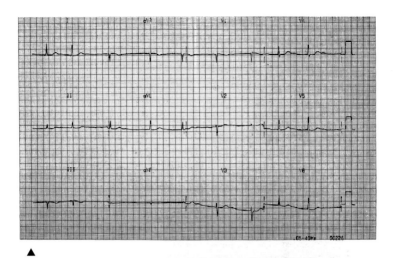

▲

Fig 8.1 Electrocardiograph showing slow atrial fibrillation.

TABLE 8.1   Baseline tests for most patients with a transient ischaemic attack or ischaemic stroke

Investigation	Treatable disorders detected
Full blood count	Anaemia, polycythaemia, leukaemia, thrombocythaemia
ESR	Vasculitis, infective endocarditis, hyperviscosity, myxoma
Electrolytes	Hyponatraemia, hypokalaemia
Urea	Renal impairment
Plasma glucose	Diabetes, hypoglycaemia
Plasma cholesterol	High cholesterol
Urine analysis	Diabetes, renal disease, vasculitis
Electrocardiogram	Left ventricular hypertrophy, arrhythmia, conduction block, myocardial infarction
CT brain scan	Subdural haematoma, meningioma, encephalitis
Carotid ultrasound	Severe stenosis of the symptomatic carotid artery

IMAGING

8.2   What is the role of duplex carotid ultrasound?

Duplex carotid ultrasound (*Fig. 8.2*) aims to non-invasively image the lumen and wall of the origin of the internal carotid artery and identify any

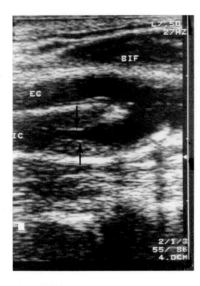

◀ **Fig 8.2** Duplex carotid ultrasound, B-mode image, showing severe stenosis of the origin of the internal carotid artery. BIF, carotid bifurcation; EC, external carotid artery; IC, internal carotid artery. With permission from Hankey & Warlow.[2]

disturbance of flow (by means of Doppler studies) and image any structural lesion, such as atherosclerotic plaque, or dissection (by means of B-mode imaging).

Doppler studies of the ophthalmic arteries can detect the direction of blood flow in the ophthalmic arteries, which may be reversed if the ipsilateral carotid artery is occluded or severely stenosed and the ipsilateral eye and cerebral hemisphere receive some of their blood supply via the external carotid artery.

Ultrasound studies of the neck vessels can also evaluate blood flow patterns and velocities at the origins of the vertebral arteries and estimate the degree of vertebral artery stenosis.

8.3 In which patients is duplex carotid ultrasound indicated?

Duplex carotid ultrasound is indicated for:

■ All patients with a non-disabling carotid ischaemic event (i.e. carotid TIA or mild ischaemic stroke) who are fit and willing for carotid endarterectomy (or stent), should the ultrasound reveal at least about 50% stenosis of the origin of the internal carotid artery on the symptomatic side. (Sometimes an operable ≥ 70% stenosis is reported by ultrasound to be only a 50% or 60% stenosis.)
Ultrasound should be performed as soon as possible because, if the patient does have severe symptomatic carotid stenosis, he/she is at risk of a major ischaemic stroke unless the artery is operated upon.

■ Patients with a disabling carotid ischaemic event, to help ascertain the cause of the stroke and appropriate strategies of secondary prevention of a recurrent stroke. Ultrasound is less urgent in these patients.

8.4   What is the role of cerebral angiography?

The traditional method of imaging the lumen of cerebral arteries has been by means of catheter contrast cerebral angiography. This involves catheterisation of the femoral artery (previously the carotid or brachial artery), directing the catheter into the aortic arch or carotid and vertebral arteries, and injecting contrast while taking X-rays of the head and neck. The images produced are of very good quality but they only image the lumen of the vessel (not the wall) and there is a small risk (about 0.5–4%) of the procedure actually causing a stroke.[3,4] Although this technique is still used to image the small intracranial blood vessels in patients with suspected cerebral aneurysms, arteriovenous malformations and arteritis, its role in the imaging of extracranial carotid and vertebral artery disease (for atheroma, dissection, etc.) has been superseded by magnetic resonance angiography (or repeated carotid ultrasound examinations by two different observers), because they are non-invasive and safe, even though the images are of inferior resolution.

8.5   In which patients is cerebral angiography indicated?

Magnetic resonance angiography (MRA) or intra-arterial digital subtraction angiography (IA-DSA; *Fig. 8.3*) is indicated for patients with a non-disabling carotid ischaemic event, *and* duplex ultrasound evidence of more than 70% stenosis of symptomatic carotid artery (and possibly more than 50% stenosis, depending on local accuracy of ultrasound), who are also fit and willing for carotid surgery (or stent). However, many surgeons are now prepared to perform carotid endarterectomy on the basis of the results of the clinical evaluation and carotid ultrasound alone. Because carotid ultrasound is not very reliable (reproducible), it is preferable at least to have the carotid ultrasound result verified by another independent carotid ultrasonographer (both blinded to the clinical history and suspected side of the symptomatic carotid). If both independent ultrasounds show more than 70% stenosis of the symptomatic carotid artery, it is probably acceptable to avoid angiography and proceed straight to carotid surgery.

Catheter cerebral angiography is indicated for patients with suspected aneurysmal subarachnoid haemorrhage (to image the aneurysm), arteriovenous malformation and cerebral vasculitis.

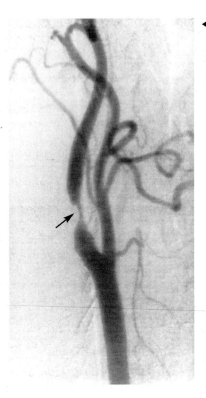

◀ **Fig 8.3** Digital subtraction angiogram showing a severe stenosis of the origin of the internal carotid artery.

8.6 What is the role of echocardiography?

Echocardiography relies on ultrasound to image the heart and measure by Doppler blood flow velocity (*Figs 8.4 & 8.5*).

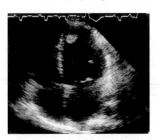
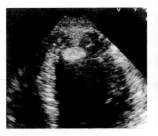

▲

Fig 8.4 Transthoracic two-dimensional echocardiogram, apical four-chamber view, showing a thrombus in the apex of the left ventricle. Adapted with permission from Hankey and Warlow.[2]

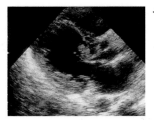

Fig 8.5 Transthoracic two-dimensional echocardiograph, parasternal long axis view, showing vegetations on the anterior leaflet of the mitral valve, which is situated behind the aortic valve. With permission from Hankey and Warlow.[2]

The main roles of echocardiography in patients with suspected TIA or ischaemic stroke are to:

■ Identify a source of embolism in the heart
■ Evaluate left ventricular function in patients with atrial fibrillation to help stratify the patient's risk of thromboembolism.

8.7 What is the difference between transthoracic and transoesophageal echocardiography?

Transthoracic echocardiography is undertaken by placing the ultrasound probe on the chest and recording ultrasound beams reflected from the anterior structures of the heart, such as the left ventricle.

Transoesophageal echocardiography is undertaken by placing the ultrasound probe in the oesophagus by endoscopy (a more invasive procedure) and recording ultrasound beams reflected from the posterior structures of the heart, such as the left atrium. Transoesophageal echocardiography also images the ascending aorta and arch of the aorta, which is increasingly recognised as an important source of atherothromboembolism to the brain.

8.8 In which patients is echocardiography indicated?

Transthoracic echocardiography (TTE) is indicated:

■ To identify a potential cardioembolic source if:
  – The patient has a non-lacunar stroke syndrome (e.g. total anterior circulation infarction, partial anterior circulation infarct or posterior circulation infarct, which are all commonly caused by embolic occlusion of a cerebral artery), and
  – The patient's heart is abnormal clinically or by ECG or chest X ray, and
  – CT brain scan shows wedge-shaped cortical/subcortical cerebral infarction (and particularly if there are multiple brain infarcts and in different arterial territories).
■ To evaluate left ventricular function, if patient is in atrial fibrillation and it is uncertain whether to anticoagulate with warfarin because of uncertainty of risk of stroke (left ventricular systolic dysfunction is a

---

TABLE 8.2 Preferred echocardiographic technique for detecting various cardiac disorders

Transthoracic echocardiography	Transoesophageal echocardiography
Left ventricular thrombus	Atrial thrombus
Left ventricular dyskinesis	Atrial appendage thrombus
Mitral stenosis	Spontaneous echo contrast
Mitral annulus calcification	Intracardiac tumours
Aortic stenosis	Atrial septal defect
	Atrial septal aneurysm
	Patent foramen ovale
	Mitral and aortic valve vegetations
	Prosthetic heart valve malfunction
	Aortic arch atherothrombosis/dissection
	Mitral leaflet prolapse

---

poor prognostic factor, as is a large left atrium and left atrial spontaneous echo contrast).

■ If TTE is negative but there is still a suspected embolic source in the heart, and particularly in:
  – The venous system (i.e. via a right-to-left shunt, such as a patent foramen ovale),
  – The inter-atrial septum (e.g. atrial septal aneurysm)
  – The left atrium or left atrial appendage, or
  – The aortic arch (*Table 8.2*).

8.9 What are the indications for MRI of the brain in patients with TIA and stroke?

Magnetic resonance imaging (with or without diffusion and perfusion weighted imaging) of the brain is indicated if:

■ CT scan performed more than 10 days after stroke shows a low-density area that could be infarction or resolving haemorrhage and it is essential to distinguish them
■ CT scan is negative and it is crucial to be able to localise the infarct (MRI is more sensitive)
■ Arterial dissection is suspected (NB. Catheter angiography remains the gold standard).

LABORATORY TESTS

8.10 When should serum cholesterol be measured after stroke?

Serum cholesterol should ideally be performed within 24 hours of onset of stroke and again more than 3 months after onset. Otherwise, falsely low readings may be obtained – acute stroke tends to lower serum cholesterol concentrations in the interval between about 24 hours and 6–12 weeks after onset.

8.11 What tests screen for a procoagulant state (thrombophilia)?

COAGULATION ASSAYS FOR LUPUS ANTICOAGULANT

- Activated partial thromboplastin time (APTT) – lacks sensitivity but remains the most appropriate screening test for the lupus anticoagulant. A prolonged APTT that fails to correct when affected plasma is mixed with normal plasma implies inhibition of the clotting system rather than deficiency of a component, and is the laboratory hallmark of the lupus anticoagulant.
- Dilute Russell's viper venom time (dRVVT) – prolongation of the dRVVT will not correct with the addition of normal plasma in the presence of lupus anticoagulant (in contrast to the clotting factor deficiency). For confirmation, a platelet neutralisation procedure should be performed to show the dependence of phospholipid inhibitors.
- Kaolin clotting time test – also detects lupus anticoagulant but it is not as sensitive as the dRVVT and sensitivity is highly reagent-dependent.
- Tissue thromboplastin inhibition test.

These are indirect coagulation assays sensitive to the phospholipid-dependent steps of blood coagulation. At least two assays, with sensitive reagents and techniques, must be used – most commonly the APTT with another test.

IMMUNOLOGICAL ASSAYS

- Anticardiolipin antibody – detected by means of solid-phase immunoassay, such as enzyme-linked immunosorbent assay (ELISA) or radioimmunoassay (RIA), employing cardiolipin or other negatively-charged phospholipids as the antigen to measure antibody concentration and binding avidity
- Other phospholipids, e.g. phosphatidyl serine
- Antibodies to β_2 glycoprotein I (β_2 GpI).

OTHER THROMBOPHILIA DIAGNOSTIC BLOOD TESTS

- Prothrombin time
- Antithrombin activity (NB. Heparin reduces antithrombin antigen and activity by 10–15%)
- Protein C activity (NB. Warfarin reduces protein C and protein S levels by 30% – these tests must be conducted prior to, or at least 2 weeks after, cessation of warfarin)

■ Protein S antigen level
■ Factor V Leiden genetic analysis or activated protein C resistance functional analysis
■ Prothrombin G20210A mutation
■ Antinuclear antibodies
■ Serum protein levels, serum protein electrophoresis and plasma viscosity – indicated in patients with elevated ESR or suspected hyperviscosity syndrome
■ Haemoglobin electrophoresis/sickle test – indicated in appropriate racial groups (e.g. Afro-Caribbean patients) to detect sickle-cell trait or disease
■ Fibrinogen
■ Platelet aggregation
■ Fasting plasma homocysteine (before and after a methionine load if possible).

8.12 What are the indications for thrombophilia screening?

■ Young patient (< 50 years) and no other cause found for TIA or ischaemic stroke
■ Past history or family history of premature arterial or venous thrombosis, especially if unusual sites (cerebral, mesenteric, hepatic veins)
■ Past history of recurrent miscarriage
■ Abnormal full blood picture or blood film (e.g. thrombocytopenia)
■ VDRL/RPR-positive – may be a false positive in the presence of anticardiolipin antibodies because cardiolipin is the antigen used in the VDRL assay. However, the VDRL is positive in only about 25% of patients with antiphospholipid antibody (APLAb).

8.13 How is the antiphospholipid antibody syndrome diagnosed?

The antiphospholipid antibody syndrome cannot be diagnosed on the basis of a single raised titre of anticardiolipin in the serum. The titre must be substantially raised on several occasions and associated not just with cerebral ischaemia but also with some combination of deep venous thrombosis, recurrent miscarriage, livedo reticularis, cardiac valvular vegetations, thrombocytopenia and migraine.

8.14 How is the lupus anticoagulant diagnosed?

Four sequential steps are necessary to establish the diagnosis of the lupus anticoagulant:

1. Demonstration of an abnormal phospholipid-dependent coagulation test (e.g. APTT, dRVVT)

2. Proof that the abnormality in step 1 is due to an inhibitor (synonym: anticoagulant)
3. Establishing the phospholipid-dependence of the inhibitor
4. Ruling out other coagulopathies.

8.15 How is the diagnosis of activated protein C resistance established?

The diagnosis of activated protein C resistance (APCR) is established through a functional APC resistance test, which has a functional clotting endpoint. It is a modified APTT in which the anticoagulant response to APC is measured. APCR is expressed as a ratio and a positive diagnosis usually requires a value of less than or equal to 2.0. In general, APCR is an effective screening test for the much more expensive genetic analysis to identify the factor V Leiden mutation, which is performed by polymerase chain reaction (PCR).

8.16 What other blood tests should be considered if the cause of the TIA or stroke remains uncertain?

■ Haemoglobin A1C – if fasting plasma glucose is elevated
■ Fasting plasma homocysteine – a possible risk factor
■ Antinuclear antibody assay – if vasculitis is suspected (e.g. elevated ESR)
■ Blood cultures – if infective endocarditis is suspected
■ Thyroid function tests – if there is atrial fibrillation, bradycardia or hypercholesterolaemia
■ HIV serology – if human immunodeficiency virus (HIV) is suspected.

The second-line investigations for TIA and ischaemic stroke are listed in *Table 8.3*.

TABLE 8.3 Second-line investigations for selected ischaemic stroke/TIA patients

Investigation	Indications
Blood	
Liver function	Fever, malaise, raised erythrocyte sedimentation rate (ESR), suspected malignancy
Calcium	Recurrent focal neurological symptoms very rarely due to hypercalcaemia
Thyroid function tests	Atrial fibrillation
Activated partial thromboplastin time, dilute Russell's viper venom	Young (< 50 years) and no other cause found, past history or family history of venous thrombosis, especially if unusual site (cerebral, mesenteric,

TABLE 8.3 (*Cont'd*)

Investigation	Indications
time anticardiolipin antibody*, antinuclear and other autoantibodies	hepatic veins) recurrent miscarriage, thrombocytopenia, cardiac valve vegetations, livedo reticularis, raised ESR, malaise, etc., positive syphilis serology
Serum proteins, serum protein electrophoresis, plasma viscosity	Raised ESR
Haemoglobin electrophoresis	Afro-Caribbean patients
Protein C and S, antithrombin III, activated protein C resistance, thrombin time†	Personal or family history of thrombosis (usually venous, particularly in unusual sites such as hepatic vein) at unusually young age
Blood cultures	Fever, cardiac murmur, haematuria, deranged liver function, raised ESR, malaise unexplained stroke in the young
Human immunodeficiency virus serology	Young (< 40 years), drug addict, homosexual, blood products transfusion, systemically unwell, lymphadenopathy, pneumonia, cytomegalovirus retinitis, etc.
Lipoprotein fractionation	Elevated cholesterol or strong family history Hyperlipoproteinaemia
Serum homocysteine (after methionine load)	Marfanoid habitus, high myopia, dislocated lenses, osteoporosis, mental retardation, young patient
Leukocyte alpha-galactosidase A	Corneal opacities, cutaneous angiokeratomas, paraesthesias and pain, renal failure
Blood/cerebrospinal fluid lactate	Young patient, basal ganglia calcification, epilepsy, MELAS/mitochondrial cytopathy, parieto-occipital ischaemia
Syphilis serology	Young patient, high risk of sexually transmitted diseases
Cardiac enzymes	History or electrocardiographic (ECG) evidence of recent myocardial infarction
Drug screen	Young patient, no other obvious cause, induced by cocaine/amphetamine, etc.
Urine	
Amino acids	Marfanoid habitus, high myopia, dislocated lenses, osteoporosis, mental retardation, young patient
Drug screen	Young patient, no other obvious cause, induced by cocaine/amphetamine, etc.

TABLE 8.3 *(Cont'd)*

Investigation	Indications
Imaging	
Chest X-ray	Hypertension, finger-clubbing, cardiac murmur or abnormal electrocardiogram, young patient, ill patient
Brain computed tomography	Continuing carotid transient ischaemic attacks of the brain, carotid endarterectomy being considered, thrombolysis being considered, taking or due to take anticoagulants or perhaps antiplatelet drugs, deteriorating stroke patient
Magnetic resonance imaging	Suggestion of arterial dissection, uncertain diagnosis of stroke
Carotid ultrasound with a view to carotid angiography	Carotid transient ischaemic attack or mild ischaemic stroke
Cerebral angiography	Carotid ultrasound suggests about 70% stenosis or more of recently symptomatic internal carotid artery and patient fit and willing for surgery, suspected arterial dissection, arteritis, arteriovenous malformation or aneurysm
Arch aortography	Symptoms of subclavian steal and unequal brachial pulses and blood pressures
Cardiac	
ECG (transthoracic or transoesophageal)	Possible cardiac source of embolism and young (< 50 years), or clinical, ECG or chest X-ray evidence of emboligenic heart disease, aortic arch dissection
24-hour ECG	Palpitations or loss of consciousness during a suspected transient ischaemic attack, suspicious resting ECG
Others	
Electroencephalogram	Doubt about diagnosis of transient ischaemic attack or stroke: ?epilepsy
Cerebrospinal fluid	Positive blood syphilis serology, young patient, ?infective endocarditis, possibility of multiple sclerosis
Body red cell mass	Raised haematocrit
Temporal artery biopsy	Older (> 60 years), jaw claudication, headache, polymyalgia, malaise, anaemia, raised ESR.

* Repeat to ensure persistently raised
† Transient falls occur after stroke so must be repeated if low

8.17 What are the indications for lumbar puncture in patients with TIA or stroke?

Lumbar puncture, to examine the cerebrospinal fluid (CSF) is indicated if:

- Subarachnoid haemorrhage (SAH) is still suspected despite a normal CT scan (must wait until at least 12 hours have elapsed since onset of stroke symptoms before performing lumbar puncture)
- Cerebral vasculitis is suspected
- Blood Venereal Diseases Research Laboratories (VDRL) or *Treponema pallidum* haemagglutination (TPHA) test is positive and tertiary syphilis is possible.

8.18 What are the indications for temporal artery biopsy?

Temporal artery biopsy is indicated if temporal/giant cell arteritis is suspected (*see Q. 6.46*), particularly in patients with the following features:

- Visual impairment (25–50% of cases of temporal arteritis) – usually sudden, painless deterioration of vision in one eye, often on waking in the morning, due to anterior ischaemic optic neuropathy
- TIA of the brain or stroke – 7% of cases of temporal arteritis
- TIA of the eye (amaurosis fugax) – 10% of cases of temporal arteritis
- Age more than 50 years
- New onset of localised headache
- Jaw or tongue claudication (pain on chewing)
- Systemic symptoms – fever, malaise, fatigue, anorexia, weight loss, night sweats, arthralgias
- Proximal, symmetrical muscle pain and stiffness of polymyalgia rheumatica
- Abnormal temporal artery clinically – tenderness or decreased pulse
- Elevated ESR (> 50 mm/h).

Temporal artery biopsy should be performed as soon as possible but should not delay the commencement of steroid treatment. Although steroid treatment will reduce the chance of a positive biopsy result, positive results have been reported up to a week, and even 3–6 months in some cases, after starting steroids.

- The biopsy should be taken from the clinically abnormal side
- The biopsy is positive in 60–80% of patients with temporal arteritis (and 15–20% of patients with polymyalgia rheumatica)
- The sensitivity of the biopsy depends on its quality, particularly its length and its preparation for histological examination
- If temporal arteries on both sides appear normal, remove a 4–5 cm length of artery from one side and examine it histologically by serial sections – arterial lesions can be segmental

■ If the biopsy is negative and the diagnosis of giant cell arteritis is still suspected, the other superficial temporal artery should be biopsied

■ If both biopsies are negative, the diagnosis of giant cell arteritis still cannot be ruled out; in these cases, the diagnosis is clinical.

8.19 What are the indications for biopsy of the leptomeninges and cerebral cortex?

Biopsy of the leptomeninges and cerebral cortex is indicated if cerebral vasculitis is suspected to be the cause of the TIA or stroke.

Most patients with cerebral vasculitis present with an acute or subacute focal or diffuse encephalopathy or meningoencephalopathy with headache, altered mentation, seizures and cognitive and behavioural abnormalities, and with multifocal neurological signs. Systemic symptoms and signs, such as fever, headache, malaise, weight loss, joint aches and pains, facial rash and livido reticularis, may be present (*see* Q. 6.45).

The decision to biopsy is made on an individual basis. If an extended period of treatment with potentially hazardous immunosuppressant drugs is being considered, the need to establish an unequivocal tissue diagnosis is of primary importance.

Biopsy of the leptomeninges and a wedge of cerebral cortex from the non-dominant temporal lobe establishes the diagnosis in about 70% of cases. False-negative biopsies occur in about 30% of autopsy-proven patients.

The risk of serious morbidity from brain biopsy is 0.5–2.0%.

PATIENT QUESTIONS

8.20 What tests will the doctors do after a TIA or stroke?

After asking about the onset and nature of your symptoms (the history) and examining your head, eyes, neck, chest, heart and limbs (physical examination), the doctor will arrange for some tests to be done to define the nature and cause of the stroke further, as described below.

Blood tests

Blood tests are to check the concentration of red blood cells, glucose (sugar) and cholesterol (fat) in the blood. A high blood glucose or cholesterol concentration may indicate underlying diabetes mellitus or high cholesterol levels, which may predispose to hardening of the arteries (atheroma). The test involves a needle being inserted into a vein in the arm.

Electrocardiography (ECG)

This is a test to check the rhythm of the heart – whether it is regular or irregular (e.g. atrial fibrillation) – and whether there is evidence of a previous heart attack or the effect of high blood pressure on the heart. It involves placing a series of electrodes on to the skin of the chest and recording the electrical activity in the heart, and is not at all painful.

Echocardiography

This is usually performed when the stroke is caused by a blocked artery to the brain (an ischaemic stroke) and when the cause of the blocked artery is thought to be a problem with the heart (i.e. a blood clot has formed in a chamber of the heart or on a valve in the heart, and has broken off and lodged downstream in a blood vessel in the neck or the brain). The doctor is usually suspicious of the heart as a source of the blood clot if the heart is beating irregularly (e.g. atrial fibrillation), if there is an abnormal sound when the doctor listens to the heart (e.g. a heart murmur), or if the ECG is abnormal.

The test involves putting some jelly on the chest and then placing a probe on the chest which emits sound waves. The jelly is to ensure good contact between the probe and the skin. The sound waves bounce off the heart and are recorded by the probe; they are then converted into images of the structure of the heart. The test is therefore an ultrasound examination of the heart. It is safe, non-invasive and painless.

CT brain scan

Computed tomography (CT) of the brain is a special kind of X-ray imaging of the brain. Its main role is to exclude other possible causes of a stroke (e.g. a brain tumour) and to distinguish between stroke caused by a blocked blood vessel and that due to a burst blood vessel. The test involves lying still on a bed while the scanner emits X-rays at your head. It does not usually involve any injections and takes only 10–15 minutes.

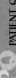

MRI brain scan

Magnetic resonance imaging (MRI) is sometimes required to obtain a more detailed image of the brain (particularly the back part of the brain) or to image the blood vessels in the brain without the need for an injection of contrast into the blood vessels. The test involves lying still on a bed while the scanner uses magnetism to image the brain. It does not use X-rays or usually involve any injections. About 5–10% of people cannot tolerate the test because they find it too claustrophobic or noisy. It usually takes 15–30 minutes.

Carotid ultrasonography

This examination is usually performed when the TIA or stroke is caused by a blocked artery to the brain (an ischaemic stroke) and the cause of the blockage is thought to be a problem with the carotid artery at the front of the neck (i.e. a blood clot has formed in a major blood vessel in the neck, and has broken off and lodged downstream in a blood vessel in the brain). The doctor is usually suspicious of the artery in the neck as a source of the clot if the stroke is caused by a blocked artery in the brain that is a branch of the carotid artery in the neck (a carotid territory TIA or ischaemic stroke) and if there is an abnormal sound when the doctor listens to the neck (a bruit).

The test involves putting some jelly on the neck and then placing a probe on the neck which emits sound waves. The sound waves bounce off the carotid artery in the neck and are recorded by the probe, and are then converted into images of the structure of the carotid artery and the inside of the carotid artery. It detects any narrowing of the artery that takes blood to the eye and brain. It is a useful test not only to determine the cause of the ischaemic stroke but also for deciding whether to perform an operation that cleans out the artery in the neck (carotid endarterectomy) to reduce the risk of future strokes.

Angiography

An angiogram is an image of the inside of the blood vessels and can be obtained non-invasively by means of magnetic resonance imaging (MRI), often at the time of an MRI scan of the brain (see above). However, the resolution of the images is not optimal. The best quality image of the inside of blood vessels is obtained by contrast catheter angiography. This involves injecting a local anaesthetic into the skin of the groin, then inserting a fine plastic tube (catheter) into the major blood vessel in the groin (femoral artery) and passing the catheter up the femoral artery into the aorta in the abdomen and chest, and then up the carotid arteries in the neck. A special dye (radio-opaque contrast) is then injected into the blood vessels in the neck and a rapid sequence of X-ray images is taken of the skull.

The angiogram shows not only the bones of the skull but also the dye (contrast) in the vessels, as it passes quickly though the brain (to be excreted in the urine). Because a catheter is inserted into the main blood vessels to the brain, and contrast dye is injected into these arteries, there is a very small risk (0.5%) that the catheter could damage the inside of one of the arteries or the contrast could irritate the inside lining of the arteries, and lead to a stroke.

Prognosis (what does the future hold for the patient?)

After the diagnosis of stroke has been made and the stroke syndrome, pathology and likely aetiology have been ascertained, the stroke patient should be assessed immediately and completely by all members of the multidisciplinary stroke team to identify his/her impairments, disabilities and handicaps and the prognosis for survival free of handicap and recurrent stroke. This forms the foundation of an ongoing problem- and goal-orientated management plan.

PROGNOSIS OF STROKE

9.1   What is the risk of dying after a stroke?

The case fatality rates after a first-ever stroke (all types combined) are about 12% at 7 days, 19% at 30 days, 31% at 1 year and 60% at 5 years.[1,2]

The relative risk of death in stroke survivors is about twice the risk of people in the general population, and the risk persists for several years.

9.2   What are the usual causes of death after stroke?

- ■ Death within a few hours of stroke onset is not common but is usually due to the direct effects of intracerebral or subarachnoid haemorrhage, and rarely massive brainstem infarction, causing brain herniation.
- ■ Death occurring within the first week after stroke is also most frequently due to the direct effects of the brain damage but the cause is as likely to be cerebral infarction as cerebral haemorrhage; ischaemic cerebral oedema is maximal about day 3.
- ■ Later on, the complications of immobility (e.g. bronchopneumonia, venous thromboembolism) and recurrent vascular events of the brain and, even more so, the heart are the common causes of death (*Fig. 9.1*).

The importance of anticipating and implementing appropriate and effective strategies targeted at these potentially preventable events is emphasised.

9.3   What is the single best predictor of early death after stroke?

The single best predictor of early death is impaired consciousness.

9.4   What other adverse prognostic factors predict a patient's prognosis for survival after stroke?

The outcome after stroke depends on the location, size and pathology of the stroke lesion, the patient's age, and other comorbidities (i.e. handicap) present before the stroke.

Indicators of poor survival are listed in *Box 9.1*.

Another major adverse prognostic factor is haemorrhagic stroke. In the first 30 days, haemorrhagic stroke (intracerebral and subarachnoid

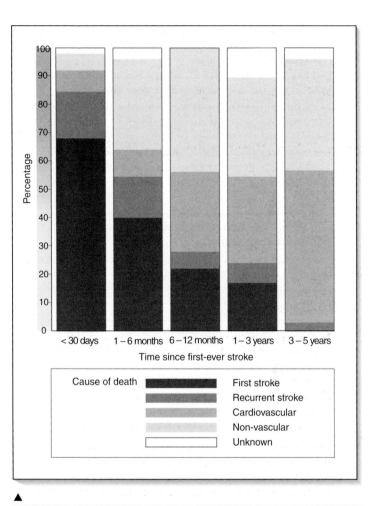

Fig 9.1 The causes of death at different time intervals after stroke. Note how most deaths in the first 30 days after stroke are due to its direct effects whereas cardiovascular disease causes most deaths in subsequent years. Adapted with permission from Hankey et al.[2]

BOX 9.1 Indicators of poor survival after stroke

- Depression of consciousness
- Urinary incontinence
- Pupillary abnormalities
- Gaze paresis
- Severe limb weakness
- Bilateral extensor plantar responses
- Cardiac failure
- Atrial fibrillation

haemorrhage) carries a much higher risk of death (50%) than ischaemic stroke (10%). However, the distinction requires early computed tomography (CT) of the brain.[3,4]

9.5 What is the usual clinical course after stroke?

Among stroke survivors, neurological function begins to improve within the first few days and continues most rapidly in the first 3 months and more slowly over the next 6–12 months, with some gains still being realised 1–2 years after stroke (not all of which are functional adaptations).

The pattern of recovery varies among patients, and in individuals, and rarely follows that implied by grouped data. Only repeated assessments in individual patients can indicate their pattern of recovery.

9.6 What is the risk of being physically or cognitively dependent at one year after a stroke?

The risk is about 20–30%. At 12 months after first-ever stroke, about one-third of all stroke patients have died, about 20–30% are dependent on another person for everyday activities (e.g. washing, dressing, mobilising) and 40–50% are independent.[3,4]

9.7 What factors determine whether a patient will make a good functional recovery after stroke?

> ## Major clinical factors predictive of independence 6 months after a stroke
>
> ■ Age
> ■ Living alone (nobody permanently living with the patient before the stroke)
> ■ Independent in activities of daily living before the stroke (Oxford Handicap score < 2 before stroke)
> ■ Normal verbal Glasgow Coma Scale score (= 5)
> ■ Arm strength – can lift both arms to horizontal
> ■ Able to walk without the help of another person (can use stick/Zimmer frame).
>
> These factors seem to be equally predictive whether they are assessed within 48 hours of stroke onset or later, whether the stroke is ischaemic or haemorrhagic and whether the patient has had a previous stroke or not.[5]
>
> ## Indicators for poor functional recovery
>
> ■ Urinary incontinence
> ■ Poor postural control
> ■ Cognitive dysfunction

- Poor motivation
- Visual–spatial-perceptual dysfunction
- Proprioceptive loss
- Severe motor loss
- Initially complete dependence in activities of daily living.

Of course, the patient's chances of staying at home or returning home from hospital depend not only on the severity of their stroke but also on other factors such as premorbid disability, whether they were living alone previously, and their social support and access to community services.

9.8 What is the risk of a recurrent stroke?

The risk of a recurrent stroke among survivors of stroke in the community, treated with best medical and surgical therapy to prevent a recurrence, is about 2–4% in the first month, 6–12% in the first months, and 10% to 16% within the first year. Thereafter, the risk falls to about 4–5% per year, so that, by 5 years, about 30% (19–42%) will have suffered a recurrent stroke.[6]

9.9 What factors influence the risk of recurrent stroke?

Intuitively, it would be expected that the main factor increasing the risk of recurrent stroke would be failure to treat the underlying cause of the initial stroke. This is supported by the fact that about 90% of recurrent strokes are of the same pathological type as the initial stroke, and that many of the factors associated with an increased risk of recurrent stroke in epidemiological studies (see below) reflect a lack of persistent control of underlying causal risk factors or diseases. These factors are listed in *Box 9.2*.

BOX 9.2 Factors influencing the risk of recurrent stroke

- Advanced age
- Clinical stroke syndrome of ischaemic strokes – partial anterior circulation infarcts and posterior circulation infarcts have a 4.9% and 4.8% risk of recurrent stroke within the first 30 days compared with lacunar infarcts, which have a 0.3% risk of recurrent stroke in the first 30 days
- Haemorrhagic initial stroke
- History of previous transient ischaemic attack (TIA)
- Hypertension
- Diabetes mellitus and elevated blood glucose (e.g. uncontrolled diabetes)
- Cigarette smoking
- Atrial fibrillation, valvular heart disease and congestive heart failure
- Severe carotid stenosis
- Dementia after stroke.

PROGNOSIS OF TIA

9.10 What is the risk of a stroke and other serious vascular events after a TIA?

As a group, patients who have had a TIA have an increased stroke risk of about 4–5% in the first month, 12% in the first year and 29% over 5 years (*see Q. 7.12 & Q. 7.13*).[7]

The risk of a coronary event after a TIA is steady (without an initially higher risk, as with risk of stroke after TIA) at about 3% per year (*see Q. 7.15*).

The risk of a stroke or other serious vascular event (myocardial infarction or death due to vascular causes) after a TIA is about 8–10% per year.

9.11 Which factors predict which patients with TIA are increased risk of stroke?

As individuals, TIA patients have a variable prognosis; some have a stroke within days and others never have another vascular event.

Independent predictors of an increased risk of stroke

- TIA of the brain (rather than the eye)
- Increasing age
- Increasing number of TIAs in the previous 3 months (i.e. multiple attacks)
- Peripheral vascular disease
- Carotid stenosis > 80%
- Other adverse prognostic factors – past history of any TIA, left ventricular hypertrophy, carotid plaque morphology (e.g. ulceration), and impaired cerebrovascular reserve (*see Q. 7.14*).[8–11]

PROGNOSIS OF SUBARACHNOID HAEMORRHAGE

9.12 What is the risk of death and dependency after subarachnoid haemorrhage?

The case-fatality rate after subarachnoid haemorrhage (SAH) is about 40%. Another 10–20% of patients remain functionally dependent.[4]

9.13 Has there been a decline in the case-fatality rate after SAH?

Yes, the past 30 years has seen a decrease in the risk of a fatal outcome of approximately 15%, presumably through improved medical and surgical management.[4] Early referral to a specialist centre seems therefore to be in the patient's best interests.

9.14 What is the risk of rebleeding after subarachnoid haemorrhage?

If patients with SAH due to a ruptured aneurysm do not undergo clipping or coiling, about:

■ 10% rebleed within hours
■ 30% rebleed within a few hours to a few weeks and thereafter
■ 2–3% rebleed every year.

During the first few weeks, there is no particular time where the risk of rebleeding is higher, nor are they any known factors that predict rebleeding, which is more likely to be fatal than the first bleed.[12,13]

In patients with SAH due to a ruptured arteriovenous malformation, the chance of survival is higher and the chance of rebleed is lower, certainly in the early period after the initial haemorrhage.[14] Exactly which features of the vascular anatomy, or other factors, are associated with particularly high risks of bleeding or epilepsy is not clear.[15]

9.15 How is rebleeding after SAH diagnosed?

Rebleeding usually causes a sudden deterioration in neurological status, with reduced consciousness level. Like the original bleed, there are few if any focal neurological features. However, if the patient is being ventilated at the time of rebleed, the only clue may be sudden fixed dilatation of the pupils.[12]

Rebleeding can only be diagnosed by repeat CT scan to show fresh haemorrhage, and even then it can be difficult to be sure. Repeat lumbar puncture is not helpful and is sometimes dangerous (if deterioration is actually due to intracerebral haematoma).

9.16 What is the risk of delayed cerebral ischaemia after subarachnoid haemorrhage?

Delayed cerebral ischaemia appears 4–14 days after onset in about 25% of patients. It is important because it implies a bad prognosis.

9.17 What are the risk factors for delayed cerebral ischaemia after subarachnoid haemorrhage?

These include:

■ Poor initial clinical state
■ Large quantities of subarachnoid or intraventricular blood on CT
■ Hyponatraemia
■ The use of antifibrinolytic drugs.[16]

9.18 What is the cause of delayed cerebral ischaemia after subarachnoid haemorrhage?

Delayed cerebral ischaemia after SAH is probably caused by the combination of vasospasm and structural changes in the wall of one or more cerebral arteries, but not necessarily the one bearing the ruptured aneurysm.

The onset of neurological symptoms and signs is usually gradual, with deteriorating consciousness level and evolving focal neurological signs.

PATIENT QUESTIONS

9.19 What are the chances of surviving after a stroke?

Overall, about 70% of people survive a stroke.

Among the different types of stroke, about 85% of those with an ischaemic stroke (due to a blocked artery) survive and about 50% of those with a haemorrhagic stroke (due to a burst artery) survive.

9.20 What are the chances of recovering after a stroke?

Among the survivors of stroke, about half make a good functional recovery and about half are left with some residual disability or handicap.

Recovery after stroke takes time, however. It is maximal in the first few months, and begins to plateau between 3 and 6 months, but small gains are still going to be made over the next 1–2 years.

Of course, some patients recover fully within hours, some within days and some within months. The rate and degree of recovery depends on the size, location and type of the stroke, as well as the nature of the body deficit, the patient's general health and their motivation.

9.21 What are the risks of a future stroke?

The risk of a future stroke after a TIA or stroke is greatest in the first year, indeed in the first few weeks and months. In general, about 1 in 10, or 10%, of individuals who have a TIA or stroke will have a stroke during the following year. After the first year, the risk falls to about 1 in 20, or 5%, each year. After a stroke also, about 5–10% of patients each year suffer a heart attack. The risk of heart attack is quite constant each year.

It is difficult to predict which individuals are likely to experience a recurrent stroke (and heart attack), but generally the risk is increased among individuals who are older, have had a recent TIA or stroke, have had numerous recent TIAs or stroke and have evidence of disease in the blood vessels of other organs (e.g. ischaemic heart disease and peripheral arterial disease).

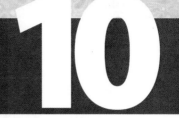

Early management (should patients be referred to hospital?)

10.1 What are the principles of the pre-hospital management of patients with suspected stroke?

Principles of pre-hospital management of suspected stroke

■ Make an accurate diagnosis of stroke, its pathological type (infarct or haemorrhage) and aetiological subtype (cause of the infarct or haemorrhage)

■ Accurately assess the patient's impairments, disabilities and handicaps, particularly in comparison with previous impairments, disabilities and handicaps

■ Estimate the prognosis for survival, and future handicap

■ Discuss the prognosis with the patient and family (if possible) and set shared short- and long-term goals

■ Consider which services are required to meet the shared goals and how to access and deliver them.

10.2 Why admit stroke patients to hospital?

Most patients with stroke are admitted to hospital. The proportion varies from one country to another – it is more than 90% in Sweden, 80% in Italy and Australia, 40–70% in the UK and fewer in other countries with less resources or different policies.

The reasons for hospital admission are varied but include the opportunity to establish the diagnosis of stroke and its pathological and aetiological subtypes (using CT imaging), to administer safe and effective therapies, to access coordinated multidisciplinary care in a stroke unit and to nurse the disabled patient.

Patients who have had a mild, non-disabling stroke may not require inpatient care but nevertheless need rapid assessment, except perhaps for very infirm or elderly patients and those already in institutional care.

The widespread introduction of thrombolytic therapy for acute ischaemic stroke, with its narrow time window, will demand much improved organisation of prehospital care and 'fast-tracking' within hospitals to avoid delays.

10.3 Is stroke a medical emergency?

Yes, in most cases stroke is a medical emergency.

Medical emergencies are defined by various criteria, such as rapidity of onset, poor prognosis and requirement for prompt effective intervention to improve outcome. Stroke meets all these criteria. Although stroke has traditionally been considered to be less of an emergency than many other conditions fulfilling one or more of these criteria (e.g. meningitis, acute myocardial infarction), it is no longer tenable to regard it as anything other than a medical emergency, except in patients who were already severely handicapped.

10.4 Should acute stroke patients be sent urgently to hospital?

Yes, most acute stroke patients should be sent urgently to hospital.

There are several reasons why most (but not all) patients with acute stroke require urgent inpatient assessment and care (over and above the need to establish an accurate diagnosis of stroke, its pathology, underlying cause and likely prognosis).

First, within hours of a stroke, various life-threatening, preventable or treatable complications may occur, such as:

- Airway obstruction and respiratory failure
- Swallowing problems causing aspiration, dehydration and malnutrition
- Epileptic seizures
- Venous thromboembolism
- Infections.

Early assessment and anticipation coupled with appropriate intervention can minimise these and improve outcome.

Second, the patient may benefit from appropriate and effective acute medical and surgical therapies (besides aspirin), such as intravenous thrombolysis (ischaemic stroke within 3 hours of onset) or suboccipital craniectomy (cerebellar infarction and oedema).

10.5 Is there evidence that care in hospital is better than care at home?

Yes, there is some evidence, but it mainly applies to hospital care by multidisciplinary stroke teams in stroke units.

There have been six randomised controlled trials comparing the effect of caring for stroke patients in hospital with the effect of caring for them in their own home by means of multidisciplinary domiciliary teams aiming to provide the equivalent of hospital care. The trials used a range of services to serve as their control (or comparison) group: three trials (of a total of about 900 patients) used care in a general medical ward, one (of about 300 patients) used a mobile stroke team in the hospital, and two (total of about 350 patients) used care in a stroke ward. When all the studies were combined there was no overall significant difference in the proportion of patients who had died or were in institutional care at 1 year after stroke onset among the hospital or home-based care groups. However, among the three trials of home care versus care in a general ward, and the one trial of home care versus care in several wards by a mobile stroke team, there was a non-significant trend toward a better outcome in the group treated at home. On the other hand, in the two trials of home care versus care in a stroke unit, there was a significant reduction in death and institutionalisation at 1 year after stroke in the patients treated in a stroke unit.

There were also several practical problems with these trials. In two of them, the actual number of hospital bed days used by the patients randomised to care at home was as great as the number used by the patients randomised to care in hospital. In other words, many of the patients ended up going to hospital anyway, and so the home-based care plan was far more expensive than the hospital plan. In another trial, one-third of the patients allocated at random to care at home had eventually to be admitted to the stroke unit.[1]

10.6 Which patients should be referred to hospital?

Most patients with suspected acute stroke should be referred to hospital, especially those patients who are likely to benefit most from the opportunities offered by hospital treatment that are listed in *Box 10.1*.

> **BOX 10.1 Advantages of hospital treatment for stroke**
> - Formulation of an accurate and early diagnosis (stroke is primarily a clinical diagnosis and the sooner a history can be elicited the more likely it is to be reliable)
> - Organisation of relevant and cost-effective investigations
> - Implementation of appropriate interventions to restore cerebral perfusion (ischaemic stroke), prevent complications, prevent recurrent stroke and facilitate recovery
> - Nursing care for sick and disabled patients
> - Provision of relevant and helpful information and support for the patient and family

10.7 Which patients can be managed at home?

Some patients can be managed successfully at home or in their residential nursing home. Admission to hospital is generally not necessary for TIA patients, or patients with mild non-disabling stroke, provided they can be accurately diagnosed (including stroke pathology and aetiology) and cared for at home with rapid back-up from a hospital-based stroke service for:

- Help with diagnosis
- Cardiological and neuroradiological investigations (which, apart from catheter angiography, can all be done on an outpatient basis)

■ Appropriate secondary prevention
■ Possibly domiciliary rehabilitation.

Also, elderly people and those who were already dependent through physical or cognitive disability and have now had a severe stroke may be better off out of hospital, particularly if they are already being well cared for in a nursing home.

Clearly, hospital admission rates vary depending on local custom and practice, geography, patient expectations and how well organised the primary care and hospital-based care are. However, admission rates are likely to be driven up by the increasing realisation that not only should stroke patients be treated by experts in their disease but that emerging new treatments – such as thrombolysis – must be given in hospital, and given very rapidly indeed to have any chance of success. This will require education of the public to recognise stroke, better organisation of emergency services and fast-tracking of stroke patients once they get to hospital.

PATIENT QUESTIONS

10.8 What should you do if you or someone else has a stroke?

If someone suddenly loses function of a particular part of the body, which is thought to be a stroke, you should immediately call for an ambulance to transport the person to the nearest hospital. At the onset of a stroke it is uncertain whether the symptoms will resolve quickly within a few hours (a TIA) or whether they will persist (a stroke).

If the symptoms have resolved by the time the person arrives at the hospital, he/she can be assessed and discharged home with appropriate investigations, treatment and follow-up. If the symptoms persist, the person should be assessed as a medical emergency and considered for treatments that rescue damaged brain cells, prevent complications of stroke (e.g. swallowing fluid and food down the wrong way and into the lungs, causing pneumonia) and minimise a recurrence of stroke (and the occurrence of heart attack).

Sometimes, the symptoms are not due to a stroke or TIA but to another medical condition such as migraine, epileptic seizure, fainting attack, or inflammation or tumour of the brain.

Hospital management (where and how should the patient be managed?)

11

THE STROKE UNIT

11.1 Where, in hospitals, should stroke patients be managed?

Patients with stroke should ideally be managed in a geographically defined stroke unit staffed by a coordinated, multidisciplinary team that is interested and has expertise in the care of stroke patients (*see* Q. 11.2). In addition, there is some evidence to suggest that patients cared for in comprehensive stroke units that aim to accelerate discharge from hospital and provide rehabilitation in the home setting (i.e. stroke units with early supported discharge services) have a better outcome than patients managed by conventional stroke unit care with discharge planning and postdischarge care.

11.2 What is an acute stroke unit?

A stroke unit is an area where patients with acute stroke are admitted directly and may remain for a variable time to be diagnosed, treated and rehabilitated by a multidisciplinary team.

It combines the functions of an acute stroke assessment area and a stroke rehabilitation unit. It is not a stroke intensive care unit.

11.3 What is the evidence that care in a stroke unit is more effective than care in a general ward?

There is now good evidence from 23 randomised trials in eight countries that organised multidisciplinary care in a stroke unit is more effective than care in a general medical ward; there are fewer deaths (22% stroke unit vs 26% general medical ward), fewer patients remaining in an institution (18% stroke unit vs 20% general medical ward), and more independent survivors (44% stroke unit vs 38% general medical ward), all without lengthening hospital stay. Overall, compared with conventional care in a general ward, organised and coordinated care by an interested and trained multidisciplinary team in a stroke unit reduces death and dependency at 1 year after stroke from 62.0% to 56.36% (odds ratio, OR 0.71, 95% confidence interval, CI 0.65–0.87).[1] This is an odds reduction of 29% (95% CI 13–35%), relative risk reduction of 10% (95% CI 5–15%) and absolute risk reduction of 5.64%. Therefore, treating 1000 patients in a stroke unit rather than in a general ward prevents 56 patients from dying or becoming dependent. The number of patients that must be treated in a stroke unit to prevent one from dying or becoming dependent is 18 (95% CI 12–45).

There were no detrimental effects reported that were attributable to stroke units.

Overall, the length of stay in the stroke unit group was reduced by about 2–11 days.

Prospective observational data of more than 14 000 patients admitted to 80 Swedish hospitals indicate that patients admitted to a stroke unit had reduced dependence at 3 months (relative risk reduction: 6%, 95% CI 1–11%).[2] Although biases are inherent in such observational data, the findings suggest that the results of the systematic review of randomised trials outlined above may be reproducible in routine clinical settings.

11.4 Is there more than one model of organised coordinated stroke care by a multidisciplinary team?

There are three main models of organised stroke care:

- Care in a geographically dedicated stroke ward (stroke unit) by a multidisciplinary team
- Care in several wards by a mobile stroke team
- Care in a mixed rehabilitation ward.

Within the geographically dedicated stroke ward there are also three models:

- Acute intensive care
- Comprehensive (acute and rehabilitation) care
- Rehabilitation.

11.5 Which model of organised coordinated stroke care is most effective?

Compared with care in a general medical ward, patients who were randomised to comprehensive (acute and rehabilitation) care in a stroke ward had the greatest reduction in death and dependency at one year ($p = 0.008$), followed by patients randomised to care in a rehabilitation ward ($p = 0.04$), followed by patients cared for by a mobile stroke team.[1]

11.6 Is a geographically dedicated stroke unit necessary?

Although it is preferable, and probably more effective (*see Q. 11.5*), a geographically dedicated stroke unit is not as important as having a multidisciplinary stroke team that meets regularly and follows the principles of regular patient assessment, goal-setting, intervention, reassessment and reintervention. Indeed, the rural general practitioner can provide an excellent stroke service if he/she is interested in transient ischaemic attack (TIA)/stroke patients, enthusiastic about teaching and coordinating nurses and any available allied health professionals, and motivated to lobby for essential resources such as a computed tomography (CT) scanner.

11.7 What are the advantages of a geographically dedicated stroke unit?

The advantages of a geographically defined stroke unit are:

- Nursing staff can play a greater part in the rehabilitation process
- Patients in acute areas with urgent needs (e.g. chest pain) do not take up nursing time from stroke patients, who may have less urgent but important needs (e.g. regular toileting, which maintains continence and dignity).

11.8 What are the disadvantages of a geographically dedicated stroke unit?

A disadvantage of a geographically defined stroke unit is that there is an inevitable limit on places. However, this can be overcome by ensuring that the unit is part of a larger area coordinated by the stroke team, so that it can expand and contract with demand.

11.9 Why is care in a stroke unit more effective?

The specific components of care in a stroke unit that save lives (mainly between 1 and 4 weeks after stroke) and reduce dependency remain uncertain. However, they probably include awareness and anticipation of complications of stroke in high-risk individuals (e.g. aspiration pneumonia, pulmonary embolism, pressure sores) and adopting appropriate interventions *before* the complications develop to prevent them from occurring.[3]

Descriptive studies also indicate that some of the benefits of stroke unit care may also be due to early mobilisation of patients, routine use of intravenous saline and selective use of antipyretic and antibiotic medication, oxygen and insulin.[4] Furthermore, there is increasing evidence that stroke patients who manage to maintain key physiological variables (blood pressure, osmolarity, temperature, oxygen saturation, blood glucose) within a narrow physiological range are more likely to enjoy an early recovery and better functional outcome.[5]

The crucial ingredients, therefore, appear to be not more intensive medical care (e.g. cardiac monitoring) but:

- Coordinated multidisciplinary assessment, intervention and maintenance of physiological homeostasis
- Measures to risk-stratify, record and prevent complications
- Active rehabilitation
- Education and training in stroke care
- Specialisation of all staff in the team.

Although intensive medical and nursing care is seldom needed (except in patients being treated with thrombolysis or those with a severe life-threatening condition such as cerebellar stroke), patients should ideally be admitted to a designated area of the hospital and their acute care should be seamlessly integrated with their rehabilitation.[1]

THE STROKE TEAM

11.10 What comprises a multidisciplinary stroke team?

A multidisciplinary stroke team is made up of one or more doctors (e.g. stroke consultant, registrar and resident), nurses (including specialist stroke liaison nurse), physiotherapists, occupational therapists, a speech and language therapist, social worker and dietitian, and ideally a pharmacist, clinical neuropsychologist and specialist in orthotics/prosthetics.

11.11 What is the role of the doctors?

The doctors in the stroke unit:

- Respond immediately to any referral for the assessment and management of suspected acute stroke patients
- Clinically assess each patient by means of a relevant and targeted clinical history and examination, documenting the nature of the symptoms and physical impairments, the timing of the onset, any precipitating factors and the subsequent course – in addition, relevant aetiological (e.g. vascular risk factors), social, vocational and emotional factors are sought
- Order appropriate initial investigations, which includes (in almost all cases) a cranial CT scan, full blood count, erythrocyte sedimentation rate, creatinine, electrolytes, glucose, electrocardiogram and urine analysis.
- Formulate, on the basis of the assessment, an answer to each of the following questions:
  - Is it a stroke (*clinical diagnosis*)?
  - Where is the stroke – which part of the brain is affected and what vascular territory (*anatomical diagnosis*)?
  - What is the cause of the stroke (ischaemic or haemorrhagic, and causes of the ischaemia or haemorrhage)?
  - What are the patient's impairments, disabilities and handicaps?
  - What is the patient's prognosis and goals?
  - How should the patient be treated (acute specific treatment to minimise brain damage and prevent recurrent stroke, general treatment to prevent complications)?

■ Discuss the diagnosis and its implications with the patient and a family spokesperson
■ Reassess the patient at least once daily, noting particularly any change in his/her clinical status, the possible reasons for any change and whether prespecified goals are being achieved
■ Coordinate rehabilitation in hospital and at discharge liaise with the general practitioner, who is particularly important for reinforcing rehabilitation strategies and monitoring progress after discharge
■ Educate patient and family
■ Educate undergraduate and postgraduate students and initiate or participate in clinical research.

11.12 What is the role of the nurses?

The nursing staff provide 24-hour continuous care, aiming to:

■ Repeatedly assess the patient's neurological status and function, swallowing function, bladder and bowel function, skin care and psychosocial status
■ Detect possible adverse effects of medications
■ Support and assist basic physiological needs and self care activities, providing fall and safety protection
■ Prevent/minimise complications of impairment/disability
■ Encourage and promote functional independence
■ Reinforce techniques learnt during formal physiotherapy, occupational therapy and speech and swallowing therapy
■ Liaise with the patient's family and educate patient/carers/family members to enable them to adapt to an altered life pattern, if appropriate.

The stroke liaison nurse provides support and education for patients and their families, and aims to help patients and family members to adjust to stroke illness.

11.13 What is the role of the speech and language therapist?

The speech and language therapist, also known as the speech pathologist, is responsible for assessing and treating swallowing and communication difficulties.

Swallowing function, and risk of aspiration, is assessed immediately using clinical skills, which are sometimes supplemented by videofluoroscopy.

A screen of receptive and expressive language skills, identifying dysphasia, dyspraxia and dysarthria, is later followed by a more formal language assessment.

11.14 What is the role of the dietitian?

The dietitian aims to assess the nutritional needs of patients and provide adequate nutrition to meet their needs. The dietitian will also provide written and verbal information to patients and their carers regarding specific therapeutic diets and/or diet principles for good health, and how the diet should be adapted to meet specific needs.

When the patient is being fed by a tube (enteral feeding), the dietitian's role is to:

■ Calculate nutrient and fluid requirements to maintain or improve the nutrition and hydration status of referred patients
■ Develop enteral feeding regimes and inform nursing staff of these
■ Order enteral feeds and provide a feeding pump if necessary
■ Review the patient's tolerance of feeds, hydration status and biochemistry results, daily if possible
■ Alter the enteral feeding regimen as necessary
■ Liaise with the speech and language therapist regarding plans for the patient's transitional feeding
■ Document nutrition intervention in the patient's medical notes.

11.15 What is the role of the physiotherapist?

The physiotherapist assesses the patient's muscle tone, movement and mobility, and aims to assist him/her to achieve the highest level of functional independence possible through specific exercises and education.

The initial review assesses respiratory function, the recovery level of the arm and leg and the assistance required with bed mobility and sitting up from a lying position. Sitting balance is evaluated with the patient sitting on the edge of the bed. If the patient is medically stable and not drowsy then standing balance, ability to transfer (e.g. to commode and chair) and ambulation are evaluated if appropriate.

Treatment aims to facilitate normal movement of the affected muscles and to inhibit overcompensation by the unaffected side (*see Q. 15.30 & Box 15.2*). This is achieved by repetitive exercises based on a problem-solving approach to improve motor function.[6] Supplementary medical therapies, such as levodopa, may be complementary.[7]

11.16 What is the role of the occupational therapist?

The occupational therapist aims to maximise the patient's occupational performance, i.e. his/her function in activities of daily living, work and leisure. Specific goals are to develop functional use of the arms for activities of daily living, to prevent contractures in the upper limb at the fingers, wrist and shoulder. In the later stages of rehabilitation the occupational therapist examines employment and the feasibility of returning to work (or other alternatives) and assesses the home together with the physiotherapist from the point of view of access and safety (e.g. bathroom, kitchen, steps). This is achieved through the use of standardised assessments, graded activities, specific strategies/techniques and provision of appropriate assistive equipment.

Small clinical trials have shown that domiciliary occupational therapy may enhance recovery, and reduce disability and the risk of deterioration, in stroke patients in the community who have not been admitted to hospital[8] or who have been hospitalised and returned home.[9,10]

11.17 What is the role of the social worker?

The social worker:

■ Assists with financial and accommodation needs
■ Arranges access to appropriate social benefits
■ Performs a psychosocial assessment of the patient and family and provides psychological and emotional support for them
■ Provides vocational guidance and assistance with return to work
■ Provides a link with and access to community resources (e.g. home help, meals on wheels).

11.18 What is the role of the pharmacist?

The pharmacist reviews medication charts daily to promote safe, rational and cost-effective therapy.

THE WORK OF THE STROKE TEAM

11.19 How does a multidisciplinary stroke team operate?

The method of operation of my own mutidisciplinary stroke team is described in *Box 11.1*.

BOX 11.1 Operation of a multidisciplinary stroke team

The team is coordinated by a leader (usually the senior doctor) and meets at least once a week to discuss all the patients. The meeting is structured such that a doctor summarises the key features of each patient (age, date of stroke, clinical syndrome, pathology, aetiology, key treatments, major problems, goals) and then a brief report (1–2 minutes) on the progress of each patient in the preceding few days or week is given by the nurse, speech and language therapist, physiotherapist, occupational therapist and social worker. If relevant, the dietitian and pharmacist also report.

BOX 11.1 (*Cont'd*)

The patient's progress is matched with the original short- and long-term goals. If progress is not as good as expected, reasons for the failure to achieve goals are sought, such as recurrent stroke, intercurrent medical problems, depression, incorrect original diagnosis, inaccurate team assessment, etc. Goals are reset and a detailed future management plan is drawn up.

Besides a formal weekly meeting, which normally lasts about 60–90 minutes for 15 patients, team members communicate with each other during the week about their patients, directly on the ward or through the written medical record . Key decisions are not made without widespread team consultation and approval.

In addition to weekly meetings, my own team also has a monthly 'Stroke Unit administration meeting' to discuss general management issues, how the team is working, what the problems are and any changes that might be made in the way we work.

11.20 Does the stroke team have meetings with the family?

When all members of the team have assessed the patient, an initial family meeting is arranged and coordinated by the social worker and/or stroke liaison nurse. The aim of the meeting is to:

- Provide an opportunity for family members to meet the team, debrief about the stroke event and ask questions
- Discuss the nature and cause of the stroke, and the patients disabilities.
- Discuss the prognosis and goals of therapy
- Discuss specific treatment plans and the patient progress in meeting rehabilitation goals
- Discuss discharge planning and discharge destination.

11.21 Why set goals?

In every stroke patient, intermediate and long-term goals should be agreed and described so that progress towards them can be measured. Moreover, everyone will feel a sense of achievement when the goals are met.

Where a patient is failing to achieve his or her goals (or milestones) then it is crucial to identify the cause and, if possible, to do something about it.

11.22 How are goals developed and described?

Goal setting may sometimes involve just one individual professional but more often requires involvement from the rest of the team, the patient and sometimes the patient's family.

It is just as important to know the home and social circumstances of a stroke patient for early decision-making (such as the desirability of emergency operation) and for later rehabilitation and discharge from hospital.

Goals should be meaningful, challenging but achievable.

11.23 What are the reasons for failure to achieve goals?

There can be many different reasons for failure. However, they tend to be medical (e.g. a recurrent stroke or other serious vascular event has occurred, a medical complication has developed – pneumonia, pulmonary embolism – or the patient has become depressed and lost interest and motivation) or to reflect an inaccuracy in the team's understanding of the patient's pathology and likely clinical course (e.g. being over-optimistic about progress).

11.24 How big should a stroke unit be?

This varies according to the incidence of stroke in the catchment population of the service.

A stroke unit should generally be large enough to be flexible in accommodating fluctuating demands – the number, gender ratio, severity and length of stay of patients will not be constant throughout the year.

The stroke unit in which I myself work has 14 beds (as part of a 28-bed neurology ward), of which seven are controlled by a neurologist (myself) and seven by one of four internal medicine specialists with an interest in vascular disease who rotate every 3 months.

We each share two full-time dedicated junior doctors (a stroke unit registrar and resident), several full-time nurses, three full-time physiotherapists, two full-time occupational therapists, a full-time speech/language/swallowing therapist, a full-time social worker, a full-time stroke-liaison nurse and a pharmacist who has other ward duties.

We manage about 300 acute stroke patients per year, and I continue their rehabilitation in a separate specialist neurological rehabilitation ward, which is a part of the hospital.

However, there is no reason why a general practitioner cannot run a smaller stroke unit of only one to four beds, as long as there is an interested and dedicated multidisciplinary team to support it.

11.25 Who should run a stroke unit?

Whoever has the necessary knowledge, training, interest and enthusiasm. This tends to be predominantly neurologists in Australia, Italy and North America, and geriatricians and general physicians (internists) in the UK. Rehabilitation specialists are also increasingly involved in running active stroke units.

11.26 Should age be a criterion for admission to a stroke unit?

No, need rather than age should determine management.

Local conditions often dictate whether or not a geriatric service might be a better option.

Our stroke unit accepts patients of any age, although some older patients with other diseases, prior severe disability or a complex social situation are managed by geriatric services.

11.27 What is rehabilitation?

Rehabilitation is a reiterative, educational, problem-solving process focused on disability (behaviour). It aims to minimise handicap and to minimise stress on/distress of the patient and family.

11.28 When does rehabilitation begin?

Rehabilitation begins on the first day of the stroke, provided the patient is conscious enough to participate. There is a seamless integration between acute care and rehabilitation; any distinction is artificial. Problems arising during one so-called 'phase' can also arise in the other (e.g. pneumonia, recurrent stroke, pulmonary embolism). Indeed, there is evidence that beginning rehabilitation as soon as possible after stroke produces better results than when rehabilitation is started later.[4]

11.29 How long should patients remain in stroke units?

A defined maximum length of stay should not be needed if the unit:

- Is of sufficient size for the population needs
- Works flexibly
- Is efficient in discharging patients.

If a maximum length of stay is established, facilities and staff must be able to deliver appropriate continuing/ongoing care.

PATIENT QUESTIONS

11.30 Where are stroke patients treated?

This depends on the nature and severity of the symptoms and the realistic goals of the patient and family. However, most patients with a stroke will be admitted to hospital for initial assessment and care. They should be cared for in either:

- A stroke unit, which is a ward dedicated to the care of patients with stroke by a multidisciplinary team of health professionals who are trained specifically in the care of stroke patients
- A general medical ward caring for patients with a wide range of medical conditions, but organised to meet the needs of stroke patients. Although not all staff will have specialist training in stroke care, the stroke patients have access to the staff on the stroke unit, who do have specialist expertise in caring for stroke.

Some patients are cared for at home or in their nursing home, particularly if the TIA or stroke has not affected the patient functionally (i.e. they can still care for themselves) or if the patient is disabled but already has appropriate care at home (or in a nursing home). Of course, patients with TIA or stroke who remain at home (or in a nursing home) still require access to the multidisciplinary members of a stroke team to assess them and confirm the diagnosis of stroke, the type of stroke, its cause, the likely outcome, the goals towards which the patient and family should be aiming, the appropriate treatment to realise these, and repeated reassessment of progress, goals and therapy.

11.31 Who treats stroke patients?

Stroke patients are no longer assessed and cared for by just a doctor and nurse, but by a multidisciplinary team of health professionals who are trained specifically in the care of stroke patients (doctors, nurses, speech therapists, physiotherapists, occupational therapists, social workers, dietitians, etc.) and who adopt a coordinated goal-orientated plan to rehabilitating the patient.

Once a stroke has been diagnosed, the trained staff assess the effects of the stroke on the individual and then work out a plan of care. There are many aspects of the assessment and interventions, and different staff members of the team focus on different things.

Doctors

Doctors assess the patient to determine the nature and severity of the symptoms and whether they are indeed caused by a stroke (rather than another condition). If so, they try to ascertain the type of stroke (i.e. is it an ischaemic stroke due to a blocked artery or a haemorrhagic stroke due to one that has burst?), usually with the help of a CT brain scan. They then try to find out the underlying cause of the blocked or burst artery (usually with some additional tests). This not only helps the doctor understand why the stroke has occurred but, more importantly, it directs the doctor in choosing the most appropriate treatment to control or remove the underlying cause, and thus minimise the brain damage caused by the stroke and also the patient's risk of having another.

Doctors, like all members of the team (see below), reassess the patient at least daily to monitor their progress.

The doctor is also generally the leader or coordinator of the team, particularly at weekly meetings, when all patients are discussed by all members of the team.

Nurses

Nurses perform many important functions in a stroke unit. These include:

- Assessment of the patient's ability to function (e.g. to speak, move, sit, transfer from bed to chair and chair to toilet, and walk)
- Reassessment of the patient regularly, and sometimes constantly, for any evidence of deterioration of consciousness (level of alertness) or ability to respond with appropriate speech and limb movements – the patient's level of consciousness (i.e. whether they are awake and alert or not) is crucial to being able to further assess if there are any problems with awareness, orientation (in time, place and person), communication, memory, intellect and mood
- Monitoring of the patient's vital body functions (e.g. heart rate, blood pressure, body temperature, pupil reactions, fluid input and output, bowel action)
- Measuring the volume of urine remaining in the bladder (by ultrasound or catheterisation) after an attempt by the patient to empty it
- Anticipating potential complications of the stroke and implementing appropriate measures to prevent them (e.g. teaching the patient to lie in appropriate postures and regularly turning him/her to prevent pressure sores on the skin)
- Caring for the needs of patients and their families
- Comforting patients and their families
- Providing information for patients and their families
- Helping patients and families 'carry over' what they have learnt in their therapy sessions by practising the techniques in everyday activities on the ward.

Speech and language therapists

Speech and language therapists assess and treat communication difficulties caused by disorders of speech and language (i.e. the understanding and expression of spoken and written language, which includes reading and writing). In addition, they also assess and treat disorders of swallowing.

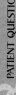

Physiotherapists

Physiotherapists mainly assess the presence and effects of muscle weakness and stiffness (tone), and incoordination. They aim to facilitate normal recovery of movement of the trunk and limbs, and optimise walking. They teach the patient and carer exercise programmes and techniques to help the patient regain as much movement as possible and move safely in the bed and around the home.

Physiotherapists determine whether the patient might benefit from aids to walking, such as injections of botulinum toxin into muscles of the feet that are causing foot spasm, or a foot support. They ultimately decide whether it is safe for the patient to attempt to walk, and whether they can try to walk alone or with support from staff or a carer.

Physiotherapists also have a major role in helping stroke patients with chest infections to drain their lungs of abnormal secretions, which keeps the patient comfortable and facilitates recovery.

Occupational therapists

Occupational therapists assess an individual's ability to carry out important functional tasks such as those concerned with activities of daily living (e.g. dressing, bathing, grooming, toileting, walking) as well as vocational skills and hobbies. They help stroke patients adapt to any disability they may have by raising their awareness of the problem, teaching them new strategies in carrying out a task, and providing specials aids or tools. They also usually visit patients' homes and arrange helpful adaptations such as hand rails, bath seats and stair lifts.

Social workers

Social workers help the patient and family access social resources, where appropriate. These include pensions, home help and accommodation in hostels and nursing homes.

Dietitians

Dietitians assess patients' dietary requirements and advise them about the healthiest diet for them.

11.32 What is rehabilitation?

Rehabilitation is active physical therapy, which aims to:

■ Help the patient regain the functional abilities that they have lost as a result of the stroke (e.g. helping them to talk, walk or use an arm functionally again)
■ Discover new ways of adapting to disabilities that are slow to recover (e.g. learning to write with the opposite hand)

■ Independently engage in personal activities of daily living (e.g. dressing, bathing, toileting), domestic activities (e.g. cooking), community activities (e.g. shopping), hobbies and return to employment if they want to

■ Support the patient and their family physically, socially and emotionally.

The precise nature of a patient's rehabilitation varies according to their needs.

11.33 When should rehabilitation begin?

Rehabilitation should begin immediately after a stroke, provided the patient is conscious and therefore able to be assessed by the members of the team, cooperate and learn from the interventions. Sometimes, severely affected stroke patients are only able to participate in an active therapy session for a short time, but their tolerance usually increases gradually.

11.34 Where should rehabilitation take place?

Rehabilitation begins where the patient is first cared for and continues until they have achieved their long-term goals.

During this time, the patient may be transferred to another hospital or unit that is more specialised in rehabilitation, or be discharged home, in which case specialist stroke rehabilitation may be provided at home, at a hospital outpatient department, at a day hospital or in the community.

11.35 How long should rehabilitation continue?

The duration (and nature) of rehabilitation depends on the patient's needs, goals and response to rehabilitation. For patients who have a mild stroke and recover fully in a short period of time, rehabilitation is only needed for a brief period. However, although recovery tends to be most rapid in the first few weeks to months after stroke, rehabilitation may continue for several months to help facilitate normal recovery (e.g. to prevent 'bad habits' from arising) and to maximise function. When rehabilitation no longer produces any important benefits then it is usually stopped. Even then, it is important to maintain a regular rehabilitation programme at home in order to maintain the function that has been achieved and hopefully to achieve further increase in function. Patients should also be reassessed intermittently to see if a further course of formal rehabilitation might help.

General management (what is basic stroke care?)

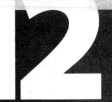

12.1 What is the general approach to early management of stroke of any type?

> **General approach to management of stroke**
> ■ Make the correct diagnosis of stroke versus not-stroke as rapidly as possible (*see Chapter 3*)
> ■ Establish the cause of stroke in terms of pathological type (infarct or haemorrhage, *see Chapter 4*) and underlying cause, particularly if directly treatable (atherothromboembolism, cardiogenic embolism, vascular malformation, etc.)
> ■ Establish the prognosis and goals for the individual patient, as far as it is possible to do so (*see Chapter 9*)
> ■ Initiate appropriate specific treatment for acute ischaemic stroke, primary intracerebral haemorrhage or subarachnoid haemorrhage
> ■ Unless the patient is very elderly, seriously handicapped or expected to die rapidly, aim to reduce early mortality and later disability by: maintenance of pulmonary, cardiovascular, fluid, electrolyte and nutritional homeostasis; and avoidance, recognition and treatment of any cause of neurological deterioration and of general complications
> ■ Initiate rehabilitation
> ■ Initiate secondary prevention in patients who might benefit
> ■ Treat coincidental disorders such as cardiac failure, angina, claudication and abdominal aortic aneurysm.

12.2 How should the airway and breathing be managed?

Maintenance of a patent airway and adequate oxygenation are fundamental to good stroke care. Abnormal patterns of respiration, such as hyperventilation and periodic breathing, are common after stroke, particularly severe stroke, but if they are present in a stroke patient with depressed consciousness it is crucial to ensure that the patient does not have an intermittently obstructed airway.[1]

Pulse oximetry is being used increasingly in the acute phase of stroke to alert the stroke team to significant oxygen desaturation.

12.3 Should stroke patients routinely receive supplemental oxygen?

No, if patients are breathing normally and maintaining good oxygenation, routine supplemental oxygen is not necessary. However, if hypoxia is present, it should be corrected with supplemental oxygen and all possible causes of the hypoxia (e.g. pulmonary oedema, embolism or infection) should be sought and treated.[2]

12.4 How should the blood pressure be managed in the acute phase after stroke?

This has not been established (*see Q. 13.33*).

Normally, blood flow to the brain is maintained at a constant level by the process of cerebral autoregulation, whereby cerebral blood vessels dilate in response to a fall in blood pressure and constrict in response to a rise in blood pressure. However, after a stroke, cerebral autoregulation is disturbed in the region of focal brain infarction or haemorrhage such that cerebral blood flow is no longer maintained and is directly dependent on systemic blood pressure. So, if the systemic blood pressure falls, so does the blood flow to the affected part of the brain. It is therefore essential to avoid systemic hypotension in acute stroke patients.

Hypotension is uncommon in stroke patients but may occur, usually because of hypovolaemia due to excessive fluid loss through sweating and by insufficient fluid intake by mouth or tube (i.e. dehydration). This can be ascertained by examining the patient and the fluid balance chart. However, hypotension may also reflect underlying sepsis or coexistent heart disease (arrhythmias, acute myocardial infarction, heart failure). It must be recognised and corrected promptly by raising the foot of the bed, replacing fluids via a safe route and treating the underlying cause (*see Box 13.2*).

Hypertension is very common after stroke, even in patients without pre-existing hypertension. This is because blood pressure rises transiently after stroke, especially haemorrhagic stroke, and falls during the first 7 days.[3,4] Current empirical policy is not to initiate new antihypertensive therapy for the first 7 days after stroke, because a reduction in blood pressure may substantially lower cerebral blood flow in the ischaemic penumbra surrounding an infarct (as a result of loss of autoregulation in ischaemic brain) and lead to further ischaemic brain damage, particularly if there is a tight stenosis of the feeding artery. However, it remains uncertain just how blood pressure should be managed after stroke.[5–7]

I usually continue any currently prescribed antihypertensive medication that the patient was taking before the stroke, provided s/he is not hypotensive and can swallow the tablets safely. Any decisions about long-term antihypertensive therapy are not made until at least a week after stroke.

Blood pressure should only be lowered actively within the first 72 hours after stroke, and cautiously at that (by about 15% over 24 hours), if there is a hypertensive crisis (such as hypertensive encephalopathy, left ventricular failure, acute aortic dissection or intracerebral bleeding) or if the blood pressure is very high and poses a real risk of cerebral haemorrhage. It is not known what level of blood pressure is too high but I would recommend treatment if:

■ Systolic BP   > 200–220 mmHg (ischaemic stroke) or
                     > 180–200 mmHg (haemorrhagic stroke)
or
■ Diastolic BP   > 120–130 mmHg (ischaemic stroke) or
                     > 100–110 mmHg (haemorrhagic stroke).

Oral antihypertensive agents are recommended, such as a diuretic, beta-blocker or calcium-channel blocker (*see Box 13.2*). Nifedipine capsules and parenteral medications should be avoided because of the rapid and sometimes precipitous fall in blood pressure that they produce.

12.5   How should pyrexia after stroke be managed?

Pyrexia after stroke may be due to:

■ Preceding infection (e.g. encephalitis, infective endocarditis)
■ The effects of the stroke itself
■ A complication of the stroke such as chest or urinary infection or venous thromboembolism.

The underlying cause must be identified and treated – but in the meantime the temperature can be lowered by simple measures (e.g. antipyretic drugs) in order to make the patient feel more comfortable and perhaps to improve outcome. Raised temperature after stroke has been associated with poor outcome, perhaps by exacerbating ischaemic brain damage, but this remains unproven and is the subject of ongoing research studies.[8,9]

Paracetamol (acetaminophen), given in a dose of 1000 mg 4-hourly (6000 mg/d) has recently been shown in a randomised trial to lower body temperature by 0.4°C (95% confidence interval, CI 0.1–0.7°C), even in normothermic and subfebrile patients.[10] However, it remains uncertain whether or not such treatment improves patient outcome.

12.6   How should swallowing, hydration and nutrition be managed after stroke?

Swallowing dysfunction and poor hydration and nutrition are common after stroke and may lead to further complications (e.g. aspiration pneumonia) and a poor outcome.[11–13]

Acute stroke patients must not be given any fluid or food by mouth until they have undergone a bedside assessment of swallowing function by a clinician or suitably trained member of the multidisciplinary stroke team (usually a trained nurse or speech pathologist) and any potential swallowing disorder has been excluded.[12,14,15] In the meantime, however, it is vital to maintain fluid and nutritional intake by intravenous catheter (saline, not glucose) or nasogastric tube.

The clinical assessment of swallowing should include a general examination of the patient (consciousness, cooperation, language function, verbal and oral praxis, and articulation), followed by an assessment of oral preparation, the oral phase and the pharyngeal phase of swallowing.[13] The gag reflex should not be used to assess swallowing function because it is not a valid or reliable sign of this. Further information about swallowing function can be obtained from videofluoroscopy. The videofluoroscopic features at presentation that are important predictors of subsequent swallowing and complications are delayed oral transit, a delayed or absent swallow reflex and penetration of contrast beyond the false vocal cords.[12]

After the bedside swallowing assessment, patients are classified as either safe to swallow or not, and this must be communicated clearly to the patient, relatives and staff (and written at the head of the patient's bed and in the hospital notes, if the patient is hospitalised). Patients with an unsafe swallow should continue to be prescribed fluids (by nasogastric tube or intravenous catheter). The type of food allowed will depend on the severity of the swallowing dysfunction, as assessed by the speech pathologist, and the patient's dietary requirements, as determined by the dietitian.

The timing, nature and role of early enteral tube feeding remains uncertain and is the subject of an ongoing clinical trial.[16] Percutaneous endoscopic gastrostomy tube feeding is preferred for patients who are likely to require prolonged feeding by tube (i.e. for more than a few weeks).

12.7 How should bladder function be assessed and managed after stroke?

Bladder function should be assessed soon after stroke onset. Ideally, after attempted voiding, the residual volume of urine in the bladder is estimated by a nurse trained in the use of bladder ultrasound. If this is more than 100 ml, the bladder should be emptied by an 'in and out' urinary catheter and the process should be repeated every 6–8 hours until the residual urine volume after voiding is less than 100 ml.

The most common cause of bladder dysfunction after stroke is detrusor hyperreflexia as a direct result of the stroke, which may be compounded by immobility (e.g. inability to sit or stand), urinary tract infection and prestroke bladder outflow obstruction (e.g. prostatomegaly, gynaecological problem). Detrusor hyperreflexia tends to cause urge incontinence and frequency of micturition.

Incontinence of urine is common in the first few days after stroke and provokes considerable distress among patients and their carers. It is usually due to a combination of factors such as detrusor hyperreflexia, impaired sphincter control, pre-existing bladder outflow obstruction, constipation, immobility, inability to communicate, inadequate response (e.g. inadequate nursing), confusion, impaired consciousness and urinary tract infection.[17]

Management of incontinence aims to identify and rectify the underlying cause(s), anticipate and prevent episodes of incontinence (e.g. regular bladder assessment and emptying by catheterisation, or toileting regimes) or institute appropriate drainage and absorption (e.g. external urinary device, absorbent pad).

The risks of an indwelling catheter include urinary tract trauma and infection. Indwelling catheters should therefore be restricted to patients in whom the measures just detailed are impractical, such as those in whom it is difficult to transfer and in whom pressure areas are a cause for concern. However, because incontinence of urine frequently resolves spontaneously during the first week or two after stroke, it is important to remove the catheter for a 'trial of voiding' and re-assessment of bladder function as soon as the patient's condition begins to improve.

For patients with persisting incontinence, cystoscopy and urodynamic investigation may be indicated to assess bladder contractility and outflow.

Urinary retention is common, especially in men, and must be systematically anticipated and excluded in patients with impaired consciousness or communication difficulties.

12.8 What potential complications of immobility are avoidable after stroke?

Avoidable complications of immobility are listed in *Box 12.1.*

> **BOX 12.1 Avoidable complications of immobility:**
> - Decubitus ulcers (pressure sores)
> - Joint contractures, pneumonia
> - Painful 'frozen' shoulder
> - Deep venous thrombosis
> - Pulmonary embolism.

Proper positioning and early mobilisation by nurses and physiotherapists help to prevent joint contractures, pneumonia and painful 'frozen' shoulder.

12.9 How can pressure areas be avoided?

Pressure sores or decubitus ulcers are avoidable. If allowed to develop, they cause the patient considerable pain and slow recovery (or are sometimes fatal). Prevention relies on an early and accurate assessment of the patient's risk, expert and interested nursing care, regular turning (e.g. every 2 hours) and the judicious use of specialised cushions and mattresses.[18]

12.10 How can venous thromboembolism be prevented?

Deep venous thrombosis (DVT) and pulmonary embolism are probably more common in immobilised stroke patients than was previously suspected – DVT, diagnosed by means of radiolabelled fibrinogen leg scanning, is present in more than half of patients with hemiparesis, but is clinically evident in less than 5% (*see Q. 15.16*).[19–21] Pulmonary embolism, diagnosed at autopsy, is present in a substantial proportion of patients with fatal stroke but is clinically evident in less than 2% of patients (*see Q. 15.21*).[22–25]

Strategies for prevention of DVT and venous thromboembolism (VTE) include physical measures (e.g. early mobilisation, including regular passive and active joint movement, and compression stockings) and antithrombotic drug therapy (aspirin, heparin).

Randomised controlled trials of compression stockings in the perioperative period suggest that they reduce the risk of venous thromboembolism by about two-thirds.[26] However, it is not known if these results can be generalised to stroke patients, in whom stockings are applied after the onset of limb paresis and in whom immobilisation is frequently prolonged. Furthermore, there are several potential drawbacks of compression stockings. These include the time taken to apply them, the discomfort to the patient (particularly in hot environments) and the occasional case of gangrene in patients with peripheral vascular disease.

In the absence of further evidence, it is recommended that immobile stroke patients are mobilised as early as possible after stroke and that compression stockings are reserved for patients at high risk of DVT, such as those who are immobile or who have a history of previous DVT.

Aspirin is prescribed immediately in all patients with acute ischaemic stroke, unless contraindicated, because it is associated with a modest but significant reduction in long-term death and dependency. It also probably reduces the risk of DVT, as it does in several other clinical scenarios.[27]

Although low-dose subcutaneous heparin significantly reduces the risk of DVT and pulmonary embolism, this favourable effect is offset by an excess risk of haemorrhagic transformation of the cerebral infarct and extracranial haemorrhage, such that at 6 months post-stroke the risk of death and dependency is the same whether or not the patient is treated with subcutaneous heparin within the first 14 days of acute ischaemic stroke.[28] However, there are probably patients at particularly high risk of VTE (e.g. immobile and a history of previous VTE) and low risk of haemorrhagic transformation (e.g. lacunar infarction) who benefit if treated with subcutaneous heparin (e.g. standard unfractionated heparin, 5000 units twice daily).

12.11 How should blood glucose be managed immediately after stroke?

Hypoglycaemia is an important treatable state that must be excluded immediately in any patient with suspected TIA or stroke because it may be the underlying cause of the focal neurological symptoms and signs (e.g. hemiparesis) and thus mimic a TIA or stroke. If not corrected promptly, permanent disability and death may ensue.

Hyperglycaemia is far more common after stroke than hypoglycaemia and may be due to diabetes (known or occult) or an acute stress response. Whatever its cause, hyperglycaemia after stroke is associated with a poor outcome. Experimental data from animal models suggests that the association may be causal, but further research is required to determine whether the association between hyperglycaemia and a poor outcome is confounded by hyperglycaemia simply being a marker of the severity of the stroke or underlying vascular disease.

Because of this uncertainty, it is presently not known how aggressively hyperglycaemia should be corrected. However, this issue may be resolved after the completion of ongoing randomised controlled trials.[29,30] In the meantime, an empirical recommendation is to try to maintain the blood glucose within normal limits and to actively correct blood glucose levels above 15 mmol/l with an infusion of insulin, glucose and potassium (and even lower levels of hyperglycaemia if there are adequate facilities for closely monitoring blood glucose, to minimise any risk of hypoglycaemia).

12.12 What is the general management of patients with aneurysmal subarachnoid haemorrhage?

This is set out in *Box 12.2*.

BOX 12.2 General management of aneurysmal subarachnoid haemorrhage

Nursing
- Continuous observation (Glasgow Coma Scale, temperature, ECG monitoring, pupils, any focal neurological deficits)

Nutrition
- Oral route preferred, but only if the patient has an intact cough and swallowing reflexes
- If nasogastric tube is necessary:
  - Deflate endotracheal cuff (if present) on insertion
  - Confirm correct placement by X-ray
  - Begin with small tests feeds of 5% dextrose
  - Prevent aspiration by feeding in sitting position and by checking gastric residue every hour
- Tablets should be crushed and flushed down (phenytoin levels will not be adequate in conventional doses)
- Total parenteral nutrition should be used only as a last resort
- Keep stools soft by adequate fluid intake and by restriction of milk content; if necessary add laxatives

Blood pressure
- Do not treat hypertension unless there is evidence of progressive end-organ damage

Fluid and electrolytes
- Intravenous line is essential
- Give at least 3 litres/day (normal saline)
- Insert an indwelling bladder catheter if voiding is involuntary
- Compensate for a negative fluid balance and for fever
- Monitor electrolytes and leukocyte count at least every other day

Pain
- Avoid aspirin
- Begin with paracetamol (acetaminophen) and/or dextropropoxyphene
- If pain is accompanied by anxiety, use midazolam (5 mg intramuscularly or infusion pump)
- If pain is severe, use codeine or, as a last resort, opiates

Prevention of DVT and pulmonary embolism
- Before occlusion of aneurysm: apply compression stockings
- After treatment of aneurysm: fractionated heparin

Medical treatment to prevent secondary ischaemia
- Nimodipine 60 mg orally every 4 hours; to be continued for 3 weeks.[31]

PATIENT QUESTIONS

12.13 What are the principles of treating stroke patients?

Each member of the stroke team has specific expertise and roles, but the main principles of their management of any patient with a TIA or stroke are to assess the patient and:

- Confirm the diagnosis of TIA or stroke and ensure that the cause of the patient's symptoms is not another medical condition
- Determine the type of stroke – was it a blocked blood vessel to the brain or a bleed into the brain?
- Determine the underlying cause of the stroke – was it a disease of the heart, blood vessels or blood?
- Determine the patient's impairments (what functions of the body are not working), disabilities (what activities of daily living the patient cannot do) and handicaps (how any disabilities might affect the patient in light of their interests, occupation, culture and personal values). For example, the same impairment (e.g. weakness of the left hand) might cause the same disabilities but be more of a handicap to a professional pianist (who could no longer work) than a politician (who could continue to do so).
- Determine the likely outcome of the patient, in terms of chances of survival, and survival free of handicap
- Establish the goals of the patient, family and stroke team
- Commence the appropriate interventions to realise those goals, minimise disability and prevent complications
- Repeatedly (at least daily) re-assess the patient's progress, review the goals and reintervene, based on the repeat assessment.

12.14 What problems may arise after a stroke?

Swallowing difficulties

About half of all stroke patients have difficulties swallowing food or fluids (dysphagia) at the time of the stroke. This is potentially very serious if patients are given something to eat or drink soon after a stroke, because the food or fluid can 'go down the wrong way' into the lungs and cause pneumonia. Also, some patients who can swallow are not given sufficient food and liquid and become malnourished and dehydrated, which may also be associated with a worse outcome.

Consequently, swallowing should be assessed immediately after a stroke by a trained nurse, speech/swallowing therapist or doctor. If problems with swallowing are present, food and fluid can be given via a small plastic tube (a nasogastric tube) that is passed into the nose through one nostril and down the gullet (oesophagus) into the stomach. Training in techniques of safe swallowing also ensues. As swallowing function recovers, foods of thick consistency are gradually introduced, followed by thinner foods and then liquids. The speech/swallowing therapist works closely with the dietitian and nurses in monitoring the total intake of fluid and calories, because it is vitally important that the patient is adequately hydrated and nourished during this time of stress.

Swallowing difficulties recover after a few days to a few weeks in most (but not all) patients.

Urinary incontinence

After a stroke at least half of patients have difficulty controlling their bladder and may leak urine. This usually recovers after a few weeks, particularly with regular toileting, but sometimes it persists.

Constipation

Constipation is common after stroke, mainly because of a inadequate intake of fluids and fibre-rich foods, combined with immobility. It usually resolves when the diet is improved and the patient is upright and mobilising. In the meantime, drug treatment may help (together with dietary modification).

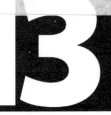

Specific management (what therapy for stroke is effective?)

13

MANAGEMENT PRINCIPLES

13.1 What is the pathogenesis of ischaemic stroke?

About 80% of all strokes are caused by occlusion of a cerebral artery, or less often a reduction in perfusion distal to a severe stenosis, resulting in focal brain infarction (ischaemic stroke).

Normally, cerebral blood flow is about 50 ml blood/100 g brain/min but, as it falls, the lack of oxygen and glucose delivered to the brain results in a time- and flow-dependent cascade characterised by a fall in energy (ATP) production. Neuronal function is affected in two stages. The first threshold is at a blood flow of about 20 ml blood/100 g brain/min, below which neuronal electrical function is compromised but is recoverable. If blood flow falls below the second critical threshold of 10 ml blood/100 g brain/min, neuronal glutamate receptors are overstimulated (excitotoxicity), free radicals are generated, spreading damage occurs, aerobic mitochondrial metabolism fails, inefficient anaerobic metabolism of glucose takes over, and lactic acidosis evolves. Energy-dependent homeostatic mechanisms of maintaining cellular ions begin to fail, potassium leaks out of the cell and sodium, water and calcium enter the cell, leading to cytotoxic oedema and calcium-induced mitochondrial failure respectively.[1] If severe ischaemia (blood flow below 10 ml blood/100 g brain/min) is maintained, irreversible damage occurs and neuronal cell apoptosis and necrosis ensue.

The recognition of these two thresholds of cerebral blood flow and stages of neuronal failure has led to the concept of the ischaemic penumbra.

13.2 What is the ischaemic penumbra?

The ischaemic penumbra is an area of brain that has reached the reversible stage of neuronal electrical failure but has not yet passed into the second irreversible stage of failure of cellular homeostasis. In theory, therefore, this tissue is potentially salvageable and could be rescued by early reperfusion or supported by neuroprotective agents.

It remains unknown, however, how long ischaemic human brain may survive and therefore what the time window is for therapeutic intervention. It probably varies among individual patients and is influenced by several factors, not just the severity of the ischaemia.

13.3 What is the aim of the medical management of acute ischaemic stroke?

The aim of management of acute ischaemic stroke is to minimise mortality and morbidity by rapidly restoring and maintaining blood flow to the ischaemic brain (penumbra), minimising brain damage, preventing recurrent stroke and preventing secondary complications of stroke.[2]

THROMBOLYSIS IN ACUTE ISCHAEMIC STROKE

13.4   What is the rationale for early reperfusion by thrombolysis?

In acute ischaemic stroke, a cerebral artery is most commonly occluded by an embolus from a proximal source, or thrombosis in situ. Some emboli are fresh thrombus but others are non-lysable substances such as organised thrombus, calcium, bacteria, tumour and prosthetic material.

When an artery is occluded by thrombus, endogenous tissue plasminogen activator (tPA) is released from the endothelium. It attaches to and activates fibrin-bound plasminogen. This mediates lysis of the thrombus and recanalisation of the occluded artery. However, all too often, such spontaneous recanalisation does not occur until after the ischaemic brain has become infarcted.

Exogenous thrombolysis (or perhaps more correctly fibrinolysis) aims to rapidly restore blood flow by lysing fresh thrombi (embolic or in-situ), which underpin many – but not all – ischaemic strokes.

13.5   What is the evidence for the safety and effectiveness of thrombolysis in the treatment of acute ischaemic stroke?

Thrombolysis has been used sporadically for more than 40 years in the treatment of acute ischaemic stroke (indeed, in the pre-computed tomography – CT – era, for the treatment of acute stroke of uncertain pathological type). However, evidence for its effectiveness and safety has only recently become available.

A total of 17 randomised controlled trials have compared thrombolytic treatment with placebo given up to 6 hours after stroke onset in 5216 highly selected patients, all of whom underwent CT or magnetic resonance imaging (MRI) of the brain before randomisation to exclude non-stroke disorders and haemorrhagic stroke.[3]

Thrombolysis was administered by the intravenous route in all but two trials (which studied intra-arterial thrombolysis). The thrombolytic agents compared with placebo were streptokinase, urokinase, recombinant tPA (r-tPA) and recombinant pro-urokinase. About 50% of the data come from trials testing intravenous r-tPA.

Direct comparisons of different thrombolytic drugs were not possible because of lack of appropriate studies. Indirect comparisons revealed no significant qualitative difference in the effect of the different thrombolytic agents, so they have been considered together in order to maximise statistical power. However, there was some heterogeneity among the trials, which could have been due to the severity of the stroke, the time to treatment, the thrombolytic drug used and variation in the concomitant use of aspirin and heparin. When heterogeneity between trials was demonstrated, the results for subgroups are stated.

13.6 What is the effect of thrombolysis on early mortality?

Compared with placebo, random allocation to thrombolytic therapy was associated with a significant increase in early death, within the first 10 days of treatment (16.6% thrombolysis, 9.8% control: OR 1.85; 95% confidence interval, CI 1.48–2.32; $2p < 0.000001$). This represents an excess of 68 (95% CI 44–93) early deaths per 1000 patients treated with thrombolysis (*Table 13.1*).[3]

TABLE 13.1 Effect of thrombolysis on outcome after ischaemic stroke

Outcome events	Thrombolysis within 6 h (%)	Control (%)	OR	95% CI of OR	Absolute risk per 1000 patients treated (95% CI)
Early (< 10 days)					
Death	16.6	9.8	1.85	1.48–2.32	+ 68 (44–93)
Fatal Intracranial Haemorrhage	5.4	1.0	4.15	2.96–5.84	+ 44
Symptomatic Intracranial Haemorrhage	9.4	2.5	3.53	2.79–4.45	+ 70 (58–83)
At final follow-up (3–6 months)					
Death	19.0	15.4	1.31	1.13–1.52	+ 36 (17–56)
Death or dependency	55.2	59.6	0.83	0.73–0.94	− 44 (−15 to − 73)

Outcome events	Thrombolysis within 3 h (%)	Control (%)	OR	95% CI of OR	Absolute risk per 1000 patients treated (95% CI)
At final follow-up (3–6 months)					
Death	22.0	20.7	1.11	0.84–1.47	+ 17 (− 28 to + 62)
Death or dependency	55.2	67.8	0.58	0.46–0.74	− 126 (− 71 to − 181)

CI, confidence interval; OR, odds ratio.

13.7 What are the risks of thrombolysis?

 FATAL INTRACRANIAL HAEMORRHAGE

The major cause of the increase in early deaths after thrombolysis was a fivefold increase in fatal intracranial haemorrhage (5.4% thrombolysis, 1.0%

control; OR 4.15, 95% CI 2.9–5.84; $2p < 0.000001$). However, there was an excess of only 29 (95% CI 17–41) fatal intracranial haemorrhages per 1000 patients treated with r-tPA (OR 3.2, 95% CI 2.0–5.2) compared with 92 (95% CI 65–120) extra fatal intracranial haemorrhages per 1000 patients treated with streptokinase (OR 6.03, 95% CI 3.47–10.47). Furthermore, compared with streptokinase (alone), the combination of streptokinase and aspirin was associated with an excess of fatal intracranial haemorrhage (OR 2.2, 95% CI 1.0–5.5).[3]

SYMPTOMATIC INTRACRANIAL HAEMORRHAGE

Thrombolytic therapy was also associated with a highly significant fourfold increase in symptomatic intracranial haemorrhage (9.4% thrombolysis, 2.5% control; OR 3.53, 95% CI 2.79–4.45; $2p < 0.000001$), equivalent to an excess of 70 (95% CI 58–83) symptomatic intracranial haemorrhages per 1000 patients treated. There was no heterogeneity between thrombolytic agents or trials.[3]

13.8 What is the effect of early thrombolysis on case fatality at 3–6 months after stroke?

At the end of patient follow-up (usually 3–6 months), patients allocated thrombolytic therapy also had an increased risk of death (19% thrombolysis, 15.4% control; OR 1.31, 95% CI 1.13–1.52), representing an extra 36 (95% CI 17–56) deaths per 1000 patients treated with thrombolysis. There was a trend toward increased case fatality the earlier concomitant antithrombotic drug therapy was introduced:

- OR 1.93 when all patients received antithrombotic drugs within 24 hours of thrombolysis
- OR 1.27 when some patients received antithrombotic drugs within 24 hours
- OR 1.14 when no patients received antithrombotic drugs within 24 hours but some thereafter
- OR 0.89 when no patients received antithrombotic drugs within the first 10–14 days.[3]

Although these data are mainly non-randomised comparisons they suggest an adverse (haemorrhagic) interaction between thrombolytic and antithrombotic therapies.

13.9 What is the effect of early thrombolysis on death and dependency at 3–6 months after stroke?

Despite an excess early hazard, thrombolysis (administered up to 6 hours after ischaemic stroke) was associated with a significant reduction in death or dependency (modified Rankin score 3–6) at the end of follow-up (55.2% thrombolysis, 59.6% control; OR 0.83, 95% CI 0.73–0.94; $2p = 0.003$). This represents 44 (95% CI 15–73) fewer dead or dependent patients per 1000 treated with thrombolysis. There was no significant heterogeneity of treatment effect among the trials, indicating that the favourable treatment effect was qualitatively the same (i.e. in the same direction) in all trials. This is reflected in the subgroup of trials using intravenous r-tPA, where there was a similar reduction in death or dependency (OR 0.79, 95% CI 0.68–0.92; $2p = 0.002$), equivalent to 57 (95% CI 20–93) fewer dead or dependent patients per 1000 treated.[3]

13.10 What is the effect of thrombolysis administered very early, within 3 hours of stroke onset?

For patients treated within 3 hours of ischaemic stroke, allocation to thrombolytic therapy was associated with a greater reduction in death or dependency (55.2% thrombolysis, 67.8% control; OR 0.58, 95% CI 0.46–0.74, $2p = 0.00002$), equivalent to 126 (95% CI 71–181) fewer dead or dependent patients per 1000 patients treated within 3 hours with thrombolysis. Thrombolysis within 3 hours was also associated with a lower excess risk of death (22.3% thrombolysis, 20.7% control; OR 1.11, 95% CI 0.84–1.47), equivalent to 17 extra deaths per 1000 patients treated (95% CI 28 less to 62 more). In trials using r-tPA within 3 hours, the equivalent estimate was 12 fewer deaths per 1000 (95% CI 61 fewer to 38 more).[3]

13.11 How should the evidence for thrombolysis be interpreted?

It seems that thrombolytic therapy for acute ischaemic stroke is very much like carotid endarterectomy for symptomatic severe carotid stenosis; both are associated with an early hazard yet a greater long-term net benefit. The burning question is no longer whether thrombolysis (and carotid endarterectomy) is effective, but in whom it is effective, in whom it is ineffective and in whom it is dangerous. At present it is not known exactly which combinations of clinical and imaging features reliably identify patients who will benefit or be harmed by thrombolysis. Nor is it clear what is the optimal thrombolytic agent, dose, half-life and route of administration. Furthermore, the most effective concomitant neuroprotective, antithrombotic and antihypertensive regime, if any, remains to be established.

13.12 What early brain imaging findings have potential for refining patient selection for thrombolysis?

Plain CT imaging signs of major infarction involving more than one-third of the territory perfused by the middle cerebral artery predicts an increased risk of symptomatic intracranial haemorrhage after thrombolysis.[4]

However, this is neither sensitive nor specific, and the interrater reliability among physicians involved in acute stroke care is less than ideal. A new CT scoring system (ASPECTS) is reported to be a simple and reliable method of quantifying early ischaemic changes on CT imaging – like an 'ECG of the brain' – that accurately predicts risk of symptomatic intracranial haemorrhage and functional outcome in ischaemic stroke patients treated with intravenous thrombolytic therapy.[5] However, its external validity and reliability has been challenged.[6]

Magnetic resonance imaging can provide a perfusion-weighted image (PWI), which reveals the region of brain that is underperfused and 'at risk', and a diffusion-weighted image (DWI), which probably identifies the core of early infarction. A mismatch between the acute PWI lesion and the (smaller) DWI lesion may represent the ischaemic penumbra of potentially salvageable brain. Clinical trials are evaluating whether patients with a PWI/DWI mismatch are likely to benefit clinically from early reperfusion.[7] If confirmed, a further challenge will be to optimise the availability and feasibility of undertaking MRI imaging of the brain within the first few hours of stroke onset in sick, dysphasic, disorientated and claustrophobic patients with acute stroke.

Finally, patient selection for thrombolysis may also be improved by proof of arterial occlusion by means of non-invasive imaging (e.g. magnetic resonance angiography, transcranial Doppler ultrasound).

Clearly, further studies are required to refine patient selection and to establish the balance of risks and benefits of thrombolysis in a broader range of patients presenting at different stages, with differing types and severities of stroke, different risk factors and different brain imaging findings.

13.13 Should tPA be licensed throughout the world?

While awaiting the results of these studies, it remains controversial whether r-tPA should be licensed for use in Australia and Asia, as it has been in the United States (1997), Canada (1999) and Germany (August 2000) for patients presenting within 3 hours of acute ischaemic stroke who are similar to the patients included in the trials, provided there is a stroke service that can ensure its safe administration (*Box 13.1*).[8]

> **BOX 13.1 Current guidelines for the use of intravenous r-tPA in ischaemic stroke**
>
> ■ Thrombolysis with intravenous r-tPA should be considered in all patients with a definite ischaemic stroke who present within 3 hours of onset
>
> ■ Thrombolytic therapy should only be administered by physicians with expertise in stroke medicine who have access to a suitable stroke service with facilities for immediately identifying and managing haemorrhagic complications

BOX 13.1 (*Cont'd*)

■ Thrombolysis should be avoided in cases where CT brain imaging suggests the early changes of major infarction (e.g. oedema, sulcal effacement, mass effect)

■ Other exclusion criteria – past history
  – Any intracranial haemorrhage
  – Stroke, serious head injury or myocardial infarction in previous 3 months
  – Gastrointestinal or urinary bleeding within previous 21 days
  – Major surgery within previous 14 days
  – Arterial puncture of non-compressible site within previous 7 days
  – Heparin exposure in preceding 48 hours and partial thromboplastin time not normal

■ Other exclusion criteria – current (i.e. pretreatment)
  – Seizure at stroke onset
  – Neurological deficits mild
  – Neurological condition improving rapidly
  – Systolic blood pressure > 185 mmHg or diastolic blood pressure > 110 mmHg
  – Oral anticoagulant use or international normalised ratio (INR) > 1.7.
  – Platelet count < 100×10^9/l
  – Prolonged partial thromboplastin time
  – Blood glucose < 2.8 mmol/l (50 mg/dl) or > 22 mmol/l (400 mg/dl).

■ Caution in patients with severe stroke (NIH stroke scale score > 22)

■ Discuss treatment and adverse effects with patient and family before treatment

■ The recommended dose of r-tPA is 0.9 mg/kg up to a maximum of 90 mg, the first 10% of the dose as a bolus over 1 min, the rest as an infusion over 60 min

■ Perform neurologic assessments every 15 min during infusion of r-tPA, every 30 min for the next 6 hours and every 60 min for the next 16 hours; if severe headache, acute hypertension or nausea and vomiting occur, discontinue the infusion and obtain an emergency CT brain scan

■ Measure blood pressure every 15 min for 2 hours, every 30 min for 6 hours and every 60 min for 16 hours; repeat measurements more frequently if systolic blood pressure is above 180 mmHg or diastolic blood pressure above 105 mmHg, and administer antihypertensive drugs as needed to maintain blood pressure at or below those levels.[10,11]

One lesson learnt from the North American experience is that treating patients who do not come within the guidelines outlined in *Box 13.1* is associated with excess risk and poor patient outcome.[9] If r-tPA is to be licensed in Australia, Asia and elsewhere in Europe, it is essential that its use is restricted, at least initially, to dedicated stroke units that are appropriately equipped and prepared to respond to demand, adhere strictly to current guidelines and undertake prospective, systematic and rigorous audit as part of a national register. This will ensure that stroke patients have access to this effective (yet risky) treatment, that stroke physicians gain experience and expertise in its use, and that quality control and patient selection continue to be optimised by correlation of baseline demographic, clinical, imaging and treatment data with early and long-term patient outcome.

13.14 Should general practitioners be treating stroke patients with r-tPA?

Not at this stage, when there is no evidence of it being administered safely and effectively in general practice.

13.15 What are the current suggested guidelines for the use of intravenous r-tPA in ischaemic stroke?

These are listed in *Box 13.1*.

ASPIRIN THERAPY

13.16 What acute medical treatment should general practitioners be giving for acute ischaemic stroke?

> All patients with acute ischaemic stroke should be given aspirin 300 mg immediately (unless allergic to/intolerant of aspirin or entering a trial of thrombolysis), and this should be continued for 14 days before changing the patient to a maintenance dose of 75–150 mg/day.

13.17 How effective and safe is aspirin when given in acute ischaemic stroke?

Aspirin 160–300 mg given orally or rectally as soon as possible within the first 48 hours of acute ischaemic stroke and daily for the next 2–4 weeks (and continued thereafter) reduces death and dependency from 47.0% to 45.8%.[12-15] This is an odds reduction of 5% (95% CI 2–9%), relative risk reduction (RRR) of 3% (95% CI 1–5%)

and absolute risk reduction (ARR) of 1.2%. Therefore, treating 1000 patients with aspirin in the first 2–4 weeks post-stroke prevents about 12 dying or becoming dependent. The number of patients needed to treat each year to prevent one adverse event each year (NNT) is 77 (43–333).

13.18 Why is early aspirin therapy in acute ischaemic stroke effective?

It is uncertain exactly why early aspirin in acute ischaemic stroke is effective in preventing death and dependency several months after stroke. However, it probably reflects early initiation of secondary prevention of stroke and other thrombotic complications rather than a direct neuroprotective effect on the ischaemic brain itself. This is because early initiation of aspirin within the first 2–4 weeks of acute ischaemic stroke is associated with a highly significant reduction in the risk of early recurrent ischaemic stroke of 7 (SD ± 1) per 1000 (1.6% aspirin vs 2.3% control, $2p < 0.000001$).[16]

The proportional and absolute benefits of aspirin in acute ischaemic stroke were similar in a wide range of patients irrespective of age, gender, delay between symptom onset and randomisation, presence or absence of atrial fibrillation, consciousness level, systolic blood pressure, stroke subtype, CT brain imaging findings or concomitant heparin use. Among the 9000 patients (22%) randomised without a prior CT brain scan, aspirin appeared to be of net benefit, with no unusual excess of haemorrhagic stroke; moreover, even among the 800 (2%) who had inadvertently been randomised after a haemorrhagic stroke, there was no evidence of net hazard (further stroke or death, 63 aspirin vs 67 control).

13.19 Is there any hazard associated with early aspirin therapy in acute ischaemic stroke?

Early aspirin therapy is associated with an excess of about 2 intracranial haemorrhages (1.0% vs 0.8%, $2p = 0.07$) and 4 extracranial haemorrhages (0.97% vs 0.57%, OR 1.7, 95% CI 1.3–2.1) per 1000 patients treated, but these small risks are more than offset by the greater reductions in recurrent ischaemic stroke (7 per 1000 patients treated) and in death and disability from other causes both in the short term[15] and the long term.[17]

Common adverse effects of aspirin (e.g. dyspepsia and constipation) are dose-related (*see Q. 14.29–Q. 14.32*).[18,19]

13.20 What is the optimal dose of aspirin for acute ischaemic stroke?

There is no clear evidence that any one dose of aspirin between 160 mg and 300 mg is more effective than another in the treatment of acute ischaemic stroke.

13.21 What if the patient cannot swallow aspirin safely?

People unable to swallow safely after a stroke can be given aspirin as a suppository or by nasogastric tube.

ANTICOAGULATION THERAPY

13.22 Is there a role for immediate systemic anticoagulation with heparin or heparinoids in acute ischaemic stroke?

No. At present, there is no level 1 evidence from randomised trials to support any role for immediate systemic anticoagulation with heparin or heparinoids in acute ischaemic stroke. There is reasonably reliable evidence from 21 randomised controlled trials in 23 427 people with acute ischaemic stroke that unfractionated heparin, low-molecular-weight heparins and heparinoids in acute ischaemic stroke have no net effect on death or dependency 3–6 months after stroke (59.7% anticoagulation vs 60.1% control, OR 0.99, 95% CI 0.94–1.05; RRR 1%, 95% CI −2 to +3%; ARR 0.4%, 95% CI −0.9 to +1.7%).

Despite significantly reducing the odds of:

- Deep vein thrombosis after stroke (15% anticoagulation vs 44% control, OR 0.21, 95% CI 0.15–0.39; RRR 64%, 95% CI 54–71%; ARR 29%, 95% CI 24–35%; NNT 3, 95% CI 2–4)
- Symptomatic pulmonary embolism (0.6% anticoagulation vs 0.9% control, OR 0.61, 95% CI 0.45–0.83; RRR 38%, 95% CI 16–54%; ARR 0.3%, 95% CI 0.1–0.6%; NNT 333, 95% CI 167–1000) and
- Recurrent ischaemic stroke (2.8% anticoagulation vs 36% control, OR 0.76, 95% CI 0.65–0.88, ARR 0.9%, NNT III)),

the benefit is offset by an equivalent increase in the risk of intracranial (1.4% anticoagulation vs 0.5% control, OR 1.52, 95% CI 0.92–2.3, ARI 0.9%, NNH 108) and extracranial bleeding (see Q. 13.24).[15,20]

13.23 Is there a role for immediate systemic anticoagulation with heparin or heparinoids in any subgroup of patients with acute ischaemic stroke?

There appear to be no clear short- or long-term benefits of anticoagulants in any prespecified subgroup of patients, including those with stroke of presumed cardioembolic origin, or with any of the types of anticoagulant that have been studied, although the number of patients studied in randomised trials of anticoagulants other than subcutaneous unfractionated heparin are small (so that random error may have obscured any real differences between anticoagulant regimens).

Even for patients with acute ischaemic stroke and atrial fibrillation, who have an increased absolute risk of early stroke recurrence, heparin is not effective because any reduction in recurrent ischaemic stroke is offset by an equal increase in haemorrhagic stroke.[21]

13.24 How harmful is immediate systemic anticoagulation for acute ischaemic stroke?

 Immediate systemic anticoagulation in patients with acute ischaemic stroke increases the rate of symptomatic intracranial haemorrhage within 14 days of starting treatment (1.4% anticoagulation vs 0.5% control absolute risk increase, ARI 0.93%, 95% CI 0.68–1.18%; relative risk increase, RRI 163%, 95% CI 95–255%; number of patients treated to harm one, NNH 108, 95% CI 85–147).[15]

13.25 Is the risk of immediate systemic anticoagulation for acute ischaemic stroke related to the dose?

 Yes, probably. The largest trial of subcutaneous heparin found that this effect was dose-dependent.

The RRI in *symptomatic intracranial haemorrhage* of using medium-dose (12 500 U) compared with low-dose (5000 U) heparin twice daily for 14 days was 143%, 95% CI 82–204%; NNH 97, 95% CI 68–169).[13]

The RRI in *major extracranial haemorrhage* after 14 days of treatment with anticoagulants was 231%, 95% CI 136–365%; ARI 0.91%, 95% CI 0.67–1.15%; NNH 109, 95% CI 87–149).[15]

13.26 How should an acute ischaemic stroke patient who is in atrial fibrillation be treated immediately?

> Patients with acute ischaemic stroke who are in atrial fibrillation and who are thought to have a cardioembolic ischaemic stroke should be treated immediately with aspirin (or thrombolysis). After 3–14 days, they can be changed over to warfarin. The decision to switch to warfarin and the timing of the change are determined by several factors. Because the risk of haemorrhagic transformation of a brain infarct seems to be greater if the infarct is large and if the blood pressure is poorly controlled, it is prudent to withhold warfarin in patients with large brain infarcts or uncontrolled hypertension until about 10–14 days after the stroke. However, for patients with small infarcts and well-controlled blood pressure, it is generally safe to resume warfarin anticoagulation sooner (i.e. as soon as 3 days after stroke). Ultimately, the decision is determined by a balance between the risk of haemorrhagic transformation of the infarct and the risk of re-embolisation from the heart. If the cardiological (+ echocardiographic) assessment indicates that the patient is at very high risk of re-embolisation of thrombus to the brain within the first week or so after stroke, then the clinician's 'hand is forced', sometimes to begin warfarin sooner than may have otherwise been intended.

PREVENTION OF DEEP VEIN THROMBOSIS

13.27 Are there any alternative treatments to prevent deep vein thrombosis and pulmonary embolism after acute ischaemic stroke?

Yes, there are alternative treatments to heparin for the prevention of deep vein thrombosis (DVT) and pulmonary embolism after acute ischaemic stroke. These include aspirin and compression stockings, both of which have been shown to prevent DVT and pulmonary embolism in controlled clinical trials (*see Q. 13.28–Q. 13.30*).

13.28 What is the evidence that aspirin is effective in preventing DVT?

A systematic review of the randomised trials available up to 1994, including a total of about 9000 patients, showed that antiplatelet agents (chiefly aspirin) significantly reduced the risk of DVT by about 39% and pulmonary embolism by 64% in a wide variety of patients at high risk of venous thromboembolism.[17] Some clinicians were not persuaded, so a large-scale trial was established to confirm or refute these results. The Pulmonary Embolism Prevention Trial randomised 13 356 patients undergoing surgery for hip fracture to low-dose aspirin or placebo. Allocation to aspirin significantly reduced the odds of pulmonary embolism by 43% (95% CI 18–60%) and symptomatic DVT by 29% (95% CI 3–48%).[22]

13.29 What is the evidence that aspirin is effective in preventing DVT after acute stroke?

Eight randomised trials of antiplatelet therapy in patients with acute ischaemic stroke show that allocation to aspirin significantly reduces the odds of pulmonary embolism by 29% (95% CI 4–47%, $p = 0.03$), and two trials show that aspirin is associated with a 22% reduction in the odds of DVT (95% CI 64% reduction to 67% increase).[15]

Taken with the evidence of benefit in other categories of patient, and given the established safety of aspirin in stroke, it seems reasonable to conclude that aspirin does reduce the risk of DVT and pulmonary embolism after stroke.

For patients with ischaemic stroke, aspirin has many advantages as a first-line agent for thromboprophylaxis: it is inexpensive, needs only once-daily administration, does not require injections and is associated with a low risk of bleeding.

The research question is now whether heparin (probably in low dose and combined with aspirin) can add to the benefit of aspirin alone and remain safe.[23]

13.30 What is the evidence that graded compression stockings are effective in preventing DVT after acute stroke?

The value of graded compression stockings (and the choice of full-length or below-knee stockings) for the prevention of DVT and pulmonary embolism after stroke is not well established. A Cochrane review on this topic is in preparation. Furthermore, the Scottish Executive has just funded the Clots in Legs or TED Stockings (CLOTS) collaborative group to undertake a multicentre, randomised controlled trial to evaluate the benefit of graded compression stockings after stroke; the study is a small 'family' of two trials, one comparing long stockings with no stockings and the other long stockings with short stockings. Details of the protocol are available at the trial website: http://www.dcn.ed.ac.uk/clots.

OTHER TREATMENTS

13.31 What is the role of neuroprotective agents?

Trials of neuroprotective agents (e.g. selfotel, aptiganel, clomethiazole, tirilazad, lubeluzole) have failed to identify a favourable treatment effect, and some have revealed dose-limiting intolerance and systemic adverse effects, such as excessive sedation and hypertension.[24] Trials of other agents (e.g. magnesium – IMAGES – and benzodiazepines – EGASIS) are in progress.

13.32 What other treatments have been tried unsuccessfully in acute ischaemic stroke?

Haemodilution, corticosteroids and glycerol have not been proved to be effective in small trials. Whether these are true or false-negative effects remain uncertain but the evidence of a lack of effect is more robust for haemodilution.

13.33 How should blood pressure be managed in acute stroke?

Blood pressure rises transiently after hemispheric stroke, especially haemorrhagic stroke, and falls during the first 7 days (*see Q. 12.4*).[25]

One systematic review of three randomised controlled trials comparing blood-pressure-lowering treatment (by various antihypertensive agents) versus placebo in 113 patients with acute stroke was inconclusive.[26] Another systematic review of 24 randomised controlled trials of calcium antagonists in 6894 people found a non-significant increase in the risk of death (RRI: 8%, 95% CI 1% reduction to 18% increase).[27] Although treatment with calcium antagonists in these trials was intended for neuroprotection, blood pressure was lower in the treatment group in most trials.

Overall, one systematic review of randomised controlled trials provides no evidence that blood-pressure-lowering treatment has benefits in people with acute ischaemic stroke and suggests that treatment in the immediate acute phase may be harmful. Further studies are required.

In the meantime, current policy is to not initiate new antihypertensive therapy for the first 7 days after stroke unless the blood pressure is very high (e.g. > 220 mmHg systolic and > 120 mmHg diastolic) and hypertensive encephalopathy, left ventricular failure, aortic dissection or intracerebral bleeding is present.

13.34 How should blood pressure be managed in acute intracerebral haemorrhage?

Although not evidence-based (*see Q. 13.33*), the general recommendations for the treatment of elevated blood pressure in patients with intracerebral haemorrhage are more aggressive than those for patients with ischaemic stroke.

The theoretical rationale for lowering blood pressure is to decrease the risk of ongoing bleeding from ruptured small arteries and arterioles.

The optimal level of a patient's blood pressure is uncertain and is determined by several individual factors, such as chronic hypertension, elevated intracranial pressure, age, presumed cause of haemorrhage and interval since onset.

The writing group of the Stroke Council, the American Heart Association, recommends that blood pressure levels be maintained below a mean arterial pressure of 130 mmHg in persons with a history of hypertension. In patients with elevated intracranial pressure who have an intracranial pressure monitor, cerebral perfusion pressure (mean arterial pressure minus intracranial pressure) should be kept above 70 mmHg. Mean arterial blood pressure above 110 mmHg should be avoided in the immediate postoperative period. If systolic arterial blood pressure falls below 90 mmHg, pressors should be given (*Box 13.2*).

BOX 13.2 Blood pressure management in the first few hours of intracerebral haemorrhage[28]

High blood pressure

Systolic BP > 230 mmHg or diastolic BP > 140 mmHg on two readings 5 min apart
■ Intravenous nitroprusside 0.5–10 µg/kg per minute

Systolic BP 180–230 mmHg or diastolic BP 105–140 mmHg or mean arterial BP > 130 mmHg on two readings 20 min apart
■ Intravenous labetalol 5–100 mg/h by intermittent bolus doses of 10–40 mg or continuous infusion (2–8 mg/min)

BOX 13.2 *(Cont'd)*

■ Intravenous esmolol 500 µg/kg as a load, followed by maintenance use of 50–200 µg/kg per minute

■ Intravenous enalapril 0.625–1.2 mg every 6 h as needed, or

■ Intravenous hydralazine 10–20 mg every 4–6 h

Systolic BP < 180 mmHg and diastolic BP < 105 mmHg

■ Defer antihypertensive therapy – choice of medication depends on other medical contraindications (e.g. avoid labetalol in patients with asthma)

If intracranial pressure monitoring is available

■ Maintain cerebral perfusion pressure above 70 mmHg

Low blood pressure

■ Volume replenishment is the first line of approach; isotonic saline or colloids can be used and monitored with central venous pressure or pulmonary artery wedge pressure

■ If hypotension persists after correction of volume deficit, continuous infusions of pressors should be considered, particularly if the systolic BP < 90 mmHg:

  – Phenylephrine 2–10 µg/kg per minute

  – Dopamine 2–20 µg/kg per minute

  – Noradrenaline (norepinephrine) titrate from 0.05–0.2 µg/kg per minute.

13.35 Is there a role for surgery in the treatment of supratentorial intracerebral haemorrhage?

The balance between benefit and harm is not clearly established for the evacuation of supratentorial haematomas.

A systematic review of all four randomised controlled trials of surgery for primary intracranial haemorrhage indicates that surgery is associated with a non-significant increase in risk of death and dependency at 6 months (OR 1.23, 95% CI 0.77–1.98; RRI: 5%, 95% CI –7% to +19%; ARI 3.3%, 95% CI –5.9% to +12.5%).[29] Open surgical drainage via a craniotomy was harmful but safer surgical techniques, such as stereotactic aspiration, are promising. For patients randomised to evacuation by neuroendoscopy rather than best medical practice there was a non-significant trend toward a favourable effect on death and disability (RRR 24%, 95% CI –2% to +44%). Further evidence from ongoing trials is awaited. In the meantime, surgery should probably be considered in a previously fit patient with a large lobar intracerebral haematoma whose consciousness level is falling and who will probably die without drainage of the haematoma. It is less clear how to manage patients with haemorrhage deep in the brain and those with severe impairments but no impairment of consciousness. These patients are usually managed conservatively or entered into a randomised trial of surgical treatment, such as the Surgical Trial in Intracerebral Haemorrhage (STICH). (Email: stich@ncl.ac.uk).

13.36 What is the role of surgery in the treatment of infratentorial intracerebral haemorrhage?

There is no evidence from randomised controlled trials of the role of evacuation in people with infratentorial haematoma whose consciousness level is declining.

Current practice is based on consensus opinion that surgical intervention may be life-saving in patients with infratentorial (cerebellar) intracranial haemorrhage whose consciousness level is declining, and so a randomised trial evaluating this policy is unlikely to take place. However, it is uncertain exactly which patients might benefit most and which is the optimal procedure (haematoma evacuation vs ventricular decompression via a ventriculostomy, or both).[30] Generally, surgical intervention is considered in any patient who is comatose or whose consciousness level is deteriorating progressively, and in whom other exacerbating causes have been excluded (e.g. neurological, non-neurological – see above). Once brainstem reflexes have been absent for several hours, death is inevitable.

13.37 What is the treatment of subarachnoid haemorrhage?

- Early aneurysm surgery is now usual practice for patients in good clinical condition but this has not been supported by a randomised controlled trial[31]
- Antifibrinolytic drugs prevent rebleeding but increase the risk of cerebral ischaemia and have no net effect on overall outcome[32]
- Oral nimodipine helps to prevent delayed cerebral ischaemia and significantly reduces the risk of a poor outcome (RR: 0.69, 95% CI 0.58–0.84).[33] (*See Box 12.2*)

PATIENT QUESTIONS

13.38 What is tPA?

tPA is tissue plasminogen activator, which is a drug that dissolves blood clots. It has been shown to be effective in improving the outcome of patients with ischaemic stroke (caused by a blocked artery to the brain) who receive the treatment within 3 hours of onset of the stroke.

If patients with ischaemic stroke of less than 3 hours duration are treated with tPA, the proportion who are ultimately either dead or dependent on another person to care for them 6 months after the stroke took place is reduced from 65% to 51%. This is a reduction in death and dependency after stroke of 14%. This means that out of every 100 patients treated in this way with tPA, the number of those who are either dead or dependent on another person 6 months after the stroke is reduced by 14, from 65 to 51.

However, tPA can also be harmful in some patients. By dissolving the blood clot that is blocking the artery, tPA restores blood flow to the part of the brain that has been cut off. If that part of the brain is still alive, it usually recovers, and so the patient recovers. However, if some of that part of the brain has already died, the blood vessel beyond the blockage may also have died. If blood flow is restored to this area of dead brain, blood may burst through the dead/weakened blood vessel, causing substantial bleeding into the brain. This can be fatal. Such bleeding occurs in about 6% of patients treated with tPA and is fatal in about 3–4%. Further research is needed to identify which patients are likely to benefit from tPA and which patients are likely to be harmed, so that doctors can make sure that tPA is only given to the former.

13.39 Why is aspirin given to all patients as soon as possible after an ischaemic stroke?

If patients with ischaemic stroke (due to a blocked artery) are not treated with tPA, then they are given aspirin immediately. This is because aspirin thins the blood a little and helps to prevents another ischaemic stroke.

Secondary prevention (how can recurrence be prevented?)

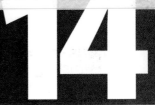

14.1 What is secondary prevention of stroke and other serious vascular events?

Secondary prevention is the immediate and ongoing long-term management of people with prior stroke and transient ischaemic attack (TIA), which aims to minimise the risk of a recurrent stroke or other serious vascular event such as a myocardial infarction or death from vascular causes.

14.2 What is the principle of secondary stroke prevention?

The principle of secondary stroke prevention is to identify and treat (or control) the underlying cause of the index vascular event of the brain as soon as possible, so as to prevent a recurrent vascular event. Because the risk of recurrent stroke is greatest immediately after stroke, the emphasis is on early as well as appropriate intervention.

14.3 Which underlying causes of stroke can be treated specifically and how?

The most common underlying causes of stroke are atherothromboembolism and cardiogenic embolism.

■ *Atherothromboembolism* should be treated by control of causal vascular risk factors (high blood pressure and cholesterol, cigarette smoking, diabetes mellitus), antiplatelet therapy, and, in the appropriate patient, carotid endarterectomy (or perhaps carotid artery stenting)

■ *Cardiogenic embolism* should be treated by treatment of the underlying cause (e.g. reversion of atrial fibrillation to sinus rhythm, replacement of diseased heart valve) and, generally, by anticoagulation with warfarin.

■ Less common, but treatable causes of ischaemic stroke include *infective endocarditis* and *giant cell arteritis*, which should be treated with antibiotics and steroids respectively.

Each cause is reviewed in turn.

REDUCTION OF BLOOD PRESSURE

14.4 How effective is blood pressure reduction in hypertensive patients with TIA or ischaemic stroke due to atherothromboembolism?

Hypertension is the most important and treatable risk factor for stroke (the risk of stroke doubles for every 7.5 mmHg increase in usual diastolic blood pressure, *see Q. 7.4*).

Data from ten randomised controlled trials suggest that lowering the blood pressure of TIA/stroke patients by 5–6 mmHg diastolic and 10–12 mmHg systolic for 2–3 years, or 9/4 mmHg for 4 years, reduces their relative risk of stroke by about 28% (95% confidence interval, CI 15–39%).[1,2,3]

A preliminary report from another trial in China, in which 5665 people with a prior stroke or TIA were randomised to receive either the diuretic indapamide or placebo, a reduction of about 2 mmHg in diastolic blood pressure over 2 years was associated with a reduction in stroke incidence of 29% (95% CI 12–42%).[4]

If the average annual risk of recurrent stroke among patients with prior stroke or TIA is about 7.0%,[5] antihypertensive therapy probably reduces this risk to 5.0%; a relative risk reduction (RRR) of 28% and an absolute risk reduction (ARR) of 2.0%.[6] Treating 1000 patients prevents about 20 strokes each year. The number needed to treat per year to prevent one stroke per year (NNT) is about 50.

14.5 Is there a role for routine blood pressure reduction in all patients with TIA or ischaemic stroke due to atherothromboembolism?

Yes, blood-pressure-lowering therapy is indicated in all middle-aged and older patients who in the preceding 2 weeks to 5 years (or more) have had a TIA or stroke, whose clinical condition is stable, and in whom there is no contraindication to BP-lowering therapy.[1]

Blood pressure lowering is therefore safe and effective irrespective of the type of TIA or stroke (ischaemic or haemorrhagic), time since the previous TIA or stroke (with the exception of the first week or two), baseline blood pressure, or patient's ethnic group and country of residence.[1,2]

The benefits are greater with more intensive and prolonged blood pressure lowering.[1,2]

14.6 What are the potential hazards of routine blood pressure reduction in all patients with TIA or ischaemic stroke due to atherothromboembolism?

Among some people with a history of stroke it is possible that blood pressure reduction may actually increase the risk of recurrent stroke, perhaps because of reduced cerebral perfusion. This possibility may be of particular relevance for people with haemodynamically compromising stenoses of the extracranial carotid or vertebral arteries, and the very elderly. However, preliminary data from more than 150 000 individuals with a history of cerebrovascular or coronary events included in trials in the Antithrombotic Trialists' Collaboration showed a positive relationship between usual diastolic blood pressure and the subsequent risk of stroke;

for every 5 mmHg decrease in usual diastolic blood pressure there was about a 15% proportional reduction in stroke risk, with no evidence of any threshold below which a lower diastolic blood pressure was not associated with a lower stroke risk.[7,8,9] The randomised controlled trials also found no evidence that reducing blood pressure by about 9/4 mmHg–12/5 mmHg was hazardous, even in TIA/stroke patients with baseline blood pressures of < 140 mmHg systolic and < 80 mmHg diastolic.[1]

Nevertheless, in order to avoid adverse effects and disruption of antoregulation of cerebral blood flow, the blood pressure should be lowered gradually over several months, not over days to weeks. The target blood pressure should be < 130/85 mmHg or as low as the patient can tolerate.

14.7   When should antihypertensive therapy begin after stroke?

There is limited evidence about when to begin antihypertensive therapy after stroke (*see Chapter 12*). However, because the usual primary goal of antihypertensive therapy is to retard further atherogenesis and vascular disease, there is no immediate urgency to begin antihypertensive therapy after stroke. If the patient is a known hypertensive on treatment, I usually just continue the same treatment in the first week or so after stroke and, if the blood pressure remains elevated in the second week, then antihypertensive therapy is augmented.

The long-term follow-up of the patient, with serial blood pressure recordings, supervision and maintenance of therapy and tight blood pressure control, is more important than the exact timing of its institution in the acute phase.

14.8   Which drugs should be used to lower blood pressure?

There is increasing evidence that conventional antihypertensives (low-dose diuretics or low-dose beta blockers) and newer antihypertensives (calcium-channel antagonists and angiotensin-converting-enzyme – ACE – inhibitors) are similarly effective in preventing major events or death from cardiovascular disease.[10] In other words, it appears to be the size (intensity) of the reduction in blood pressure, rather than the type of antihypertensive drug, which is important in preventing hard clinical outcome events (*Table 14.1*).[11] A reduction of 5–6 mmHg in diastolic blood pressure and 10–12 mmHg in systolic blood pressure is associated with about a 38% (SD ±4) reduction in the risk of stroke,[12] and perhaps even greater reduction in risk of stroke among Asians.[13] Furthermore, the costs of the conventional antihypertensives are substantially lower than those of the newer antihypertensives.[14,15]

TABLE 14.1 Effects of different blood-pressure-lowering drugs from most recent updated systematic review of randomised trials[10]

	Relative risk reduction (%)	
	Stroke (95% CI)	Major cardiovascular events* (95% CI)
Comparisons with placebo		
Diuretics or beta blockers	38 (28–48)	21 (13–28)
ACE inhibitors	30 (15–43)	21 (14–27)
Calcium-antagonist-based therapy	39 (15–36)	28 (13–41)
Direct comparisons		
ACE inhibitor vs diuretic/beta-blocker	– 5(– 19 to + 8)	0 (– 8 to + 7)
Calcium antagonist vs diuretic/ beta-blocker	13 (2–23) (just favours calcium antagonist)	– 2 (– 10 to + 5)
ACE inhibitor vs calcium antagonist	– 2 (– 21 to + 15)	8 (– 1 to + 17)
More intensive vs less intensive blood-pressure-lowering strategies	20 (2–35) (favours more intensive strategies)	15 (4–24)

* Stroke, myocardial infarction, heart failure or death from any cardiovascular cause.
ACE, angiotensin-converting enzyme; CI, confidence interval.

14.9   What are the major adverse effects of different classes of antihypertensive agents?

- *Thiazide diuretics* – hypokalaemia, adverse influence on blood lipids, blood glucose and uric acid
- *Beta-blockers* – adverse influence on glucose tolerance and lipid metabolism
- *ACE inhibitors* – cough
- *Calcium-channel antagonists* – short- and intermediate-acting dihydropyridine calcium-channel blockers, such as nifedipine and isradipine, may be associated with an increased risk of cardiovascular morbidity and mortality.

Low-dose diuretics and beta blockers do not produce long-term metabolic effects likely to be of clinical importance.

OTHER MEASURES TO PREVENT RECURRENT STROKE

14.10   How effective is ACE inhibition for patients with TIA or ischaemic stroke due to atherothromboembolism?

The results of the heart outcomes prevention evaluation (HOPE) trial[16] suggest that the addition of ramipril 10 mg/day to best medical therapy (e.g. vascular risk factor control, antiplatelet therapy, carotid revascularisation) has an additional favourable effect in reducing the rate of recurrent stroke, myocardial infarction or death from vascular causes by about one-quarter. The reduction in vascular events is larger than might be expected from just lowering the blood pressure (*see Q. 7.21*). Whether this is a chance effect or a real additional effect of ACE inhibition by ramipril on atherogenesis (as well as blood pressure lowering) is controversial.[17]

14.11 Is there a role for cholesterol reduction among patients with TIA or ischaemic stroke due to atherothromboembolism?

Yes. Pravastatin and simvastatin have both been shown to be effective in reducing the risk of serious vascular events among patients with a history of previous TIA or ischaemic stroke[18,19].

Among 821 patients with a history of stroke or TIA (and CHD) who were randomised in the CARE and LIPID trials[20,21] to pravastatin (n=436) or placebo (n=385), the odds of a recurrent stroke during follow-up were reduced by 33% (95% CI: −1% to +56%) from 15.1% (placebo) to 10.6% (pravastatin) among patients assigned to pravastatin therapy.

Among 3,280 patients with a previous history of stroke who participated in the Heart Protection Study, 1,820 patients had a past history of stroke only, and 1,460 patients had a past history of CHD *and* stroke[22]. For the 1,820 patients with previous stroke only, random allocation to simvastatin 40mg/day was associated with a significant reduction in any stroke, myocardial infarction (MI), vascular death or revascularisation procedure from 23.6% (placebo) to 18.7% (simvastatin). This was a RRR of 21% (95% CI: 5 to 34%, p<0.001), and ARR of 49 serious vascular events (4.9%) per 1000 stroke patients allocated simvastatin over 5 years[22]. Among the 1,460 patients with known CHD *and* a past history of stroke, allocation to simvastatin was associated with a similar reduction in any stroke, MI, vascular death or revascularisation procedure from 37.4% (placebo) to 32.4% (simvastatin); RRR: 14% (95% CI: 0.5 to 25%), and ARR 5% over 5 years[22].

Because about one sixth (17%) of the patients allocated placebo subsequently 'crossed-over' to statin therapy during the 5 year treatment period, and about one sixth (15%) of the patients allocated simvastatin were non-compliant and discontinued statin therapy, the above 'intention-to-treat' comparisons assessed the effects of only about two-thirds (85% compliance minus 17% cross-over) taking simvastatin during the scheduled 5-year treatment period. This yielded an average LDL-cholesterol concentration of 1.0 (SE:0.02) mmol/l lower (about two-thirds of the effect of actual use of 40 mg simvastatin daily) among patients allocated simvastatin compared with placebo. In addition, mean plasma total cholesterol was reduced by 1.2 (0.02) mmol/l, and HDL cholesterol increased by 0.03 (0.01) mmol/l, with simvastatin compared with placebo.

Simvastatin was well tolerated. The annual excess risk of myopathy with simvastatin was about 0.01%. Abnormalities of liver function tests (> 4 × upper limits of normal) were reported in 0.42% of the simvastatin group and 0.31% of the placebo group[22]. There was no adverse effect of simvastatin on haemorrhagic stroke, although the number of haemorrhagic stroke events in both groups was very small.

The precision of the estimates of effectiveness and safety of statins in preventing recurrent stroke, amongst stroke patients, should be clarified further by the forthcoming results of the Stroke Prevention by Aggressive Reduction in Cholesterol Levels (SPARCL) trial, which compares atorvasatin 80 mg daily with placebo in 4,300 adult men and women with recent (1–6 months prior to randomisation) non-disabling stroke or TIA, and LDL-C concentrations ≥ 2.6 mmol (100 mg/dL) and ≤ 4.9 mmol/l (190 mg/dL), but without a history of CHD (www.neuro.wustl.edu/stroke/trials);. The primary outcome measure is the time from randomisation to the first occurrence of any (fatal or nonfatal) stroke. Recruitment was completed in early 2001, and the 5 year follow-up continues. To date, the clinical event rate has been higher than forecast, and so it is predicted that follow-up will be complete in late 2004. The Cholesterol Treatment Trialists' Collaboration is carrying out a meta-analysis of all randomised trials of cholesterol reduction that were of more than two years duration and included more than 1000 people, and the first cycle of the analyses, when combined with the BHF/MRC-HPS, will include data from 57,000 patients and 2,200 strokes[23].

14.12 Which patients with TIA or ischaemic stroke due to atherothromboembolism should be treated with a statin medication?

All patients with TIA or ischaemic stroke due to atherothromboembolism should be considered for treatment with a statin medication, irrespective of their age, gender or plasma cholesterol concentration[18,22]. This is because their absolute risk of a serious vascular event is high enough (at least 5% per year) to make it worthwhile, and probably cost-effective, to take simvastatin or pravastatin, and lower their risk by at least 25% (to less than 4% per year).

The HPS subsequently showed that the proportional (one quarter) reduction in event rate attributable to simvastatin was consistent (and significant) in each subcategory of patient studied and each sub-category of baseline total plasma cholesterol and LDL-cholesterol, even among patients who presented with target LDL levels below 3.0 mmol/l (116 mg/dL) and total cholesterol levels below 5.0 mmol/l (< 193 mg/dL)[22].

14.13 How effective is cessation of cigarette smoking among patients with TIA or ischaemic stroke due to atherothromboembolism who are still smoking?

There have been no randomised controlled trials but observational studies suggest that stopping smoking decreases the risk of stroke by at least 1.5 times, and up to three times in people under the age of 55 years (*see Q. 7.7 & Q. 7.8*).[24] If the baseline annual risk of stroke is about 7%, then stopping smoking could reduce the risk of stroke (and other serious vascular events) from about 7% to at least 4.7% per year, a RRR of at least 33% (95% CI 29–38%) and ARR of at least 2.3%. The NNT is at most 43.

14.14 How quickly do risks diminish when smokers stop smoking?

Observational studies have found that the relative risk of mortality and of cardiovascular morbidity falls after cessation of smoking. The risk can take many years to approximate to that of non-smokers, particularly in those with a history of heavy smoking (*see Q. 7.8*).

14.15 What other lifestyle interventions may reduce the risk of stroke and other serious vascular events?

- Physical exercise
- Weight loss
- Diet low in fat and high in fruit and vegetables
- Salt restriction.

14.16 What is the effect of physical activity on the risk of stroke and other serious vascular events?

There is strong observational evidence that moderate to high levels of physical activity reduce the relative risk of coronary events by about 30–50% compared with people who are sedentary.

Randomised trials show that aerobic exercise reduces blood pressure by about 4.7 mmHg systolic (95% CI 4.4–5.0 mmHg) and 3.1 mmHg diastolic (95% CI 3.0–3.3 mmHg), and body weight.

14.17 What are the potential adverse effects of physical activity?

Potential adverse effects include musculoskeletal injuries and sudden death, but the absolute risk of sudden death after strenuous activity is small (although it is greatest in people who are habitually sedentary) and does not outweigh the observed benefits.

14.18 What is the effect of weight reduction on the risk of stroke and other serious vascular events?

Randomised trials show that modest weight reductions of 3–9% body weight are achievable in motivated middle-aged and older adults and may lead to modest reductions in blood pressure by about 3 mmHg systolic and 3 mmHg diastolic in obese people with hypertension. However, many adults find it difficult to maintain weight loss.

14.19 What is the effect of eating more fruit and vegetables on the risk of stroke and other serious vascular events?

Observational studies suggest that eating more fruit and vegetables reduces the risk of heart attack and stroke. The size of any real protective effect is uncertain. The observed associations could be the result of confounding as people who eat fruit and vegetables often come from higher socioeconomic groups and adopt other healthy lifestyles. However, randomised trials show that a high fruit and vegetable diet modestly reduces blood pressure by about 2.8 mmHg systolic (97.5% CI 0.9–4.7 mmHg) and 1.1 mmHg diastolic (97.5% CI 2.4 mmHg decrease to 0.3 mmHg increase, $p = 0.07$), and a combined low fat and high fruit and vegetable diet reduces blood pressure by about 5.5 mmHg systolic (97.5% CI 3.7–4.4 mmHg) and 3.0 mmHg diastolic (97.5% CI 1.6 mmHg decrease to 4.3 mmHg increase, $p = 0.07$).

14.20 What is the effect of salt restriction on the risk of stroke and other serious vascular events?

There is evidence from systematic reviews of randomised trials that salt restriction may lead to modest reductions in blood pressure, with more benefit in people older than 45 years than in younger people.[25] A mean reduction in sodium intake of 118 mmol (6.7 g) per day for 28 days leads to reductions of 3.9 mmHg (95% CI 3.0–4.8 mmHg) in systolic blood pressure and 1.9 mmHg (95% CI 1.3–22.5 mmHg) in diastolic blood pressure.

14.21 Does dietary supplementation with antioxidants reduce the risk of stroke and other serious vascular events?

There is no evidence that dietary supplementation with potassium, calcium, magnesium, fish oil or calcium reduces the risk of stroke and mortality. There is also no evidence of benefit with beta carotene supplements, and randomised trials suggest they may be harmful. Other antioxidant supplements may be beneficial but there is insufficient evidence to support their use at present.

However, potassium, fish oil and perhaps calcium supplementation do reduce blood pressure (the major modifiable causal risk factor for stroke) a little.

There is inconclusive evidence regarding the effects of calcium supplementation, magnesium supplementation and alcohol reduction on blood pressure.

14.22 What is the effect of potassium supplementation on blood pressure?

Potassium supplementation of about 60 mmol daily (2000 mg, which is roughly the amount contained in five bananas) is feasible for most adults and reduces blood pressure a little, by about 4.4 mmHg systolic (95% CI 2.2–6.6 mmHg) and 2.5 mmHg diastolic (95% CI 0.1–4.9 mmHg).

14.23 What are the adverse effects of potassium supplementation on blood pressure?

Potassium supplementation is not harmful in people without kidney failure and in people not taking drugs that increase serum potassium.

Gastrointestinal adverse effects such as belching, flatulence, diarrhoea or abdominal discomfort occur in about 2–10% of people.

14.24 What is the effect of fish oil supplementation on blood pressure?

Fish oil supplementation in large doses of 3 g/day modestly lowers blood pressure by about 4.5 mmHg systolic (95% CI 1.2–7.8 mmHg) and 2.5 mmHg diastolic (95% CI 0.6–4.4 mmHg).

ANTIPLATELET THERAPY

14.25 How effective is antiplatelet therapy in patients with TIA or ischaemic stroke due to atherothromboembolism?

A systematic review by the Antithrombotic Trialists' Collaboration[9] showed that, among patients at high risk of vascular disease (e.g. previous symptomatic atherothrombosis of the cerebral, coronary and peripheral arteries), antiplatelet drugs reduce the odds of any serious vascular event (non-fatal stroke, non-fatal myocardial infarction or death from vascular causes) by about 25%.

Among individuals with a prior ischaemic stroke, antiplatelet drugs prevent about 38 serious vascular events for every 1000 treated for about 2.5 years (i.e. 3.8%) or about 15 serious vascular events per 1000 patients treated per year.

14.26 What are the bleeding risks associated with antiplatelet therapy?

 The risk of intracranial bleeding with antiplatelet treatment is small, at most 1–2 per 1000 people treated per year in trials of long-term antiplatelet treatment (i.e. 0.1–0.2%).

The risk of major extracranial bleeding (which is mostly non-fatal) is only about 3 per 1000 per year (0.3%).

In general therefore, the benefits of antiplatelet therapy in stroke and other high vascular risk patients (about 15 events per 1000 patients treated per year) outweigh the hazards (about 2 non-fatal extracranial haemorrhages per 1000 patients treated per year).

14.27 How effective is aspirin as an antiplatelet agent in patients with TIA or ischaemic stroke due to atherothromboembolism?

Aspirin reduces the odds of a serious vascular event (non-fatal stroke, non-fatal myocardial infarction or death due to a vascular cause) among patients with a prior TIA or ischaemic stroke by 17% ± 4.4 ($2p = 0.00009$).[9] This is a RRR of 13% (95% CI 6–19%) and an ARR of 3% over approximately 3 years, or about 1% per year (*Fig. 14.1*);[26] the risk of serious vascular events in TIA/stroke patients is reduced from an average of about 7.0% per year to 6.0% per year (an ARR of 1.0%). The NNT is therefore about 100.

14.28 What is the optimal dose of aspirin for patients with TIA or ischaemic stroke due to atherothromboembolism?

> The most reliable evidence of the relative effect of different doses of aspirin comes from direct comparisons in randomised trials, which suggest that aspirin at a dose of 75 mg daily is as effective as higher doses.[9,26–28]
>
> There is insufficient evidence to be certain that doses below 75 mg daily are as effective; the only direct randomised comparison of the effects of daily doses of 30 mg and 283 mg among around 3000 people with a recent TIA or minor ischaemic stroke found no significant difference, but the possibility of a small difference could not be excluded.[28]

14.29 How safe is aspirin for patients with TIA or ischaemic stroke due to atherothromboembolism?

 The most important adverse effect of aspirin is potentially life-threatening bleeding. However, aspirin is also associated with an increased risk of extracranial (mainly gastrointestinal) haemorrhage and upper gastrointestinal upset. Some patients are also allergic to aspirin. About 5% of patients cannot tolerate aspirin or are allergic to it.

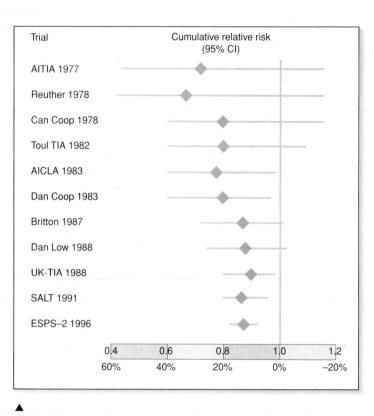

▲

Fig 14.1 Cumulative meta-analysis in chronological order (1977–1996) of 11 randomised controlled trials of aspirin vs control in almost 10 000 patients with previous TIA or ischaemic stroke, showing relative risks and corresponding relative risk reductions with 95% confidence intervals (CI). Each line represents the relative risk and 95% CI of that study combined with all previous studies. Adapted with permission from Algra and van Gijn 1999.[26]

14.30 What is the risk of intracranial haemorrhage for patients taking aspirin?

Intracranial haemorrhage, which is uncommon but can be fatal, is increased in people taking aspirin by about 1 case per 1000 cases treated for 3 years.[29]

14.31 What is the risk of extracranial (gastrointestinal) haemorrhage for patients taking aspirin?

The risk of haematemesis attributable to aspirin is about 0.2–1.0 per 1000 person-years of exposure which is a relative excess risk of about 70%.[30]

14.32 Is the risk of extracranial (gastrointestinal) haemorrhage associated with aspirin dose-related?

Yes. High-dose aspirin is associated with a trend towards an increase in odds of upper gastrointestinal haemorrhage compared with medium-dose aspirin (2.6% vs 1.9%, OR 1.4, 95% CI 0.9–2.1),[27,31] but there is no difference between medium-dose (283 mg) and low-dose (30 mg) aspirin from the limited trial data available (1.9% vs 1.8%, OR 1.2, 95% CI 0.7–2.0).[28]

14.33 Is the risk of extracranial (gastrointestinal) haemorrhage associated with aspirin related to the type of aspirin preparation?

No, not really. At average daily doses of aspirin of 325 mg or less, the relative risks of upper gastrointestinal haemorrhage for plain, enteric-coated and buffered aspirin are about 2.6, 2.7 and 3.1 respectively.[32]

14.34 What is the risk of upper gastrointestinal upset for patients taking aspirin?

Symptoms of upper gastrointestinal upset (nausea, heartburn and epigastric pain) arise in about 15–32% of individuals taking placebo, 30% of those taking aspirin 300 mg/day and 24–44% of those taking 900–1300 mg per day.[33]

14.35 Is the risk of upper gastrointestinal upset associated with aspirin dose-related?

Randomised trials involving direct comparisons of different doses of aspirin indicate that high-dose (500–1500 mg daily) aspirin significantly increases the odds of upper gastrointestinal symptoms compared with medium-dose (75–325 mg daily) aspirin (high-dose 26.2%, medium-dose 21.9%, OR 1.3, 95% CI 1.1–1.5).[27,31] Medium-dose (283 mg) aspirin is associated with a trend towards an increase in odds of upper gastrointestinal upset compared with low-dose (30 mg) aspirin (medium-dose 11.4%, low-dose 10.5%, OR 1.1, 95% CI 0.9–1.4).[28]

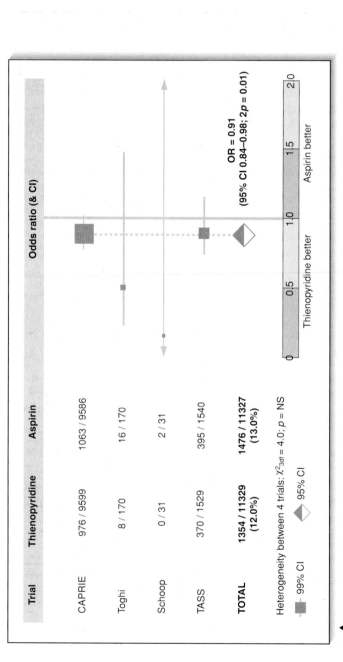

Trial	Thienopyridine	Aspirin
CAPRIE	976 / 9599	1063 / 9586
Toghi	8 / 170	16 / 170
Schoop	0 / 31	2 / 31
TASS	370 / 1529	395 / 1540
TOTAL	**1354 / 11329** **(12.0%)**	**1476 / 11327** **(13.0%)**

Heterogeneity between 4 trials: χ^2_{3df} = 4.0; p = NS

Odds ratio (& CI)

OR = 0.91
(95% CI 0.84–0.98; 2p = 0.01)

Thienopyridine better   Aspirin better

Fig 14.2 Direct comparisons of the proportional effects of the thienopyridines versus aspirin on serious vascular events (stroke, myocardial infarction or vascular death) in patients at high risk of vascular disease. Compared with aspirin, the thienopyridines (clopidogrel and ticlopidine) reduce the odds of a subsequent serious vascular event by about 9% (95% confidence interval, CI 2–16%), from 13% (aspirin) to 12% (thienopyridines) at 2 years. CAPRIE, Clopidogrel versus Aspirin in Patients at Risk of Ischemic Events; TASS, Ticlopidine Aspirin Stroke Study. Adapted with permission from Hankey et al 2000.[54]

14.36 Is any single antiplatelet agent more effective than aspirin for patients with TIA or ischaemic stroke due to atherothromboembolism?

Yes, the thienopyridine derivatives clopidogrel and ticlopidine are both marginally but significantly more effective than aspirin.

Compared with aspirin, clopidogrel and ticlopidine both reduce the risk of stroke and other important vascular events among patients with prior stroke and TIA by about 10% (95% CI 3–17%; *Fig. 14.2*).[34] If the risk of stroke is about 6.0% per year for patients taking aspirin, then it would be expected that clopidogrel or ticlopidine would reduce the risk to 5.4% per year, which is an ARR of 0.6%. The NNT is 166 compared with aspirin.

14.37 How safe are the thienopyridines compared with aspirin?

Compared with aspirin, the thienopyridines clopidogrel and ticlopidine are both associated with a significantly lower rate of:

- gastrointestinal haemorrhage (2.5% aspirin compared with 1.8% thienopyridine; OR 0.71, 95% CI 0.59–0.86)
- upper gastrointestinal upset (17.1% aspirin compared with 14.8% thienopyridine; OR 0.84, 95% CI 0.78–0.90).[34]

Compared with aspirin, clopidogrel and ticlopidine are both associated with a significantly higher rate of skin rash and diarrhoea, but the magnitude of these adverse effects of clopidogrel and ticlopidine are quantitatively different. In comparison with aspirin, ticlopidine is associated with a twofold increase in odds of skin rash (11.8% vs 5.5%) and diarrhoea (20.4% vs 9.9%), whereas clopidogrel is associated with an increase of only about one-third in odds of skin rash (6.0% vs 4.0%) and diarrhoea (4.5% vs 3.4%).[34]

Compared with aspirin, ticlopidine is also associated with a threefold increase in odds of neutropenia (2.3% vs 0.8%), whereas clopidogrel is not associated with an excess of neutropenia and thrombocytopenia.[34]

Observational studies suggest that ticlopidine is associated with a significant excess incidence of thrombotic thrombocytopenic purpura of 0.02% (95% CI 0.009–0.04%),[35] compared with the estimated incidence of 0.00037% (standardised morbidity ratio 56; 95% CI 26–107).[36] Although clopidogrel was not associated with any excess of thrombocytopenia (platelets $< 100 \times 10^9$/l) compared with aspirin (0.26% vs 0.26%; OR 1.00; 95% CI 0.57–1.74) among the 9553 patients who were allocated clopidogrel in the CAPRIE trial,[37] a report of 11 cases of thrombotic thrombocytopenic purpura associated with clopidogrel use has raised concerns about the safety of clopidogrel.[38] However, it remains uncertain whether the reported association between clopidogrel and thrombotic thrombocytopenic purpura is coincidental or causal.[39] Follow-up studies are in progress.

14.38 What is the preferred thienopyridine antiplatelet agent?

Clopidogrel is now preferred to ticlopidine because it is as effective as
ticlopidine but does not cause an excess of neutropenia and
thrombocytopenia compared with aspirin, and does not cause as much skin
rash and diarrhoea as ticlopidine. It is also associated with less
gastrointestinal haemorrhage and upper gastrointestinal upset than aspirin,
when aspirin was used in trials in a dose of about 325 mg/day.

14.39 How effective is the combination of dipyridamole with aspirin, compared with aspirin alone, in preventing recurrent stroke in patients with TIA or ischaemic stroke due to atherothromboembolism?

Compared with aspirin, the combination of aspirin and modified-release
dipyridamole is associated with a reduction of about 15% (5–26%) in the
relative risk of serious vascular events among TIA and ischaemic stroke
patients and a non-significant reduction in odds of a serious vascular
event of 6% (95% CI: –6% – +17%) in all high-vascular-risk patients[9]
(*Fig. 14.3*).[40–42] Most of this reduction appeared to be attributable to a
substantial reduction in non-fatal strokes (*Fig. 14.3*), suggesting that the
addition of dipyridamole to aspirin may be appropriate for patients at
particularly high risk of stroke. The size of this estimate continues to be
studied in the European/Australasian Stroke Prevention in Reversible
Ischaemia Trial (ESPRIT).[43]

14.40 How safe is the combination of aspirin and dipyridamole for patients with TIA or ischaemic stroke due to atherothromboembolism?

Headache and gastrointestinal events (e.g. nausea, diarrhoea) are the main
reasons that patients receiving dipyridamole-containing antiplatelet
regimens discontinue treatment prematurely. About 7–8% of patients
taking dipyridamole cease their medication because of headache, compared
with about 2% of patients given aspirin or placebo.[42] Similarly,
gastrointestinal events led to premature discontinuation of dipyridamole in
about 6–7% of patients compared with about 4% of those given aspirin or
placebo.[42] The addition of dipyridamole to aspirin does not appear to
exaggerate the excess risk of haemorrhage associated with aspirin.

14.41 Are other combinations of antiplatelet drugs safe and effective for TIA and stroke patients?

The combination of *aspirin and clopidogrel* is the treatment of choice for
preventing death and myocardial infarction after coronary artery stenting

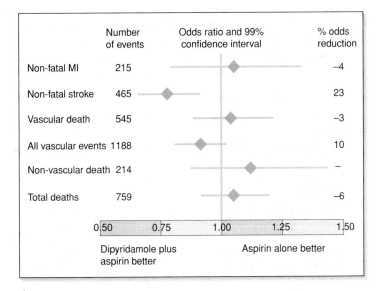

Fig 14.3 Direct comparisons of the proportional effects of the combination of aspirin and dipyridamole versus aspirin on vascular events and non-vascular deaths, derived from a total of 8616 high-vascular-risk patients studied in the Antiplatelet Trialists' Collaboration and the second European Stroke Prevention Study. Adapted with permission from Wilterdink and Easton 1998 (copyrighted 1999 American Medical Association).[41] MI: myocardial infarction.

and in patients with unstable angina. However, the long-term safety and effectiveness of the combination of clopidogrel and aspirin in patients with recent TIA and ischaemic stroke is still being compared with that of clopidogrel alone in an ongoing clinical trial.

The combination of *aspirin and a parenteral platelet glycoprotein IIb/IIIa blocker* given immediately to patients with unstable angina or non-Q-wave myocardial infarction, or undergoing percutaneous coronary interventions, is significantly more effective than aspirin alone in reducing the 30-day rate of death or nonfatal myocardial infarction (OR 0.81, 95% CI 0.75–0.88).[44] However, the combination of long-term aspirin and an oral platelet glycoprotein IIb/IIIa blocker in these patients appears to be no more effective than aspirin alone.[45] The unpublished results from a clinical trial comparing the combination of aspirin and an oral platelet glycoprotein IIb/IIIa blocker with aspirin alone in TIA and ischaemic stroke patients were similarly disappointing.

14.42 What are the relative costs of aspirin, clopidogrel and the combination of aspirin with dipyridamole?

In Australia, it costs about A$20 to treat a patient with aspirin for 1 year, A$330 to treat with aspirin and dipyridamole and about A$1000 to treat with clopidogrel. In the UK, the respective annual costs are £2 (aspirin), £117 (asasantin) and £460 (clopidogrel).

14.43 Is there a role for warfarin (coumadin) in secondary stroke prevention among patients with TIA or ischaemic stroke due to atherothromboembolism?

At present, there is no evidence that long-term anticoagulation is effective in preventing stroke and other serious vascular events with patients with TIA or ischaemic stroke due to atherothromboembolism[46]. Indeed, the use of warfarin, with a target international normalised ratio (INR) of 3.0–3.5, is associated with excess risk of haemorrhage, particularly in the elderly and those with evidence on cranial computed tomography (CT) of intracranial small-vessel disease.[47] The risks and benefits of long-term anticoagulation (INR 2.0–3.0) for patients with TIA or ischaemic stroke due to atherothromboembolism continue to be studied in the ongoing European/Australian Stroke Prevention in Reversible Ischaemia Trial.[43]

14.44 Which antiplatelet drug regime should be used in patients with TIA or ischaemic stroke due to atherothromboembolism?

- Acute ischaemic stroke patients should be immediately started on aspirin 300 mg daily (or, if possible, entered into further trials of thrombolysis and other promising acute therapies). After the acute phase, aspirin should be continued in a lower dose, 75 mg daily.
- If patients cannot tolerate aspirin or are allergic to aspirin (about 5% of patients), they should be treated with clopidogrel 75 mg/day.
- If the patient is considered to be at high absolute risk of another stroke or other serious vascular event and likely to benefit from the further 10% relative risk reduction that more costly treatments such as clopidogrel and the combination of aspirin and dipyridamole can offer, then these should be considered.
- If the patient suffers a recurrent stroke or serious vascular event while taking aspirin, and if the cause is still thought to be atherothromboembolism, then either dipyridamole should be added to aspirin or the patient should be changed to clopidogrel. Whether adding clopidogrel to aspirin is safe and effective in patients with recent TIA or ischaemic stroke due to atherothromboembolism remains the subject of an ongoing clinical trial.

SURGICAL INTERVENTIONS

14.45 How effective is carotid endarterectomy in patients with TIA or ischaemic stroke due to atherothromboembolism from an internal carotid artery stenosis?

The effectiveness of carotid endarterectomy is determined to a large extent (but not entirely) by:

■ The degree of carotid artery stenosis (the greater the degree of stenosis, the greater the benefit)
■ Whether the stenosis is symptomatic or not – carotid endarterectomy is beneficial mainly when the carotid stenosis has been the cause of recent (within the past 3–6 months) symptoms of focal neurological dysfunction due to carotid territory ischaemia (i.e. recent carotid TIA or ischaemic stroke; see Q. 7.16).

Carotid endarterectomy is effective in patients with recent carotid territory TIA or mild ischaemic stroke, who have severe carotid stenosis (70–99% of the diameter of the artery) and who are fit and willing for surgery.[48,49] It reduces the relative risk of stroke by about 48% (95% CI 27–63%).[50] If the 3-year risk of stroke is about 26.5% (8.8% per year), this is a reduction to 13.7% (4.6% per year), an ARR of 12.8% (4.2% per year). The NNT is 8 to prevent one stroke at 3 years, or 24 to prevent one stroke each year. If the absolute risk of stroke is greater, the absolute benefit of carotid endarterectomy is greater and the NNT is lower. An example of a group of patients in whom the absolute benefit of carotid endarterectomy is even greater is elderly patients, provided the patients do not have other life-threatening illnesses and the surgeon is skilled.[51,52]

Carotid endarterectomy is less effective in patients with recent carotid territory TIA or mild ischaemic stroke who have moderate carotid stenosis (> 50–69% diameter stenosis) and are fit and willing for surgery.[48,49] It reduces the relative risk of stroke by about 27% (95% CI 5–44%) but the absolute benefits are much less because the absolute risk of stroke without carotid endarterectomy is much less (i.e. there is less potential for benefit than for patients with severe symptomatic carotid stenosis).[50]

14.46 In which patients with TIA or ischaemic stroke due to atherothromboembolism from an internal carotid artery stenosis is carotid endarterectomy most effective?

Only up to 16% of patients with recent carotid territory brain ischaemia and severe carotid stenosis on the symptomatic side actually benefit from carotid endarterectomy (i.e. less than one in 6).[53]

These are patients who score 4 or more in the prognostic model in *Box 14.1*.

> **BOX 14.1 Prediction model for benefit from carotid endarterectomy among patients with recent carotid ischaemia and severe symptomatic carotid stenosis.[53]**
>
> **Independent risk factors for stroke with best medical therapy**
> Ischaemic events of the brain (as opposed to the eye)   1 point
> Recent ischaemic events (in the past two months)   1 point
> Severe degree of carotid stenosis: 80–89%   1 point
>   90–99%   2 points
> Carotid plaque irregularity   1 point
>
> **Independent risk factors for perioperative risk of stroke and death**
> Female gender   −0.5 point
> Systolic BP > 100 mmHg   −0.5 point
> Peripheral vascular disease   −0.5 point

14.47 How safe is carotid endarterectomy in patients with TIA or ischaemic stroke due to atherothromboembolism from an internal carotid artery stenosis?

 Carotid endarterectomy is associated overall with an increased relative risk of disabling stroke or death within 30 days of carotid surgery of about 2.5 (95% CI 1.6–3.8).[50]

The risk of carotid endarterectomy is not related to the degree of carotid stenosis. It varies considerably among different surgeons operating on various types of patients, from as low as 1% to as high as 30%.

Referring doctors (and patients[54]) should have access to the perioperative stroke and death rate of their prospective surgeon(s), derived from independent and rigorous audit.[55] However, interpretation of unusually high or low operative risks must take into account the effects of chance and case-mix.[56] Otherwise, over-simplistic interpretation of crude results may lead to unjustified criticism of individual surgeons and not to improvements in patient care. The decision whether or not to operate should involve consideration of all the important prognostic factors for stroke and perioperative stroke and death.

14.48 Which factors are associated with an increased risk of perioperative stroke and death associated with carotid endarterectomy?

These are listed in *Box 14.2*.

> **BOX 14.2 Factors associated with increased risk of stroke and death following carotid endarterectomy**
>
> - Female gender (perhaps because of smaller carotid arteries – perhaps more difficult to operate on)
> - Systolic blood pressure > 180 mmHg (perhaps increased risk of reperfusion injury and cerebral haemorrhage)
> - Peripheral arterial disease (a marker of atherosclerotic plaque burden)
> - Occlusion of the contralateral internal carotid artery (indicates poor collateral cerebral circulation)
> - Stenosis of the ipsilateral external carotid artery (poor collateral circulation).[57]

14.49 What are the other adverse effects of carotid endarterectomy?

 Other specific adverse effects of carotid endarterectomy, besides those inherent in any operation, include:

- Lower cranial nerve palsy (about 5–9% of patients)
- Peripheral nerve palsy (about 1% of patients)
- Major neck haematoma requiring surgery or extended hospital stay (about 5–7% of patients)
- Wound infection (3%).[58]

14.50 What determines the net effectiveness of carotid endarterectomy?

This is determined by the patient's absolute risk of another carotid territory ischaemic event (which increases with the degree of carotid stenosis), the surgical perioperative stroke and death rate (which is about 4–8%, irrespective of the degree of carotid stenosis), and the patient's life-expectancy.

14.51 How effective is carotid endarterectomy for neurologically asymptomatic carotid stenosis?

Carotid endarterectomy is rarely indicated for asymptomatic severe carotid stenosis because it only reduces the 3-year risk of stroke from 9.2% (3.1% per year) to 7.4% (2.5% per year), a RRR of 20% (odds reduction 32%, 95% CI 10–49%) and ARR of 1.8% (0.6% per year).[59] The NNT is 55 to prevent one stroke at 3 years or 166 to prevent one stroke each year.

Although the risk of perioperative stroke or death from carotid endarterectomy seems to be lower for people with asymptomatic carotid stenosis (2.7%) than for people with symptomatic carotid stenosis (generally about 6–8%), the risk of stroke or death without carotid surgery in neurologically asymptomatic people is much lower. Therefore, for most people, the overall risks and benefits from carotid surgery are quite evenly balanced and may not favour carotid surgery until several years have passed.

14.52 Is there any role for screening for asymptomatic carotid stenosis?

No. Given the low prevalence of severe carotid stenosis in the general population, screening asymptomatic people may result in more strokes than it prevents.[60]

14.53 How effective and safe is carotid angioplasty and stenting in patients with TIA or ischaemic stroke due to atherothromboembolism from an internal carotid artery stenosis?

Percutaneous transluminal angioplasty and stenting (endovascular treatment) has been shown in one clinical trial of 504 patients with carotid stenosis to have similar major risks and effectiveness in preventing stroke to carotid endarterectomy.[58] However, the estimates of risk and effectiveness remain imprecise and so further results are required before endovascular treatment becomes a standard treatment for carotid stenosis. Nevertheless, endovascular treatment does have the advantage of avoiding minor complications associated with carotid endarterectomy, such as cranial neuropathy and neck haematoma.[58]

STROKE CAUSED BY CARDIOGENIC EMBOLISM

14.54 How should atrial fibrillation be managed in patients with TIA and ischaemic stroke?

The management of atrial fibrillation (AF) has four principal objectives:

- To confirm and document the arrhythmia
- To identify and treat the underlying cause
- To relieve symptoms of decreased cardiac output by controlling the ventricular rate and restoring and maintaining sinus rhythm
- To reduce the risk of systemic thromboembolism, particularly stroke.

The arrhythmia can be confirmed by electrocardiography.

All patients, except the very elderly and infirm, should undergo investigation for underlying causes of AF, including thyroid function tests and echocardiography.

In haemodynamically stable patients, beta-blockade, verapamil or diltiazem can be used to control the heart rate. Recent-onset AF reverts spontaneously within 24 hours in at least half of patients (irrespective of digoxin).[58]

Patients who have been in AF for more than 48 hours should be considered for anticoagulation and strategies to restore and maintain sinus rhythm. The chances of successful cardioversion are higher if the AF is of recent onset and the size of the left atrium is normal.[61] However, for patients who are elderly (in whom AF is usually chronic and antiarrhythmic drug therapy may be risky), it is often reasonable to avoid attempted cardioversion, accept the AF and aim for adequate control of ventricular rate (digoxin combined with beta-blockade, verapamil or diltiazem) and long-term anticoagulation.

14.55 Is warfarin more effective than no warfarin in preventing stroke among patients with AF?

Yes, warfarin is substantially more effective than no warfarin in preventing stroke among people in AF. Irrespective of the baseline risk of stroke, warfarin reduces the risk of stroke by about two-thirds.

PRIMARY PREVENTION

Five large randomised controlled primary prevention trials have shown that, in people with chronic non-valvular AF, warfarin reduced the risk of stroke by about two-thirds (68%, 95% CI 50–79%, $p < 0.001$), from about 4.5% to 1.4% per year overall, with little increase in frequency of major bleeding (warfarin 1.2% vs control 1.0%) or intracranial haemorrhage (warfarin 0.3% per year vs control 0.1% per year).[62]

This means that warfarin will prevent about 30 strokes per 1000 patient years of treatment at a cost of at least two serious bleeding episodes per 1000 patients treated for 1 year. It must be stressed, however, that this acceptable rate of bleeding was achieved in patients who were carefully selected, screened and closely followed; 53–93% of eligible patients with AF were not included in the trials because of an increased risk of bleeding. Exclusion criteria in some or all trials included old age (> 75 years), serious illness (liver, kidney, brain or malignant disease), alcoholism, fall risk (e.g. syncope), forgetfulness, non-steroidal anti-inflammatory drugs and uncontrolled hypertension.

SECONDARY PREVENTION

One secondary prevention trial (the European Atrial Fibrillation Trial[63]) showed that, in people with chronic non-valvular AF and symptoms of previous TIA or stroke, who have a stroke risk of 12% per year, warfarin therapy (target INR 2.5–4.0) reduced the risk of stroke by about two-thirds

(66%, 95% CI 53–80%), to 4% per year. The annual incidence of major bleeding complications was 2.8% in the anticoagulant group and 0.7% in the placebo group. No intracranial bleeds were identified in patients assigned to warfarin.

These data mean that warfarin prevents about 80 strokes per 1000 patient years of treatment in patients who have had a TIA or stroke and who are in AF, at a cost of at least 20 serious bleeding episodes per 1000 patients treated for 1 year.

14.56 When should anticoagulation be started after a recent ischaemic stroke for patients in AF?

The timing of anticoagulation after recent ischaemic stroke depends on the risk of recurrent thromboembolism (*See Q. 7.11, Box 7.1 & Box 14.3*) and the risk of haemorrhagic transformation of the brain infarct (which is higher within the first 2 weeks and in patients with large brain infarcts and uncontrolled hypertension).

BOX 14.3 Risk stratification and prophylaxis in atrial fibrillation

High risk (6–12% per year risk of stroke)
- Age > 65 years and hypertension or diabetes
- Previous transient ischaemic attack (TIA) or stroke
- Valvular heart disease
- Heart failure
- Recent myocardial infarction
- Impaired left ventricular function on echocardiography
- Thyroid disease
- Left atrial thrombus or left atrial spontaneous echo contrast (transoesophageal echocardiography performed on the basis of clinical suspicion)

Treatment: Warfarin (target INR 2.0–3.0) if possible and not contraindicated

Moderate risk (3–5% per year risk of stroke)
- Age < 65 years and hypertension or diabetes
- Age > 65 years and not in high risk group

Treatment: Warfarin (target INR 2.0–3.0) or aspirin 75–300 mg daily, depending on individual case and echocardiography findings.

Low risk (< 1% per year risk of stroke)
- Age 65 and no hypertension, diabetes, TIA, stroke, or other clinical risk factors

Treatment: Nil or aspirin 75–300 mg daily.

Common empirical practice is to treat fibrillating acute ischaemic stroke patients immediately with aspirin 300 mg/day and then, depending on the above factors, begin warfarin 5 mg per day between days 3 and 14 after stroke onset, aiming to achieve an INR of 2.0. Randomised trials comparing aspirin with heparin during the first 2 weeks of acute ischaemic stroke among patients in AF show no benefit from early anticoagulation, because any net gains from reduction in recurrent ischaemic stroke are offset by the extra risk of haemorrhagic stroke.

14.57 Is aspirin more effective than no aspirin in preventing stroke among patients with AF?

Yes, aspirin is modestly more effective than no aspirin in preventing stroke among people in AF. Irrespective of the baseline risk of stroke, aspirin reduces the risk of stroke by about 20–25%.

Three primary prevention and three secondary prevention trials have shown that, in people with AF, aspirin reduces the incidence of stroke by 22% (95% CI 2–38%), from 5.2% (placebo) to 3.7% (aspirin) per year for primary prevention (ARR 1.5% per year) and from 12.9% (placebo) to 10.4% (aspirin) per year for secondary prevention (ARR 2.5% per year).[62]

Aspirin was not associated with any significant excess of intracranial haemorrhage (aspirin 0.16%, control 0.13%) or major extracranial bleeding (aspirin 0.5%, control 0.6%).[62]

This means that aspirin might prevent about 15–25 strokes per 1000 patient years of treatment, depending on the type of patient treated and their baseline risk of stroke, with no significant excess risk of major bleeding.

14.58 Do direct 'head to head' comparisons show that warfarin is more effective than aspirin in preventing stroke among patients with AF?

The relative benefits and risks of warfarin and aspirin have been studied in three trials, all of which showed that warfarin was associated with half the risk of stroke associated with aspirin (47% RRR, 95% CI 28–61%, $p < 0.01$).

14.59 Why is aspirin less effective than warfarin in preventing stroke among patients with AF?

A speculative interpretation of the above data is that the modest effect of aspirin in AF patients is in preventing strokes due to atherothromboembolism and not cardiogenic embolism. This is because the magnitude of the treatment effect (a 22% RRR) is very similar to the effect of aspirin in patients with symptomatic atherothromboembolism of the brain, heart and limbs. Whether aspirin (or another antiplatelet agent) combined with adjusted-dose warfarin (INR 2.0–3.0) would be safe and more effective than warfarin alone in AF patients (preventing both atherothrombotic and cardiogenic strokes) remains unknown.

14.60 Is the combination of low-intensity, fixed-dose warfarin and aspirin more effective than standard adjusted-dose warfarin alone in preventing stroke among patients with AF?

No. For patients with AF who are at high risk of stroke, adding aspirin 325 mg/day to low-intensity, fixed dose warfarin, adjusted to an INR of 1.2–1.5, was not as effective in preventing stroke or systemic thromboembolism as standard adjusted-dose warfarin therapy, maintaining an INR of 2.0–3.0 (event rates 7.9% per year vs 1.9% per year respectively, $p < 0.0001$).[62] Furthermore, there is no difference in the rates of major bleeding.

Three subsequent trials also showed trends toward the superiority of adjusted-dose warfarin (INR 2.0–3.0) over low-intensity anticoagulation or an aspirin-anticoagulation regimen.[62]

14.61 Are there any other antiplatelet agents that may be effective in preventing stroke among patients with AF?

The Italian SIFA study reported that a new antiplatelet agent, indobufen, 100–200 mg twice daily, was as effective as adjusted-dose warfarin (INR 2.0–3.5) in preventing stroke, systemic embolism, myocardial infarction and vascular death in 916 patients with non-valvular AF and a recent (< 15 days) TIA or non-disabling ischaemic stroke.[62] The 12-month event rates were 10% in the warfarin group and 12% in the indobufen group ($p = 0.47$). However, the numbers of patients and outcome events were quite small, follow-up was short and it is possible that a true difference was not detected.

Future studies are being planned to evaluate the safety and effectiveness of other newer antiplatelet agents (such as clopidogrel, oral glycoprotein IIb/IIIa receptor inhibitors and oral thrombin inhibitors) and combination antiplatelet therapies (such as aspirin–ticlopidine, aspirin–clopidogrel and aspirin–dipyridamole) as strategies of thromboprophylaxis in AF.

SELECTION OF PATIENTS FOR THROMBOPROPHYLAXIS

14.62 Which patients with AF should be treated with thromboprophylaxis?

Not all patients with AF benefit from thromboprophylactic treatment. The decision to treat depends on the balance between the risk of thromboembolism without treatment and the risks of thromboembolism and haemorrhage with treatment in each patient, as well as the patient's willingness to accept the potential risks, costs and inconvenience of treatment in order to possibly benefit. The current profile of individual risk of thromboembolism and bleeding complications (see below) remains imprecise and continues to be refined as new data emerge.

14.63 Who is at high risk of stroke and thromboembolism without thromboprophylactic treatment?

The important independent prognostic factors for an increased risk of stroke among individuals with AF are increasing age, a history of previous TIA or stroke, hypertension, diabetes mellitus and transthoracic echocardiographic evidence of moderate–severe left ventricular systolic dysfunction. Echocardiographic evidence of enlarged left atrial size and left atrial spontaneous echo densities/contrast ('smoke'), possibly indicative of stasis of blood, are also significant risk factors for stroke.

These risk factors are cumulative (*see Box 14.3*):

- For people younger than 65 years with no risk factors the untreated annual risk of stroke is about 1%, whereas with one or more risk factors it is about 5%
- For people aged 65–75 years with no risk factors the annual risk of stroke is about 4%, and with one or more risk factors it is about 6% per year
- For people older than 75 years with no risk factors risk of stroke is about 3–4%, whereas with one or more risk factors it is about 8%.

14.64 Who is at high risk of haemorrhage with anticoagulant treatment?

The major risk factors for anticoagulant-associated intracranial haemorrhage include:

- Fragile intracranial blood vessels (previous symptomatic cerebrovascular disease, CT evidence of small-vessel disease – 'leukoaraiosis')
- High blood pressure (poorly controlled hypertension)
- Excessive anticoagulation (INR > 3.5) or factors predisposing to it such as confusion, dementia, difficulty accessing anticoagulant monitoring, alcoholic liver disease and a tendency to falls.

Increasing age adds to the risk for all of these and is thus a potent risk factor for anticoagulant-associated haemorrhage. In the subgroup of patients (mean age 80 years) in the Stroke Prevention in Atrial Fibrillation II trial, the rate of intracranial haemorrhage was as high as 1.8% per year in those who were allocated to warfarin (target INR 2.0–4.5) and 0.8% among those who were assigned to aspirin.[62] Although the target INR in this study (2.0–4.5) was higher than that currently recommended (2.0–3.0), these data suggest that the low rate of intracranial haemorrhage documented in the five primary prevention AF trials may not apply to very elderly individuals (who were not well represented in many of these trials; the mean age of the patients studied in the AF trials was 69 years and only about one-quarter were older than 75 years).

14.65 What influences the decision to prescribe antithrombotic therapy for AF?

Current practice necessitates individualisation of therapy after an integrated clinical assessment that evaluates thromboembolic risk due to AF alone, other potential indications for anticoagulation, haemorrhagic risk and non-medical factors relevant to compliance, possibility of monitoring the INR at least monthly, gait instability, risk of other trauma, and patient values and preferences. Decision analysis can also be useful.

The role of transthoracic echocardiography (in addition to excluding structural heart disease in all patients who first present with AF) is to further refine stroke risk in the small group of patients with low risk of stroke according to clinical factors. Only rarely is transoesophageal echocardiography needed for risk stratification, despite it being the most sensitive clinical tool available to detect left atrial thrombus and spontaneous echo contrast, which are markers for increased risk of thromboembolism. In clinical practice, however, transoesophageal echocardiography may have a particular place in improving risk stratification for those individuals with a relative contraindication to warfarin or when transthoracic echocardiography is inadequate.

The choices of thromboprophylactic agents for AF include warfarin, which is the most effective but also the most risky treatment, and aspirin, which is less effective than warfarin but also safer. The combination of aspirin and low-dose warfarin is not any more effective than aspirin alone. The most appropriate treatment regimen is one in which patients at high risk of stroke and low risk of haemorrhage are treated with warfarin, and patients at low risk of stroke or high risk of haemorrhage are treated with aspirin.

14.66 Which patients with AF do not need to be treated with thromboprophylaxis?

Individuals with AF who are less than 60 years old and have no evidence of any concurrent heart disease or previous stroke or TIA have a very low risk of a thromboembolic event, about 0.6% per year. The potential benefits of aspirin in these patients (which may reduce the risk by 0.12% per year – 20% of 0.6%) may be offset by an equal potential risk of aspirin-associated haemorrhagic stroke (0.12%).

14.67 Which patients with AF should be treated with aspirin?

Aspirin is indicated for individuals in AF who are at fairly low absolute risk of stroke (about 1–2% per year), such as those without any of the independent thromboembolic risk factors (*Box 14.3*), or those at risk of an anticoagulant-related haemorrhage that exceeds the risk of stroke (more than 1% per year). For some people, such as the elderly and hypertensives, whose risk of stroke and haemorrhage are both high, the treatment decision can be difficult and may be determined ultimately by patient preference.

Patients taking aspirin should be monitored over time and their treatment changed to warfarin if risk factors emerge, which occurs in 10–15% of aspirin-treated patients per year.

14.68 Which patients with AF should be treated with warfarin?

Warfarin is indicated for individuals with chronic AF at high absolute risk of stroke (more than 4% per year), such as those with any of the independent thromboembolic risk factors listed above, and a lower risk of haemorrhage (*Box 14.3*). Similarly, anticoagulant therapy should be considered in patients with paroxysmal AF, depending on their thromboembolic risk factors, as well as the frequency and duration of the paroxysms. Although clinical trial evidence suggests that the stroke rate of patients with paroxysmal AF is similar to patients with chronic AF, the trials did not specifically examine the benefits of antithrombotic therapy in patients with paroxysmal AF. Furthermore, the range of thromboembolic risk in such patients is likely to be extremely wide, from very low for the patient with one short paroxysm once a year to considerably higher for the patent who is having daily lengthy paroxysms.

14.69 What is the optimal target INR?

The intensity of oral anticoagulant therapy that provides the best balance between the prevention of thromboembolism and the occurrence of bleeding complications appears to be an INR of 2.0–3.0 but may be lower (1.8–2.0) in patients at greater risk of bleeding (i.e. the elderly) and may be higher (3.0–4.0) in patients at greater risk of thromboembolism, such as those with prosthetic heart valves.[64,65]

It is important to emphasise that, in people in whom anticoagulant therapy is indicated, the odds of stroke increases substantially when the INR falls below 2.0; patients with an INR of 1.7 have twice (95% CI 1.6–2.4) the likelihood of stroke of those with an INR of 2.0, and patients with an INR of 1.5 have 3.3 (2.4–4.6) times the likelihood of stroke of those with an INR of 2.0.

14.70 What if warfarin needs to be ceased?

When cessation of warfarin therapy is required because of other (usually surgical) procedures, it is necessary to stratify the invasiveness of the procedure (minimal vs major) and the short-term risk of thromboembolism. Warfarin can be discontinued for 5 days before a major procedure and continued at a decreased dose for a minor procedure. Therapy should be reinstituted as soon as possible after invasive procedures. Patients at high risk of thromboembolism (e.g. severe mitral stenosis, mechanical mitral prosthesis, left ventricular dysfunction) should be admitted to hospital early for intravenous administration of heparin during warfarin cessation.

14.71 What is the 'bottom line' about anticoagulant thromboprophylaxis for TIA/ischaemic stroke patients?

Long-term oral anticoagulation is indicated for TIA/ischaemic stroke patients who have a high risk source of embolism in the heart such as recent transmural anterior myocardial infarction, dilated cardiomyopathy, valvular heart disease and atrial fibrillation.

Anticoagulating TIA/ischaemic stroke patients in atrial fibrillation reduces the annual risk of stroke from 12.0% to 4.0%, a RRR of 67% (95% CI 43–80%) and ARR of 8.0%. The NNT is 12.

The benefit of anticoagulation is even greater in atrial fibrillation patients who have a higher absolute risk of stroke, such as the elderly (age > 75 years), and those with a history of hypertension, diabetes or previous TIA or stroke, and echocardiographic evidence of impaired left ventricular function.

The target INR should be about 2.5 (range 2.0–3.0) except in the very elderly and patients with prosthetic heart valves. Because those over 75 years are at greatest risk of intracranial bleeding during warfarin therapy (as well as at higher risk of embolism if in atrial fibrillation), the target INR should be reduced to 2.0–2.5, or perhaps as low as 1.5–2.0, because some anticoagulant benefit is present with an INR of 1.5–1.9. For patients with prosthetic heart valves, an INR of at least 2.5–3.5 is needed for bileaflet or tilting disc valves, and higher for caged ball or caged disc valves (INR 3.0–4.0).

DECISION-MAKING

14.72 How should warfarin therapy be started and maintained?

In the past it was customary to use a loading dose of 10 mg. However, for most situations, a reduced starting dose of 5 mg per day will achieve an INR of 2.0 in 4–5 days. Although the warfarin is rapidly and completely absorbed, and it blocks hepatic synthesis of the functional vitamin-K-dependent haemostasis factors (II, VII, IX, X, protein C, protein S), its impact on the INR is delayed for a few days until preformed coagulation factors are removed.

The INR is measured daily or every second day during the first week of treatment, with the dose of warfarin (taken in the evening) titrated against the morning's INR. It is then measured at increasing intervals depending on the response.

Many patients, once the dose is stable, can be well controlled with 4–6 weekly testing and dose adjustment, but others need more frequent assessment.

The average maintenance dose is about 4.5 mg per day (0.5–15 mg/day) but in any individual it often fluctuates over time. Old age, reduced body weight and impaired cardiac and liver function all predict a smaller than average dose requirement.

14.73 How safe is it to discontinue anticoagulation in patients with intracranial haemorrhage who are at high thromboembolic risk (e.g. AF, prosthetic heart valve)?

The risk of thromboembolism with and without anticoagulation needs to be compared with the risk of rebleeding into the brain with and without anticoagulation.

There are few methodologically sound studies to help us. The risks of re-embolism in patients with high-risk cardiac sources of embolism (e.g. AF) range from about 2% to 20% in the first month after stopping anticoagulation, and the risks of rebleeding into the brain after starting anticoagulation are similar and vary from very low to 20% in the first month.[66]

If a patient who is taking warfarin because of a high thromboembolic risk experiences an intracranial haemorrhage, the warfarin should be stopped and its effects reversed fully with vitamin K_1 orally, subcutaneously or intravenously (very rarely, the last may cause a serious anaphylactoid reaction), and clotting factor replacement (e.g. fresh frozen plasma and Prothrombinex-HT, a factor II, IX and X concentrate).[67,68] This will minimise the risk of rebleeding. The timing of recommencing anticoagulation will depend on the risk of embolisation (which depends in turn on the nature of the underlying cardiac lesion and associated risk factors for embolisation) and on the risk of rebleeding (which depends on the blood pressure, coagulability of the blood, and size and location of the original haemorrhage).

It is possible to resume warfarin therapy quite early, even within the first 7–14 days, without high risk of recurrent bleeding in patients with a high risk of re-embolisation and a small intracranial bleed, controlled blood pressure and normal platelets and blood clotting system. The discontinuation of warfarin therapy for 1–2 weeks has a comparatively low probability of embolic events in patients at high embolic risk (e.g. AF, prosthetic heart valve).

14.74 Is there a role for treating patent foramen ovale?

Not at present (*see Q. 6.33*).

Given that secondary preventive measures (e.g. anatomical closure, warfarin, aspirin) are not without risk, the challenge is to identify patients in whom the patent foramen ovale is causative and, therefore, who may gain benefit from anatomical closure. Those in whom the patent foramen ovale is 'innocent' are unlikely to benefit from closure and the optimal therapy for this subgroup is yet to be defined.

The benefit from anatomical closure vs medical therapy or no active treatment is yet to be proven. Therefore, while a patient preference of a 'once off' mechanical solution is intuitively appealing, it cannot yet be recommended until results of randomised trials are available. After all, in some series, closing off a patent foramen ovale in individuals who have had a stroke, presumably because of it, has failed to prevent recurrent strokes in these individuals (presumably because they were due to other causes and the patent foramen ovale was an innocent bystander).[69]

14.75 What to do about recurrent TIAs?

For the patient with frequent, even daily TIAs, something must be done to stop the attacks, not only because the patient may end up with a stroke, but because the attacks may be disabling and frightening in themselves.

The first step is to exclude other non-vascular causes of recurrent focal neurological disturbances (e.g. migraine, epilepsy, structural intracranial lesions, hypoglycaemia, psychogenic) and try to ascertain the cause of the TIA. The underlying pathophysiology of the TIA is frequently uncertain but in many cases probably reflects recurrent thromboembolism from an 'active' ulcerated atherosclerotic plaque. Otherwise, recurrent but small drops in systemic blood pressure (e.g. after heavy meals, hot baths, starting a new hypotensive drug) might be enough to cause recurrent low-flow TIAs if there is severe arterial disease in the neck. Other treatable causes include cardiogenic embolism (anticoagulation), arteritis (steroids), vasospasm (calcium-channel blockers) and infective endocarditis (antibiotics).

Given the range of possible causes, it is not reasonable to expect a single intervention to be effective in the treatment of all types of TIA and in the prevention of stroke. If the likely cause of the 'crescendo' TIAs is atherothromboembolism or cardiogenic embolism, antithrombotic therapy is indicated. Aspirin (300 mg/day) is the drug of first choice. In addition, if the attacks are carotid in distribution and non-invasive ultrasound imaging shows severe stenosis of origin of the symptomatic internal carotid artery (and the patient is fit and willing to undergo surgery), then repeat carotid ultrasound or carotid angiography (magnetic resonance angiography or conventional catheter angiography) with a view to carotid endarterectomy/stenting is indicated. If carotid occlusion or severe inoperable stenosis is revealed, any antihypertensive treatment should be reviewed in case the blood pressure is too low and the continuing TIAs are due to low cerebral blood flow.

If the TIAs continue and if no 'surgical' lesion is found at the carotid bifurcation (i.e. it is normal, only mildly stenosed, or occluded), or if the attacks are vertebrobasilar in distribution, then it is reasonable to increase the dose of aspirin, switch from aspirin to clopidogrel or add dipyridamole to aspirin. If these measures fail, and if the diagnosis is still considered to be TIA due to atherothrombosis, then empirical therapy with the combination of aspirin and clopidogrel, or formal anticoagulation with heparin followed by warfarin may be tried. If the TIAs stop, then the warfarin can usually be slowly withdrawn after a few weeks and replaced by lifelong antiplatelet therapy. If the attacks still persist, the differential diagnosis of TIA should be reconsidered.

14.76 What is the role of the general practitioner in secondary stroke prevention?

General practitioners have a major role to play in secondary prevention of stroke and other serious vascular events among patients with previous TIA and stroke.

Their main role is to regularly follow the patient, ensure optimal control of the underlying disease causing the stroke (usually vascular risk factors) and medication compliance and tolerance, and assess and manage any new symptoms. The neurologist/physician should only be required if difficulties arise in controlling the underlying disease or interpreting and managing new symptoms.

14.77 When to refer to a specialist?

Refer any patient for whom you need help – e.g. diagnosis, investigation, acute management, rehabilitation and/or secondary prevention.

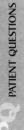

PATIENT QUESTIONS

14.78 How can the risk of another stroke be reduced?

Diet

A diet that includes all foods in moderation is advisable. Particular emphasis should be given to maintaining a diet low in saturated fat, alcohol and salt; and high in fibre, fruit and vegetables. Saturated fats increase blood cholesterol (even more than cholesterol in the diet), and alcohol and salt both increase blood pressure. High blood pressure is the strongest risk factor for stroke, and high blood cholesterol is the strongest risk factor for heart attacks.

Smoking

Cigarette smoking increases the risk of stroke as well as heart attacks, lung cancer and other cancers and diseases of blood vessels. It is absolutely crucial to stop smoking in order to minimise the risk of stroke and to maximise the benefit of other efforts to reduce it. Nicotine patches or gum, used in consultation with your doctor, improve the likelihood of successfully giving up smoking.

Blood pressure

High blood pressure is the most important causal risk factor for stroke. Fortunately, it can be lowered with a change in lifestyle and with tablets. This will substantially reduce the risk of another stroke. However, many people unfortunately do not know that they have high blood pressure until it is measured. It is therefore important that patients have their blood pressure checked regularly (e.g. every 1–6 months) by their doctor. If the blood pressure is too high (generally above 140/85) then it can be lowered by losing weight, exercising regularly and avoiding excess alcohol and salt in the diet. In addition, tablets can be taken each day that lower blood pressure, although (as with most drugs) these may sometimes also cause side-effects.

Aspirin, clopidogrel and dipyridamole

For patients with the most common type of stroke (an ischaemic stroke caused by a blood clot that has formed on an area of hardening of the arteries) it has been shown that tablets that block the formation of these blood clots can help to prevent further strokes. Because these clots are mainly formed by cells in the blood called platelets, the drugs that interfere with them are called antiplatelet drugs. The best known examples are aspirin, clopidogrel and dipyridamole.

The most widely used is aspirin, in a dose of 75 mg, 150 mg or 300 mg each day. This reduces the risk of further strokes and heart attacks by about one-quarter. It probably does not matter which dose of aspirin the doctor prescribes, because they are all effective, but lower doses may cause less indigestion. For patients who cannot tolerate aspirin, other alternatives exist, such as clopidogrel and dipyridamole. Furthermore, there is increasing evidence that combining aspirin with clopidogrel or dipyridamole may be more effective than taking aspirin alone.

Most patients with ischaemic stroke due to hardening of the arteries are advised to continue to take aspirin (and/or clopidogrel or dipyridamole) indefinitely unless they develop adverse effects.

Anticoagulants

Anticoagulants (e.g. warfarin, coumarin) are recommended for individuals with ischaemic stroke (i.e. stroke caused by a blocked artery to the brain) in which the underlying cause is a disorder of the heart that caused a blood clot to form there and then to break off and lodge in a blood vessel to the brain. The most common disorders that do this are a recent heart attack, a disease of one of the heart valves, an artificial heart valve and an abnormal irregular heart beat (atrial fibrillation). In patients with these conditions, warfarin is very effective in reducing the risk of further blood clots forming and further strokes occurring.

However, warfarin is a very potent blood thinner, and its effects on the blood need to be closely monitored by regular blood checks. Doctors aim to keep the blood about twice to three times as thin as normal. A blood test recording an INR (international normalised ratio) of 2.0–3.0 is usually advised. However, if the blood is not thin enough (INR 1.0–1.8) further blood clots and strokes may occur, and if the blood is too thin (INR more than 3.5) then there is an increased risk of bleeding happening somewhere in the body.

Many drugs can interact adversely with warfarin and make the blood too thick or thin. Alcohol is one of them. So, alcohol intake should be minimised in patients taking warfarin. Patients will be given further important information about this in discussions with their doctor.

Carotid surgery (endarterectomy) and carotid stenting

About 1 in 10 people with a stroke caused by a blocked blood vessel have a very narrow (but not completely blocked) artery in the front of the neck on one side (the carotid artery). In order to reduce the chances of this narrowing causing another stroke, there are two ways of removing it. One is by an open surgical operation called a carotid endarterectomy. This involves a surgeon making an incision (about 10 cm long) down the front of the neck on one side, opening up the artery, cleaning it out and then sewing it up again. This operation takes about $1\frac{1}{2}$ hours and patients are not usually in hospital for more than about 4–5 days afterwards. Carotid endarterectomy is associated with a small risk (about 2–3 per 100) of actually causing a stroke at the time, but for the 97 or so in every 100 patients who have no problems after the operation, it reduces the risk of another stroke by about half.

Another, as yet unproven, technique is to put a needle into the main artery in the groin, which carries blood to the leg. A catheter is passed through the needle and guided up the artery (in the opposite direction to the blood flow coming down into the leg) into the main blood vessel in the abdomen and chest, and then into the artery in the neck. A little balloon on the end of the catheter is then inflated. This process, called angioplasty, opens up the artery. However, in order to keep the artery open, a tiny cylinder of wire mesh, called a stent, is then placed over the balloon. The balloon is deflated and the catheter is withdrawn. The stent remains embedded in the inner lining of the artery and helps to keep the artery open. At present, the safety and long-term effectiveness of carotid artery stenting, compared with carotid endarterectomy, is being studied in research trials.

Research

Many of the new effective treatments for stroke have been developed and tested for their safety and effectiveness in research studies before being introduced widely into practice. Of course, there are always new ideas and treatments to be tested to see if they are any better than current best practice. The most common type of research method to evaluate the effect of new treatments is called a *randomised controlled trial*. This is a study design where a new kind of treatment is compared with the currently accepted best treatment to see if it is equally safe and whether it is any more effective. If there is no effective treatment at present, a 'dummy' pill, called a *placebo*, may be used, which looks and tastes the same as the pill being studied and is harmless but ineffective. When doctors are uncertain whether to treat a patient with the current best available treatment (or placebo) or the promising new one, they may ask the patient whether they would consent to being allocated at random to one or other treatment. If the patient agrees, they are otherwise treated exactly the same as any other patient and given the best of medical care. All patients are followed-up over a period of time and the outcome of all patients in both groups is recorded by someone who is not aware of which treatment was given to which patient. In other words, the outcome measurement is performed 'blind' to knowledge of the way the treatment was allocated. The results are then analysed, and the proportions of patients in each treatment group who did well are compared. This helps doctors decide if one treatment is better than another.

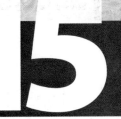

Post-stroke care (how should new problems be managed?)

PROGRESS OF STROKE

15.1 What are the causes of neurological deterioration after stroke?

NEUROLOGICAL

■ Progression/completion of the stroke
■ Extension of the stroke
■ Haemorrhagic transformation of infarcted brain
■ Raised intracranial pressure due to brain oedema
■ Raised intracranial pressure due to obstructive hydrocephalus
■ Epileptic seizures
■ Incorrect initial diagnosis (*see Differential diagnosis of stroke, Chapter 3*)
■ Recurrent stroke.

NON-NEUROLOGICAL

■ Metabolic encephalopathy – hyponatraemia, hypoglycaemia, hypoxia, hypercapnia
■ Toxic encephalopathy – infection, drugs
■ Depression.

NB. Almost all the causes of deterioration after stroke listed above are treatable and reversible if recognised promptly. Hence the importance of regular monitoring of vital signs by nursing staff (and communication of changes to medical staff), frequent repeated assessments of the patient by the stroke team, and immediate action.

15.2 What is 'progressing stroke' or 'stroke in evolution'?

Following stroke onset, some patients continue to deteriorate neurologically over the next few hours or days. This is variably referred to as evolving or progressing stroke but as often as not it is due to one of many other possible causes (see 'causes of neurological deterioration after stroke' above), and is often reversible with prompt and appropriate treatment.[1,2]

If, after excluding other causes, it is suspected that the cause is progressive thrombosis or thromboembolism, and the patient has not responded to optimal antiplatelet therapy, then intravenous heparin may be used despite the lack of evidence supporting its effectiveness (*see Qs. 13.22, 14.75*).

15.3 What is haemorrhagic transformation of infarcted brain?

This is a natural occurrence in up to 65% of stroke patients (usually about 7–14%) and up to 90% of patients with cardioembolic stroke within the first week after symptom onset (*see Q. 3.35*). However, it leads to parenchymal haematoma formation and neurological deterioration in only a minority of patients (usually about 0.5–8%).[3]

Haemorrhagic transformation of infarcted brain seems to occur in patients with acute ischaemic stroke in whom spontaneous or thrombolysis-induced recanalisation is delayed (beyond about 6 hours).[4] The mechanism is uncertain but may simply reflect ischaemia and infarction of the vessels (as well as the brain) distal to an arterial occlusion. Recanalisation leads to reperfusion of infarcted vessels that have lost their integrity (due to ischaemia – lack of blood supply via the vasa vasorum), which rupture when the reperfusing blood is pumped in at high (systemic arterial) pressure.

Risk factors for haemorrhagic transformation include delayed arterial recanalisation, increasing age, hypertension, large infarcts (severe initial neurological deficit) and embolic cause for the arterial occlusion.

15.4 How is haemorrhagic transformation of infarcted brain recognised and managed?

Clinically important haemorrhagic transformation of infarcted brain manifests as an acute or subacute deterioration in neurological function, often with an increase in severity of the focal neurological deficits caused by the initial cerebral infarct.

If a patient deteriorates neurologically, the appropriate initial investigation is an urgent plain cranial computed tomography (CT) scan. This will show haemorrhagic transformation as an area of high density (whiteness) due to blood in the region of brain infarction (*see Fig. 3.14*). Of course, the CT scan may also identify or rule out other possible causes of neurological deterioration (e.g. hydrocephalus) but not all possible causes (e.g. hypoglycaemia).

The management of haemorrhagic transformation is usually to withhold any antithrombotic therapy (e.g. warfarin and heparin definitely, aspirin probably) and consider whether neurosurgical decompression is indicated (usually only if the haemorrhage is life-threatening).

15.5 What are the causes and clinical features of raised intracranial pressure after stroke?

Haemorrhagic stroke may cause a rapid rise in intracranial pressure, due to the space occupying effects of the haemorrhage, and manifest as rapid onset headache, vomiting and loss of consciousness.

Ischaemic stroke does not so commonly cause a rise in intracranial pressure unless the infarct is large (e.g. complete middle cerebral artery territory infarction) and about 48 hours, and often longer, have evolved. Cytotoxic and vasogenic brain oedema is usually maximal about 72 hours after brain infarction. An exception is cerebellar and brainstem infarction, which may cause sufficient early oedema to compress the cerebrospinal

fluid (CSF) pathways in the posterior fossa (e.g. fourth ventricle or ce...
aqueduct) and cause raised intracranial pressure by means of an obstructive
hydrocephalus.

15.6 How should raised intracranial pressure be managed after stroke?

The management of raised intracranial pressure aims to establish and treat
the underlying cause and exacerbating factors, and to lower the pressure.

General measures include fluid restriction, elevation of the head of the
bed, treatment of fever, correction of hypoxia and hypercapnia and
avoidance of hypo-osmolar fluids.

Specific measures depend on the cause but none actually reduce the
oedema – they shrink the surrounding normal brain or decompress the
brain. If the cause is obstructive hydrocephalus, drainage of the CSF by a
ventricular drain may be all that is required. If the cause is brain oedema,
intracranial pressure can be lowered successfully with osmotic diuretics
(e.g. mannitol 20%, 0.25–0.5 g/kg every 4 hours, and glycerol, providing the
blood–brain barrier is intact), hyperventilation and even decompressive
craniectomy. However, it is unclear whether such aggressive interventions
are associated with improved survival and an acceptable quality of life.[5,6]

Selected patients who are deteriorating neurologically (e.g. deteriorating
consciousness level, new focal neurological signs) and who are considered
to have a chance of a reasonable recovery (e.g. young, otherwise healthy)
should be transferred to an intensive care unit for monitoring and
aggressive management of raised intracranial pressure. However, despite
this, early decline in conscious state remains a very poor prognostic factor
for survival and survival free of handicap.

Incidentally, steroids are not effective for the raised intracranial pressure
caused by haemorrhagic stroke or the cytotoxic oedema caused by brain
infarction (but are effective for the vasogenic oedema caused by brain
tumours, for example). Furthermore, they are associated with multiple
potential adverse effects.

COMPLICATIONS

15.7 What are the common complications after stroke and how can they be prevented?

Many of the complications that may occur after stroke are common yet
preventable (*Table 15.1*). The key is to anticipate them in high-risk patients,
implement appropriate prevention strategies and assess patients regularly
(at least daily). Patients at particular risk are the elderly, those with pre-
existing handicap or diabetes, a total anterior circulation syndrome (TACS;

...incontinence, and those who have been hospitalised ...ys.[7]

...lications after stroke

	Prevention strategy
...stroke	
Epile... ...ures	Anticipate after cortical stroke; treat after first seizure
Pneumo...	Assess swallowing function immediately and regularly
	If any risk of aspiration, feed by tube (nasogastric, percutaneous endoscopic gastrostomy, intravenous)
	Chest physiotherapy
Fever	Exclude infection (urine, chest, intravenous line, heart), infarction (chest, heart, bowel, limb), deep vein thrombosis, pulmonary embolism, drug allergy.
After first few days	
Urinary problems	Post-void bladder ultrasound – if residual urine volume (> 100 ml), empty bladder by catheter, and repeat 6–8-hourly
	Avoid indwelling catheters if possible
	Useful appliances: absorbent pads and pants, urinals + non-spill valve for men, bedside commode, penile sheath
Bowel problems	Monitor frequency of bowel movements
	Maintain fluid and fibre intake
Dehydration	Monitor and ensure adequate fluid intake
Pressure sores	Good nursing (regular turning)
	Natural sheepskin fleeces and bootees, padded/foam mattresses, Roho cushions, low-air-loss beds
Venous thromboembolism	Anticipate if immobile – mobilise early
	Full-length graduated compression stockings
	Aspirin or subcutaneous heparin 5000 U twice daily if ischaemic stroke
Spasticity and contractures	Regular physiotherapy, and exercise at home
	Baclofen, diazepam, botulinum toxin (focal spasticity)
Pain	Exclude treatable cause
	Amitriptyline for central post-stroke pain
Painful shoulder	Recognise high-risk patient (low tone, weakness, neglect, proprioceptive loss, visual field defect) and avoid pulling on shoulder when nursing and treating patient
	Physiotherapy (positioning, mobilisation, exercises)
	Support –: orthoses, sling, cuff (but may promote spasticity)
	Medication – analgesics (systemic, local)

TABLE 15.1 (Cont'd)	
Complication	Prevention strategy
	Other physical – ultrasound, acupuncture, biofeedback, transepidermal nerve stimulation
	Surgery – sympathectomy, contracture relief, humeral head suspension
Falls and fractures	Recognise high-risk patient and environment
	Regularly and systematically look for signs of fracture as patients with communication problems, sensory loss or neglect may not report injury
Low mood and anxiety	Recognise high-risk patient (previous depression, language problems, poor functional status, social isolation)
	Explain to patient nature, sequelae and prognosis of stroke
	Psychotherapy, antidepressants
Emotionalism	Amitriptyline 25 mg nocte, or fluoxetine.

15.8 Which patients are at particularly high risk of complications after stroke?

See Q. 15.7.

15.9 How common are epileptic seizures after stroke?

Epileptic seizures occur in about 5% of patients during the first 2 weeks following stroke.[8–10] The cause is usually an infarct or haemorrhage involving the cerebral cortex. Most seizures after stroke are partial in onset with or without secondary generalisation. Postictal confusion is often prolonged in elderly people and may contribute to physical injury sustained during seizure activity.

15.10 What is the management of epileptic seizures soon after stroke?

The diagnosis of a seizure following stroke can be challenging and might need a witnessed event. Once confirmed, the diagnosis of stroke should be reviewed, taking care to ensure that the focal neurological symptoms and signs are not merely a postictal phenomenon (e.g. Todd's paresis) or secondary to another intracranial pathology such as encephalitis, and that non-convulsive seizures are not misdiagnosed as a stroke. If seizures are due to stroke, the cause is usually a large infarct or haemorrhage involving the cerebral cortex.

Antiepileptic drugs are the mainstay of treatment, as in other forms of secondary epilepsy. Low-dose (but therapeutic) regimens can help keep adverse effects to a minimum. Patients, and often their spouses and children, need to be convinced of the need for lifelong treatment because of the high risk of recurrence associated with an underlying structural lesion of the brain (i.e. infarction or haemorrhage). The choice of antiepileptic drug depends on the adverse effect and drug interaction profile. A double-blind trial supported lamotrigine over carbamazepine in the elderly.[11] An acceptable alternative is sodium valproate which is also well tolerated in the elderly and undergoes fewer drug interactions than carbamazepine and phenytoin.[12] Complete seizure control can be expected in more than 70% of patients.

15.11 How common is depression after stroke?

Depression occurs commonly, and understandably, after stroke. At 4 months after stroke, about one-quarter of patients have DSM-III criteria for a depressive disorder, and more than half of these remain depressed at 12 months.[13] After stroke, a substantial proportion of patients also experience anxiety states such as agoraphobia and social phobias.

15.12 Is the risk of depression after stroke influenced by the site of the stroke in the brain?

No.[14]

15.13 Is post-stroke depression association with a poor outcome?

Yes, post-stroke depression is associated with an increased risk of death and poor functional outcome among survivors.[15–19]

15.14 Why is post-stroke depression associated with a poor outcome?

It is uncertain why post-stroke depression is associated with a poor functional outcome, but it may be due to the fact that depressed and disabled stroke survivors are not motivated to be rehabilitated and tend to remain in bed and avoid active rehabilitation. They are then prone to the common complications of stroke (e.g. deep vein thrombosis – DVT – and pulmonary embolism, chest infection, urinary tract infections and skin breaks), some of which can be fatal, and fail to maximise their potential for full functional recovery.

15.15 Can depression be treated after stroke?

Depression after stroke should be treated with psychosocial support and antidepressants if necessary. The results of four small clinical trials of the treatment of post-stroke depression with nortriptyline (up to 100 mg/day), citalopram (10–20 mg/day), or fluoxetine (20 mg/day) indicate a significant favourable effect of active treatment on depression (but the effect on long-term functional outcome requires further study).[20–22] Early socialisation may also help.

DEEP VEIN THROMBOSIS AND PULMONARY EMBOLISM

15.16 How common is DVT after acute stroke?

Studies with iodine-125 fibrinogen screening in patients with acute hemiplegic stroke have shown an incidence of DVT of about 50% within 2 weeks in the absence of heparin prophylaxis (*see Q. 12.10*). DVTs develop as early as the second day, with a peak incidence between 2 and 7 days after stroke.[23]

In a study of 150 patients admitted to a stroke rehabilitation unit at, on average, 9 weeks after stroke, bilateral venography revealed DVT in 33%.

Most DVTs after stroke affect the paralysed leg and are asymptomatic. About two-thirds are below-knee DVTs, in contrast to unselected (non-stroke) patients presenting with symptomatic DVT, in whom the majority are proximal.

15.17 What are the main risk factors for venous thromboembolism after acute stroke?

The risk of DVT correlates with the degree of paralysis and is greater in older patients and those who have atrial fibrillation. The predilection for the paralysed leg is probably explained by a combination of loss of the calf muscle pump and repeated minor trauma.

15.18 What is the clinical significance of asymptomatic proximal DVT after stroke?

The main clinical significance of asymptomatic proximal DVT is its potential to cause fatal pulmonary embolism. Indeed, most symptomatic pulmonary emboli in unselected patients are unheralded and arise from previously subclinical DVT.

15.19 What is the clinical significance of asymptomatic below-knee DVT after stroke?

Although pulmonary emboli arising from below-knee DVTs are more likely to be small and asymptomatic, the main clinical significance of asymptomatic below-knee DVT is its potential to extend proximally, as it does in about 20% of cases, and also to cause pulmonary embolism (i.e. pulmonary embolism can occur in the absence of propagation).

15.20 What is the clinical significance of pelvic vein thrombosis after stroke?

Pelvic vein thromboses may account for a significant minority of pulmonary emboli (about 11%) and thrombosis of the inferior vena cava for about 5%.

15.21 How common is pulmonary embolism after acute stroke?

The incidence of pulmonary embolism in the absence of heparin prophylaxis varies from 0.8% to 13% at 2 weeks (*see Q. 12.10*).

Autopsy studies show that half of patients who die in hospital after the first 48 hours following stroke have evidence of pulmonary embolism; pulmonary emboli account for 13–25% of early deaths after stroke.

Fatal pulmonary emboli are most common in the second, third and fourth weeks after stroke.

15.22 How is pulmonary embolism diagnosed?

The diagnosis of pulmonary embolism is frequently missed in stroke patients because the clinical symptoms and signs are non-specific and stroke patients may not complain of symptoms because of dysphasia, cognitive impairment or mental obtundation. In addition, pneumonia, the illness for which pulmonary embolism is most often mistaken, is also a common complication after stroke, and patients with pneumonia and up to two thirds of patients with pulmonary embolism both develop fever. Indeed, the two conditions not uncommonly coexist.

Stroke patients with suspected pulmonary embolism (e.g. chest pain, shortness of breath, haemoptysis or 'non-specific neurological deterioration' – there may be no chest symptoms of pulmonary embolism) should be investigated with electrocardiography (ECG), arterial blood gases and ventilation–perfusion scanning as the imaging modality of first choice.

15.23 How is DVT diagnosed?

The presently available techniques for the objective diagnosis of DVT include contrast venography, non-invasive methods (e.g. compression venous ultrasonography) and biochemical assays.

The optimal non-invasive diagnostic strategies for patients with suspected venous thrombosis are:

- Serial compression ultrasonography (i.e. a repeat study 1 week later in patients with an initial normal result)
- Clinical score combined with compression ultrasonography
- Compression ultrasonography combined with an assay for D-dimer, a fragment that is specific for the degradation of fibrin.[24]

15.24 How should symptomatic venous thromboembolism be treated?

Treatment of symptomatic venous thromboembolism (pulmonary embolism or proximal DVT) with full anticoagulation for at least 3 months is highly effective in reducing morbidity and mortality among unselected (non-stroke) patients. Among patients presenting with symptomatic pulmonary embolism, a 3-month period of full anticoagulation reduces the risk of recurrent fatal pulmonary embolism to only 1.5%.

Low-molecular-weight heparin is at least as effective as unfractionated heparin and is associated with a lower mortality.

The treatment of symptomatic venous thromboembolism should therefore begin with intravenous or subcutaneous heparin, which should continue until oral anticoagulant treatment, started concurrently, increases the international normalised ratio (INR) above 2.0 for more than 24 hours (*Box 15.1*). The optimum duration of oral anticoagulant treatment is unresolved (6 weeks, 3 months, 6 months, lifelong), but may be guided by the presence of temporary or persistent risk factors or presentation with recurrent venous thromboembolism.[24]

BOX 15.1 Initial treatment of established venous thrombosis of the legs or pulmonary embolism, without refractory hypotension

Unfractionated heparin

If unfractionated heparin is preferred initially, the dose is 5000 U intravenous bolus followed by 30 000–35 000 U/24 h by intravenous infusion or 35 000–40 000 U/24 h subcutaneously, adjusted to maintain partial thromboplastin time at 1.5–2.5 × control.

Low-molecular-weight heparin

If low-molecular-weight heparin is preferred initially, the alternative drugs and their doses are:

- Dalteparin 200 anti-Xa U/kg once daily
- Enoxaparin 100 anti-Xa U/kg twice daily
- Nadroparin 90 anti-Xa U/kg twice daily
- Reviparin 90 anti-Xa U/kg twice daily
- Tinzaparin 175 anti-Xa U/kg once daily

by subcutaneous injection without bolus injection and laboratory monitoring.

Both regimens are continued for 5–10 days with an oral anticoagulant started on day 1, then continued alone.

15.25 How should symptomatic below-knee DVT be treated?

The treatment of symptomatic below-knee DVT is controversial. The current consensus is that these patients should be either fully anticoagulated or followed up with serial non-invasive testing for 14 days, an approach shown to be safe in the absence of proximal extension.

RESIDUAL HANDICAPS

15.26 How should transient ischaemic attack and stroke patients be advised about driving a motor vehicle?

Patients who have suffered a *transient ischaemic attack* (TIA) may drive on the advice of their doctor. Individuals who are having recurrent events that could impair driving ability should not drive until medical assessment leads to effective prophylaxis.

Patients who have suffered a *stroke* should not drive for a minimum of 1 month after the stroke if there is significant neurological, perceptual or cognitive deficit that would compromise performance. Dense hemiplegia, visual field defect, visual or sensory neglect and receptive dysphasia require specialist assessment and clearance. Return to driving depends on assessment by the doctor and, where appropriate, an 'off' and 'on' road driving assessment by a registered driving assessor. A visual field defect need not necessarily exclude driving but the patient must meet all the visual criteria for driving:

- *Binocular visual acuity*, measured with both eyes open while wearing any corrective lenses usually worn for driving – must be better than 6/12. More than one error in reading the letters of the 6/12 lines is a fail.
- *Binocular visual field along the horizontal meridian* – must be more than 120° when measured with a Goldman IV4e target or its equivalent. Automated visual field tests, including the Estermann Field Test, are acceptable in the absence of clinical evidence of more peripheral visual field deficits.
- *Hemianopia* – normally fails to meet visual field requirement.
- *Quadrantanopia or scotoma* – patients should not drive until driver licensing authority has considered optometrist's or ophthalmologist's report.
- *Eye movements* – patients with diplopia within the central 20° should not drive.
- *Nystagmus* – patients should not drive if binocular visual acuity is worse than 6/12.
- *Loss of vision in one eye* – patients should not drive for 3 months after permanent loss of monocular vision. Patients may then drive if they meet visual acuity and other vision criteria. They should have mirrors on both sides of the car or motorcycle.
- *Colour vision defects* – no restriction. Patients with red (protan) colour defects should be cautioned about hazardous situations – especially traffic lights, brake lights and parked cars at night. They may not be eligible for a commercial vehicle licence.[25]

Patients who have suffered a *subarachnoid haemorrhage* should not drive for 3 months after the event. Medical and occupational therapist assessment is recommended. If appropriate, refer to an ophthalmologist or optometrist for formal assessment of visual fields.

Patients who have a *vascular malformation of the brain* should not drive until assessed by a specialist. The driver licensing authority may issue a conditional licence if the risk of complications is small and the patient is free of other conditions such as epilepsy.

15.27 How does stroke affect the patient's sexual function?

Most stroke patients and their spouses/partners experience a marked decline in sexual function (e.g. libido, sexual arousal, erectile and orgasmic ability, vaginal lubrication and coital frequency) and sexual satisfaction after their stroke. The major underlying factors are physical, psychological and social. They include general attitude toward sexuality, fear of impotence, inability to discuss sexuality, unwillingness to participate in sexual activity and degree of functional disability.[26,27] However a minority of patients (about 10%) experience an increase in libido and sexual satisfaction, which does not always appear to be related to the site of the brain lesion (as opposed to hypersexuality, which has been associated with temporal lobe lesions). It is probably explained by improved relations between the patient and the spouse or by other positive changes in psychosocial elements.

Sexual counselling after stroke is needed for many stroke patients and their spouses. However, because most patients will not disclose their sexual problems spontaneously, they must be sought by direct questioning.

15.28 What is spasticity?

Spasticity is classically defined as 'a velocity-dependent increase of tonic stretch reflexes (muscle tone) with exaggerated tendon reflexes'. However, it may be viewed as a broader syndrome not simply limited to an increase in tonic stretch reflexes and an increased resistance to passive stretch (hypertonia) but also including focal muscle hypertonia with dystonic features.

It is usually caused by an upper motor neurone (supranuclear) lesion of the corticospinal tracts, which causes a characteristic syndrome consisting of negative signs (muscle weakness, lack of dexterity and paresis) and positive signs (flexor spasms, increased tendon reflexes and 'clasp-knife' rigidity). These positive features are those of spasticity.

15.29 What are the adverse effects of spasticity?

Spasticity may be associated with painful muscle spasms, muscle contractures and even bone fractures, predispose to pressure sores and interfere with rehabilitation and the performance of activities of daily living.

It is a distinct problem that arises in many stroke patients who have damage to the corticospinal tracts. It is implicated in the formation of muscle contracture and even in the recovery of muscle strength.

15.30 How can spasticity after stroke be minimised?

Spasticity can be reduced by the methods listed in *Box 15.2*.

BOX 15.2 Methods for reducing residual spasticity after stroke

Conservative therapies
These are practised by physiotherapists (*see Q. 11.15*) and include:

- Passive and active stretching exercises through the range of motion of the muscle and joint
- Muscle heating or cooling
- Electrical stimulation of muscle.

Drug therapies
These include:

- *Neural depressants* – baclofen (oral and intrathecal), benzodiazepines, clonidine, tizanidine
- *Muscle relaxants* – dantrolene.

Such systemic treatments are only partially effective in reducing spasticity and may also have adverse effects of sedation and generalised weakness.

Botulinum toxin injection into spastic muscles
Botulinum toxin A, injected in small doses into spastic muscle(s), with or without electromyographic guidance, is effective within 7–10 days in 80–90% of patients.[28] It is taken up by peripheral nerve terminals and prevents calcium-dependent release of acetylcholine from the presynaptic axon at motor endplates, resulting in a reversible, partial chemical denervation and paralysis of the injected muscle, and reduction or abolition of the spasms. The effect lasts for about 2–4 months, after which terminal sprouting restores muscle end-plate neurotransmission. Up to 5% of initially responsive patients may subsequently not respond, because of:

- Incorrect storage of the toxin
- Underdosing
- Injection of inappropriate muscles
- A worsening or change in the pattern of spasticity (possibly with involvement of deep, inaccessible muscles)

BOX 15.2 (*Cont'd*)

- Development of contractures
- Altered perception of response
- The development of immunity.

Immunity is associated with very frequent injections, 'booster' injections and higher doses. Higher doses of botulinum toxin-F may be effective, with few adverse effects.

It is important that botulinum toxin injections are only used in conjunction with physiotherapy – i.e. they are an adjunct to an active and ongoing physiotherapy programme.

Motor point or nerve blocks

- Phenol or alcohol injections.

These neurolytic agents are painful, may produce irreversible scarring or sensory loss and have a variable duration of action. Administration of phenol can be difficult because it requires percutaneous injection into accessible nerves or surgical isolation of the nerve in less accessible targets.

Surgical interventions

- Tendon transplant or lengthening, rhizotomies, myelotomies, neural transection.

The effect of these procedures is permanent, their efficacy is variable and their morbidity significant.

PATIENT QUESTIONS

15.31 What problems may arise after a later stroke?

Depression

Depression occurs commonly, and understandably, after stroke. It usually becomes apparent in the first few weeks and may persist for several weeks to months. Because it is often associated with a lack of interest in rehabilitation, it can adversely affect the recovery and outcome of patients after stroke. It can be treated successfully with appropriate counselling and antidepressant medication.

Sometimes, stroke can lead to outbursts of uncontrollable emotion (usually crying, but sometimes laughing), called emotional lability, which also may respond to counselling and antidepressant medication.

15.32 What about life after stroke?

In general, patients are encouraged to return to their normal prestroke lifestyle, providing they feel up to it and providing features of it were not possibly responsible for the stroke (e.g. smoking, excess alcohol). Indeed, resuming physical and sexual activity and, if possible, going back to work are encouraged. They will improve recovery and will not cause another stroke; indeed, they are likely to reduce the risk.

Sport and exercise

After a stroke, patients are encouraged to resume physical activities and hobbies, as long as they are physically capable of doing so. Naturally, persistent problems with intellect, mood, speech, vision, muscle weakness and coordination, and balance may restrict these activities.

Sexual activity

Patients are encouraged to resume sexual relations after a stroke. However, some patients take some time to regain their sex drive and others find that the effects of the stroke (e.g. limb paralysis or stiffness) can make it difficult to get into positions of intimacy. However, these problems can generally be overcome with help and advice from the stroke team. Some men have problems maintaining an erection because of the effects of the stroke itself, the cause of the stroke (e.g. diabetes, smoking) or the side effects of some of the drugs used to reduce the risk of another stroke (e.g. drugs that lower blood pressure). Fortunately, there are now many successful ways of overcoming this problem, which the doctor can advise about.

Drinking alcohol

Excessive alcohol intake is strongly discouraged because it may interact adversely with some of the medications the patient may be taking to prevent another stroke (e.g. warfarin), because it raises blood pressure and thus increases the risk of another stroke, and because the effects of intoxication may alter the patient's judgement and put them at risk of injuring themselves. However, there should be no problem with consuming alcohol in moderation (i.e. 1–2 standard drinks per day).

Driving a motor vehicle

Whether or not a patient has recovered functionally after a TIA or stroke, they should not drive for at least a month. This is because the risk of having another stroke is highest in the first month or so.

Patients who have been left with some disability that would interfere with driving should not drive at all until they have been cleared by their doctor. The main disabilities after stroke that are relevant to driving are:

- Loss of vision (usually loss of one half of the visual field of each eye, so that the patient cannot see anything to the right or to the left)
- Inattention to activity in one half of the visual field of each eye
- Weakness or incoordination of limb movement
- Lack of awareness
- Slowed reaction times.

If there is any doubt about patients' fitness to drive, the doctor can refer them to a special centre that will assess their driving ability (both off the road and on the road).

In many countries, patients are legally obliged to inform the relevant Driving and Vehicle Licensing Authority (DVLA) that they have had a stroke and the effects it has had on them. In the UK the address is DVLA, Longview Road, Swansea SA99 1TU (tel: 01792 783438).

If patients do not inform the DVLA and continue to drive, their insurance company is not obliged to cover any costs incurred in the event of them having an accident. They may also be liable for any damage they cause to others.

Flying in an aeroplane

It is generally safe to fly after a stroke, but patients travelling abroad should inform their travel insurance company that they have had a stroke.

Resuming back at work

Deciding whether and when to go back to work depends on many factors, such as the type of work the patient wants to do, the persistent problems that the stroke may have caused, and the patient's desire, need and tolerance to work.

Many people feel quite tired after a stroke and experience difficulty in concentrating and carrying out any kind of physical activity for any length of time. Patients are often encouraged to resume part-time work to begin with, and then see how they are doing. Ultimately, the patient is probably the best judge of whether and when to go back to work, unless they have had a type of stroke that reduces their awareness of and insight into their disabilities; some patients think they have no problems after a stroke when indeed they do.

15.33 Is there any support for families and carers?

Stroke affects not only the patient but also their entire family. The impact of stroke on carers has been a subject of much research recently. Several organisations are now recognising the needs of carers, which include:

- A named person or contact for advice, particularly after the patient is discharged from hospital
- An information pack that tells carers how to contact and access local community services that can support the patient and carer
- A local stroke group or club, which may provide access to information, advice, practical help and involvement in activities such as speech therapy, exercise classes, social gatherings. Some local stroke groups also cater specifically for younger stroke patients.

15.34 Are there any volunteer and support groups for stroke survivors and their families and carers?

Support groups for stroke survivors are listed in Appendix A at the end of the book.

Stroke in special populations

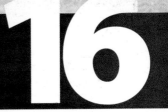

16.1 How common is stroke among children?

Stroke affects about 2.7 per 100,000 children per year, of whom about 45% are under 5 years of age.[1]

16.2 What types of stroke affect children?

Ischaemic stroke affects about 70% and haemorrhagic stroke about 30% of children with stroke.[1] Most haemorrhagic strokes are caused by intracranial vascular abnormalities such as vascular malformations and aneurysms. The majority of patients with ischaemic stroke (about 85%) have at least one detectable risk factor for stroke. Haematological (prothrombotic) and metabolic disorders cause about 25% of ischaemic strokes and frequently coexist. Cardiac disorders, particularly congenital heart disease (in the setting of cardiac surgery or catheterisation) account for about 15–20% of ischaemic strokes. Vasculopathies cause about 20% of ischaemic stroke. The most common is moyamoya syndrome.

16.3 What is the outcome of stroke among children?

About 20% of children with stroke die, about 45% experience a persistent neurological deficit or epilepsy and about 35% recover without sequelae.[1]

Recurrent stroke occurs in up to 20% and is associated with increased mortality.

16.4 What is the management of the 'young stroke'

The management of stroke and transient ischaemic attack (TIA) in young patients (i.e. less than about 40 years of age) is not very different from the management of older patients. The range of causes is similar but the probabilities differ: among patients older than 60 years atherothromboembolism and complex small-vessel disease are the most common causes of stroke (followed by embolism from the heart) whereas among patients younger than 40 years atherothromboembolism and complex small-vessel disease are most uncommon and other arterial diseases, such as dissection and inflammatory arterial disease, are more common, as are migraine and embolism from the heart.

Young patients who survive a stroke also tend to have a more favourable prognosis for functional recovery.

16.5 How common is stroke during pregnancy and the puerperium?

Stroke complicating pregnancy or the puerperium is very rare. It occurs in perhaps only 1–3 per 10 000 deliveries in developed countries.[2] Indeed, it is so rare that it is not possible to estimate the exact risk, nor even the size of any excess risk over and above what is expected in non-pregnant women of the same (childbearing) age.

16.6 What are the typical causes of stroke during pregnancy and the puerperium?

The diseases that may typically cause stroke during pregnancy and the puerperium are:

- Infective endocarditis
- Paradoxical embolism of thrombus from the legs or pelvic veins, via a right-to-left cardiac shunt (e.g. patent foramen ovale, pulmonary arteriovenous malformation) to occlude a large artery (e.g. acute middle cerebral artery occlusion)
- Metastases from haemorrhagic choriocarcinoma may cause multiple intracerebral haematomas – the diagnostic test is a raised serum human chorionic gonadotrophin concentration
- Cervical artery dissection (during labour)
- Rupture of an intracranial aneurysm or arteriovenous malformation causing intracranial haemorrhage (usually during labour)
- Low-flow infarction or disseminated intravascular coagulation complication shock associated with obstetric disasters
- Peripartum dilating cardiomyopathy and embolism of thrombus to brain
- Sickle-cell crisis
- Intracranial venous thrombosis (particularly during the puerperium)
- Ergot-type, bromocriptine and other vasoconstricting drugs causing post-partum cerebral segmental vasoconstriction (puerperal cerebral angiopathy) with headache, seizures, focal infarcts and haemorrhage.

16.7 What is eclampsia?

Eclampsia is a syndrome characterised by increasing blood pressure, proteinuria, peripheral oedema, cerebral oedema and sometimes 'vasospasm' and haemorrhage, complicated by disseminated intravascular coagulation.

It is characterised clinically by a global or multifocal encephalopathy with headache, seizures, cortical blindness and impaired consciousness.

The serum alkaline phosphatase and uric acid concentrations are raised.

Imaging of the brain by computed tomography (CT) shows bilateral hypodensities in the parieto-occipital lobes of the brain.[3] Imaging of the brain by magnetic resonance imaging (MRI), T2-weighted images, shows increased signal in the occipital and parietal lobes bilaterally, and narrowing of cerebral arteries. The differential diagnoses include intracranial venous thrombosis and focal cerebral infarction (bilateral posterior cerebral artery) and haemorrhage.

The underlying cause remains unclear. Severe hypertension may lead to narrowing of the lumen of cerebral arteries by inducing vasospasm, oedema in the vessel wall or other mechanisms. It may also impair cerebral autoregulation and promote extravasation of fluids and proteins into the brain parenchyma.

Possible effective treatments include magnesium sulphate, calcium channel blockers (e.g. nimodipine) and ketanserin (a serotonin 2 receptor blocker). Corticosteroids and non-steroidal anti-inflammatory agents are more controversial.

16.8 How should stroke in pregnancy or the puerperium be managed?

Stroke occurring during pregnancy or the puerperium should be investigated in the same way as any other stroke in a young, otherwise healthy woman, with the exception that possible exposure of a fetus to any diagnostic irradiation must be minimised, if not avoided completely.[4]

The risk of stroke recurrence in any future pregnancy is not known but must be fairly low and dependent on the underlying cause of the initial stroke.

The risk associated with future oral contraception is also not known but is probably best avoided, if alternative strategies of contraception can be adopted.

APPENDIX A
Volunteer and
support groups and websites

The Stroke Association (UK)

In England and Wales, the Stroke Association provides practical support, including telephone helplines, publications and welfare grants, to people who have had strokes, their families and carers. (see CHSS and NICHSA for Scotland and Northern Ireland.) At local levels, the Stroke Association provides:

- Family support workers –people who offer emotional support and advice to families of people who have had a stroke, and to people affected by stroke who live alone
- A community service called Dysphasia Support – volunteers work to improve communication skills with people who have lost the ability to speak, read or write.

The national headquarters of the UK Stroke Association can be contacted at:

Stroke Association
Stroke House
123–127 Whitecross Street
London EC1Y 8JJ
UK
Tel: +44 (0)20 7566 0300
Website: **http://www.stroke.org.uk**

The National Stroke Foundation (Melbourne, Australia)

Provides similar services to the UK Stroke Association.

National Stroke Foundation
Head Office, Level 11, 167 Queen Street
Melbourne, Victoria
Australia 3000
Tel: +61 3 9670 1000; fax: +61 3 9670 9300; freecall: 1800 657 007;
email: admin@strokefoundation.com.au
Website: **http://www.strokefoundation.com.au**

Chest, Heart and Stroke Scotland (CHSS)

The CHSS provides information and support in Scotland for patients, families and carers affected by chest, heart and stroke illnesses. Their volunteer stroke service offers rehabilitation and support, and the CHSS advice line provides professional advice from trained nurses.

Chest, Heart and Stroke Scotland
65 North Castle Street
Edinburgh EH2 3LT
UK
Tel: +44 (0)131 225 6963; fax: +44 (0)131 220 6313
CHSS advice line: tel: 0845 077 6000; email: admin@chss.org.uk
Website: **http://www.chss.org.uk**

Northern Ireland Chest, Heart and Stroke Association (NICHSA)

The NICHSA supports the rehabilitation of stroke and cardiac patients through, amongst other things, a network of local clubs.

NICHSA
21 Dublin Road
Belfast BT2 7HB
UK
Tel: +44 (0)28 9032 0184; fax: +44 (0)28 9033 3487
Advice helpline: tel: 084 5769 7299; cardiac liaison sister helpline: tel: 084 5601 1658
Website: **http://www.nichsa.com**

Different Strokes

Different Strokes is run by and for younger people who have had a stroke. Their helpline is staffed by young stroke survivors, and a national counselling network is available. Local branches exist organise regular exercise classes.

Different Strokes
Sir Walter Scott House
PO Box 5082
Milton Keynes MK5 7ZH
UK
Tel: +44 (0)1908 236 033
Website: **http://www.differentstrokes.co.uk**

Local stroke clubs

Local stroke clubs are emerging rapidly. They take many different forms and may be organised by local stroke survivors or carers, district nurses, general practitioners, local branches of the Stroke Association or Different Strokes. If interested, it is wise to contact the local general practitioner, members of the patient's specialist stroke team or, in the UK, the Health Information Service (freephone in UK: 0800 66 55 44).

Carer groups

- *Carers National* – Tel: +44 (0)20 7490 8818

■ *The Relatives and Residents Association* – Provides help and advice for
people in long-term care facilities. Tel: +44 (0)207 916 6055

Specific disability groups

Action for Dysphasia Adults (ADA)
1 Royal Street
London SE1 7LL
UK
Tel: +44 (0)207 262 9572

Continence Foundation
The Basement
Doughty Street
London WC1N 2PH
UK
Tel: +44 (0)207 404 6875; helpline +44 (0)207 831 9831

SPOD (The Association to Aid the Sexual and Personal Relationships
of People with a Disability)
286 Camden Road
London N7 OBJ
UK

Medical websites and other sources of information

American Heart Association
Website: http://www.americanheart.org/Heart and Stroke A Z guide/

American Stroke Association
Websites: http://www.strokeaha.org, http://www.strokeassociation.org

Asian Vascular Society
Website, sponsored by the Philippine Heart Association, the Heart
Foundation of the Philippines and the Philippine Asian Vascular
Society.
Website: http://www.asianvascular.org/index.htm

Australasian Stroke Trials Network
Website: http://www.astn.org.au/

Canadian Stroke Consortium
Website: http://www.strokeconsortium.ca

Chest, Heart and Stroke, Scotland
Website: http://www.chss.org.uk

Cochrane Collaboration
Website: http://www.cochrane.org/

Cochrane Stroke Review Group
Website: http://www.dcn.ed.ac.uk/csrg

Doctors.net
The UK's premier medical internet information portal, with more than 65,000 members. E-mail access, journal searches, discussion forums, and more – all for free – doctors.net.uk is by doctors, for doctors.
Website: http://www.doctors.net.uk

European Stroke Organisation
Websites: http://www.eurostroke.org, http://www.stroke2002.com

Heart and Stroke Foundation of Canada
Website: http://www.na.heartandstroke.ca

International Stroke Thrombolysis Register for Safe Implementation of Thrombolysis in Stroke (SITS)
Website: http://www.acutestroke.org

The Internet Stroke Center
A web resource for information about stroke care and research.
Website: http://www.strokecenter.org

National Electronic Library for Health (NELH)
A source of relevant up-to-date information on effective forms of health care.
Website: http://www.nelh.nhs.uk

National Institute of Neurological Disorders and Stroke
Website: http://www.ninds.nih.gov/

National Neuroscience Institute of Singapore
11 Jalan Tan Tock Seng
Singapore 308443
Tel (65) 357 7153; fax: (65) 256 4755
Website: http://www.nni.com.sg

National Stroke Research Institute (Australia)
Website: http://www.strokeresearch.com.au

The Royal College of Physicians of London
A source of evidence-based guidelines on stroke.
Website: http://www.rcplondon.ac.uk

The Scottish Intercollegiate Guidelines Network
A source of evidence-based guidelines on stroke
Website: http://www.show.scot.nhs.uk/sign/clinical.htm

Stroke: A Guide for Patients and Their Families
A resource for health professionals and the public for interactive
communication and information about atherothrombosis. Funded by
a pharmaceutical company (Sanofi-Synthélabo) that is active in
research and developing treatments for atherothrombosis.
Website: http://www.atherothrombosis.org/

The Stroke Information Directory
Website: http://www.stroke-info.com/

The Vitamins To Prevent Stroke (VITATOPS) Trial
Website: http://www.health.wa.gov.au/VITATOPS/

Personal accounts
On being struck by a stroke
Stroke survivor E.B. Jelks tells his story.
Website: http://www.strokesurvivor.org

Stroke and rehabilitation
People can and do make recoveries as Helen McIntosh tells in her
books.
Website: http://home.vicnet.net.au/~helenm/#stroke

APPENDIX B
Diagnostic evaluation of suspected transient ischaemic attack and stroke

First line investigations (for all patients, by doctor of first contact)

HISTORY AND EXAMINATION

■ Establish diagnosis of transient ischaemic attack (TIA) or stroke
 – Sudden loss of focal neurological function (< 24 hours TIA, > 24 hours stroke), (*see chapter 3*)
■ Seek precipitating and aetiological risk factors (*see chapter 7*)
 – Previous TIA/stroke
 – Hypertension
 – Diabetes
 – Smoking
 – Alcohol abuse
 – Drug abuse
 – Ischaemic or valvular heart disease
 – Atrial fibrillation
 – Infective endocarditis
 – Carotid stenosis
 – Neck trauma
 – Arteritis
■ Seek prognostic factors for survival, functional outcome and recurrent stroke (*see chapter 9*)
■ Obtain past, family and social history
■ Classify stroke syndrome
 – Total anterior circulation syndrome
 – Partial anterior circulation syndrome
 – Lacunar syndrome
 – Posterior circulation syndrome
■ Assess swallowing function

NEUROIMAGING

Urgent plain computed tomography (CT) brain scan to:
■ Exclude non-stroke pathologies
■ Distinguish haemorrhage from infarction
■ Ascertain likely mechanism of stroke

VASCULAR IMAGING

■ Duplex carotid ultrasound – if non-disabling carotid ischaemic event (i.e. carotid TIA or mild ischaemic stroke)

CARDIOPULMONARY

■ Electrocardiogram (ECG)
■ Chest X-ray

LABORATORY TESTS

■ Urgent blood glucose
■ Full blood count, erythrocyte sedimentation rate, serum biochemistry, lipid profile and urinalysis.

Second line investigations (for select, generally referred, patients)

VASCULAR IMAGING

■ Magnetic resonance angiography or intra-arterial digital subtraction angiography if:
  – Non-disabling carotid ischaemic event
    and
    Duplex ultrasound evidence of more than 70% stenosis of symptomatic carotid artery
    and
  – Patient fit and willing for carotid surgery
■ Duplex carotid ultrasound if: disabling carotid ischaemic event

CARDIAC IMAGING

■ Transthoracic ECG if:
  – Non-lacunar syndrome
    and
  – Abnormal heart clinically or by ECG or chest X-ray
(to identify potential embolic source in the left ventricle and evaluate left ventricular function)
■ Transoesophageal ECG if suspected embolic source in the venous system, left atrium or aortic arch

NEUROIMAGING

■ Magnetic resonance imaging (MRI; with or without diffusion- and perfusion-weighted imaging) if:
  – CT scan performed more than 10 days after stroke shows a low-density area that could be infarction or resolving haemorrhage and it is essential to distinguish them

- CT scan is negative (or shows multiple infarcts) and it is crucial to be able to localise the acute infarct (MRI is more sensitive)
- Arterial dissection is suspected (NB: catheter angiography remains the gold standard)

LABORATORY TESTS

- Coagulation profile
- Thrombophilia screen – protein C, protein S, antithrombin III, factor V Leiden (activated protein C resistance) and prothrombin G20210A mutation
- Antiphospholipid antibodies – anticardiolipin antibody, lupus anticoagulant
- Syphilis serology
- Autoimmune screen
- Fasting plasma homocysteine
- Blood cultures, thyroid function tests
- Human immunodeficiency virus serology.

REFERENCES

Chapter 1

1. Warlow CP, Dennis MS, van Gijn J et al. *Stroke: a practical guide to management.* Oxford: Blackwell Scientific Publications; 2000.
2. Oxford University Press. *A Lexicon.* Abridged from Liddell and Scott's Greek–English Lexicon. Oxford: Oxford University Press; 1963.
3. Hankey GJ, Warlow CP. *Transient ischaemic attacks of the brain and eye.* London: WB Saunders/Baillière Tindall; 1994.

Chapter 2

1. Sudlow CLM, Warlow CP. Comparable studies of the incidence of stroke and its pathological subtypes. Results from an International Collaboration. *Stroke* 1997; **28**: 491–499.
2. Hankey GJ, Warlow CP. *Transient ischaemic attacks of the brain and eye.* London: WB Saunders/Baillière Tindall; 1994.
3. MacDonald BK, Cockerell OC, Sander JWAS, Shorvon. SD. The incidence and lifetime prevalence of neurological disorders in a prospective community-based study in the UK. *Brain* 2000; **123**: 665–676.
4. Bonita R, Solomon N, Broad JB. Prevalence of stroke and stroke-related disability: estimates from the Auckland Stroke Studies. *Stroke* 1997; **28**: 1898–1902.
5. Wyller TB, Bautz-Holter E, Holmen J. Prevalence of stroke and stroke-related disability in North Trondelag County, Norway. *Cerebrovasc Dis* 1994; **4**: 421–427.
6. Bots ML, Looman SJ, Koudstaal PJ et al. Prevalence of stroke in the general population. The Rotterdam study. *Stroke* 1996; **27**: 1499–1501.
7. Geddes JML, Fear J, Tennant A et al. Prevalence of self reported stroke in a population in northern England. *J Epidemiol Comm Health* 1996; **50**: 140–143.
8. Balarajan R. Ethnic differences in mortality from ischaemic heart disease and cerebrovascular disease in England and Wales. *Br Med J* 1991; **302**: 560–564.
9. Leung SY, Ng THK, Yuen ST et al. Pattern of cerebral atherosclerosis in Hong Kong Chinese: severity in intracranial and extracranial vessels. *Stroke* 1993; **24**: 779–786.
10. Bonita R, Broad JB, Beaglehole R. Ethnic differences in stroke incidence and case fatality in Auckland, New Zealand. *Stroke* 1997; **28**: 758–761.
11. Pickle LW, Mungiole M, Gillum RF. Geographic variation in stroke mortality in blacks and whites in the United States. *Stroke* 1997; **28**: 1639–1647.
12. Elliott WJ. Circadian variation in the timing of stroke onset: a meta-analysis. *Stroke* 1998; **29**: 992–996.

13. Jakovljevic D, Salomaa V, Sivenius J, et al. Seasonal variation in the occurrence of stroke in a Finnish adult population. The FINMONICA Stroke Register. *Stroke* 1996; **27**: 1774–1779.
14. Rothwell PM, Wroe SJ, Slattery J, Warlow CP, on behalf of the Oxfordshire Community Stroke Project. Is stroke incidence related to season or temperature? *Lancet* 1996; **347**: 934–936.
15. Bonita R, Stewart A, Beaglehole R. International trends in stroke mortality 1970–1985. *Stroke* 1990; **21**: 989–992.
16. Corwin LE, Wolf PA, Kannel WB, McNamara PM. Accuracy of death certification of stroke: the Framingham study. *Stroke* 1982; **13**: 818–821.
17. Murray CJL, Lopez AD. Mortality by cause for eight regions of the world: Global burden of disease study. *Lancet* 1997; **349**: 1269–1276.
18. Gross CP, Anderson GF, Powe NR. The relation between funding by the National Institutes of Health and the burden of disease. *N Engl J Med* 1999; **340**: 1881–1887.
19. Hankey GJ. Preventing stroke-what is the real progress? *Med J Aust* 1999; **171**: 285–286.
20. Malmgren R, Bamford J, Warlow C et al. Projecting the number of patients with first-ever strokes and patients newly handicapped by stroke in England and Wales. *Br Med J* 1989; **298**: 656–660.

Chapter 3

1. Dennis MS, Bamford JM, Sandercock PAG, Warlow CP. Incidence of transient ischaemic attacks in Oxfordshire, England. *Stroke* 1989; **20**: 333–339.
2. Calanchini PR, Swanson PD, Gotshall RA et al. Cooperative study of hospital frequency and character of transient ischaemic attacks. IV. The reliability of diagnosis. *JAMA* 1977; **238**: 2029–2033.
3. Kraaijeveld CL. Van Gijn J, Schouten HJA, Staal A. Interobserver agreement for the diagnosis of transient ischaemic attacks. *Stroke* 1984; **15**: 723–725.
4. Koudstaal PJ, Gerritsma JGM, van Gijn J. Clinical disagreement on the diagnosis of transient ischaemic attack: is the patient or the doctor to blame? *Stroke* 1989; **20**: 300–301.
5. Hankey GJ, Warlow CP. Cost-effective investigation of patients with suspected transient ischaemic attacks. *J Neurol Neurosurg Psychiatry* 1992; **55**: 171–176.
6. Kingsley DPE, Radue EW, Du Boulay EPGH. Evaluation of computed tomography in vascular lesions of the vertebrobasilar territory. *J Neurol Neurosurg Psychiatry* 1980; **43**: 193–197.
7. Martin JD, Valentine J, Myers SI et al. Is routine CT scanning necessary in the preoperative evaluation of patients undergoing carotid endarterectomy? *J Vasc Surg* 1991; **14**: 267–270.
8. Faught E. Current role of electroencephalography in cerebral ischaemia. *Stroke* 1993; **24**: 609–613.
9. Allder SJ, Moody AR, Martel AL et al. Limitations of clinical diagnosis in acute stroke. *Lancet* 1999; **354**: 1523.

10. Norris JW, Hachinski VC. Misdiagnosis of stroke. *Lancet* 1982; **1**: 328–331.

11. Von Kummer R, Allen KL, Holle R et al. Acute stroke: usefulness of early CT findings before thrombolytic therapy. *Radiology* 1997; **205**: 327–333.

12. Dennis MS, Bamford JM, Molyneux AJ et al. Rapid resolution of signs of primary intracerebral haemorrhage in computed tomograms of the brain. *Br Med J* 1987; **279**: 379–381.

13. Grond M, Von Kummer R, Sobesky J et al. Early computer-tomography abnormalities in acute stroke. *Lancet* 1997; **350**: 1595–1596.

14. Gacs G, Fox AJ, Barnett HJM, Vinuela F. CT visualisation of intracranial arterial thromboembolism. *Stroke* 1982; **14**: 756–762.

15. Hankey GJ, Khangure MS, Stewart-Wynne EG. Detection of basilar artery thrombosis by computed tomography. *Clin Radiol* 1988; **39**: 140–143.

16. Barber PA, Demchuk AM, Hudon ME et al. Hyperdense sylvian fissure MCA 'dot' sign. A CT marker of acute ischemia. *Stroke* 2001; **32**: 84–88.

17. Manelfe C, Larrue V, von Kummer R et al. Association of hyperdense middle cerebral artery sign with clinical outcome in patients treated with tissue plasminogen activator. *Stroke* 1999; **30**: 769–772.

18. Hakim AM, Ryder-Cooke A, Melanson D. Sequential computerised tomographic appearance of strokes. *Stroke* 1983; **14**: 893–897.

19. Lindgren A, Norrving B, Rudling O, Johansson BO. Comparison of clinical and neuroradiological findings in first-ever stroke: a population-based study. *Stroke* 1994; **25**: 1371–1377.

20. Becker H, Desch H, Hacker H, Pencz A. CT fogging effect with ischaemic cerebral infarcts. *Neuroradiology* 1979; **18**: 185.

21. Skriver EB, Olsen TS. Transient disappearance of cerebral infarcts on CT scan, the so-called fogging effect. *Neuroradiology* 1981; **22**: 61–65.

22. Sage MR. Blood–brain barrier: a phenomenon of increasing importance to the imaging clinician. *Am J Neuroradiol* 1982; **3**: 127–138.

23. Wardlaw JM. Is routine computed tomography in strokes unnecessary? *Br Med J* 1994; **309**: 1498–1500.

24. Alberts MJ, Faulstich ME, Gray L. Stroke with negative brain magnetic resonance imaging. *Stroke* 1992; **23**: 663–667.

25. Mohr JP, Biller J, Hilal SK et al. Magnetic resonance versus computed tomographic imaging in acute stroke. *Stroke* 1995; **26**: 807–812.

26. Ida M, Mizunuma K, Tada S. Subcortical low intensity in early cortical ischaemia. *Am J Neuroradiol* 1994; **15**: 1387–1393.

27. Yuh WTC, Crain MR, Loes DJ et al. MR imaging of cerebral ischaemia: findings in the first 24 hours. *Am J Neuroradiol* 1991; **12**: 621–629.

28. Bryan RN, Levy LM, Whitlow WD et al. Diagnosis of acute cerebral infarction: comparison of CT and MR imaging. *Am J Neuroradiol* 1991; **12**: 611–620.

29. Wardlaw JM, Armitage PA, Dennis MS et al. The use of diffusion-weighted magnetic resonance imaging to identify infarctions in patients with minor strokes. *J Stroke Cerebrovasc Dis* 2000; **9**: 70–75.

30. Fisher M, Sotak CH. Diffusion weighted MR imaging and ischaemic stroke. *Am J Neuroradiol* 1992; **13**: 1103–1105.

31. Warach S, Gaa J, Siewert B et al. Acute human stroke studied by whole brain echo planar diffusion-weighted magnetic resonance imaging. *Ann Neurol* 1995; **37**: 231–241.

32. Binnie CD, Prior PF. Electroencephalography. *J Neurol Neurosurg Psychiatry* 1994; **57**: 1308–1319.

33. Kappelle LJ, van Huffelen AC, van Gijn J. Is the EEG really normal in lacunar stroke? *J Neurol Neurosurg Psychiatry* 1990; **53**: 63–66.

34. MacDonnell RAL, Donnan GA, Bladin PF et al. The electroencephalogram and acute ischaemic stroke: distinguishing cortical from lacunar infarction. *Arch Neurol* 1988; **45**: 520–524.

35. Van Gijn J, Rinkel GJE. Subarachnoid haemorrhage: diagnosis, causes and management. *Brain* 2001; **124**: 249–278.

36. Vermeulen M, van Gijn J. The diagnosis of subarachnoid haemorrhage. *J Neurol Neurosurg Psychiatry* 1990; **53**: 365–372.

37. Vermeulen M, van Gijn J, Blijenberg BG. Spectrophotometric analysis of CSF after subarachnoid haemorrhage: limitations in the diagnosis of rebleeding. *Neurology* 1983; **33**: 112–114.

38. Edlow JA, Caplan LR. Avoiding pitfalls in the diagnosis of subarachnoid hemorrhage. *N Engl J Med* 2000; **342**: 29–36.

39. Van Gijn J. Slip-ups in diagnosis of subarachnoid haemorrhage. *Lancet* 1997; **349**: 1492.

Chapter 4

1. Hankey GJ, Warlow CP. *Transient ischaemic attacks of the brain and eye.* London: WB Saunders/Baillière Tindall; 1994.

2. Kraaijeveld CL. Van Gijn J, Schouten HJA, Staal A. Interobserver agreement for the diagnosis of transient ischaemic attacks. *Stroke* 1984; **15**: 723–725.

3. Bamford J, Sandercock P, Dennis M et al. Classification and natural history of clinically identifiable subtypes of cerebral infarction. *Lancet* 1991; **337**: 1521–1526.

4. Anderson CS, Taylor BV, Hankey GJ et al. Validation of a clinical classification for subtypes of acute cerebral infarction. *J Neurol Neurosurg Psychiatry* 1994; **57**: 1173–1179.

5. Nicolai A, Lazzarino LG, Biasutti E. Large striatocapsular infarcts: clinical features and risk factors. *J Neurol* 1996; **243**: 44–50.

6. Bamford JM, Warlow CP. Evolution and testing of the lacunar hypothesis. *Stroke* 1988; **19**: 1074–1082.

7. Lodder J, Bamford J, Kappelle J, Boiten J. What causes false clinical prediction of small deep infarcts? *Stroke* 1994; **25**: 86–91.

8. Kim JS, Lee JH, Choi CG. Patterns of lateral medullary infarction. Vascular lesion–magnetic resonance imaging correlation of 34 cases. *Stroke* 1998; **29**: 645–652.

9. Huang CY, Yu YL. Small cerebellar strokes may mimic labyrinthine lesions. *J Neurol Neurosurg Psychiatry* 1985; **48**: 263–265.

10. Amarenco P. The spectrum of cerebellar infarctions. *Neurology* 1991; **41**: 973–979.

11. Mathew P, Teasdale G, Bannan A, Oluoch-Olunya D. Neurosurgical management of cerebellar haematoma and infarct. *J Neurol Neurosurg Psychiatry* 1995; **59**: 287–292.
12. Caplan LR, Tettenborn B. Vertebrobasilar occlusive disease: review of selected aspects. 1. Spontaneous dissection of extracranial and intracranial posterior circulation arteries. *Cerebrovasc Dis* 1992; **2**: 256–265.
13. Caplan LR, Tettenborn B. Vertebrobasilar occlusive disease: review of selected aspects 2. Posterior circulation embolism. *Cerebrovasc Dis* 1992; **2**: 320–326.
14. Argentino C, De Michele M, Fiorelli M et al. Posterior circulation infarcts simulating anterior circulation stroke: perspective of the acute phase. *Stroke* 1996; **27**: 1306–1309.
15. Bladin CF, Chambers BR. Frequency and pathogenesis of haemodynamic stroke. *Stroke* 1994; **25**: 2179–2182.
16. Hupperts RMM, Warlow CP, Slattery J, Rothwell PM. Severe stenosis of the internal carotid artery is not associated with borderzone infarcts in patients randomised in the European Carotid Surgery Trial. *J Neurol* 1997; **244**: 45–50.

Chapter 5

1. Bamford J, Sandercock P, Dennis M et al. A prospective study of acute cerebrovascular disease in the community: the Oxfordshire Community Stroke Project, 1981–1986. 2. Incidence, case fatality rates and overall outcome at one year of cerebral infarction, primary intracerebral and subarachnoid haemorrhage. *J Neurol Neurosurg Psychiatry* 1990; **53**: 16–22.
2. Allen CMC. Clinical diagnosis of acute stroke syndrome. *Q J Med* 1983; **43**: 515–523.
3. Celani MG, Ceravolo MG, Duca E et al. Was it infarction or haemorrhage? A clinical diagnosis by means of the Allen Score. *J Neurol* 1992; **239**: 411–413.
4. Poungvarin N, Viriyavejaku IA, Komontri C. Siriraj stroke score and validation study to distinguish supratentorial intracerebral haemorrhage from infarction. *Br Med J* 1991; **302**: 1565.
5. Besson G, Robert C, Hommel M, Perret J. Is it clinically possible to distinguish non-hemorrhagic infarct from hemorrhagic stroke? *Stroke* 1995; **26**: 1205–1209.
6. Weir CJ, Murray GD, Adams FG et al. Poor accuracy of scoring systems for differential clinical diagnosis of intracranial haemorrhage and infarction. *Lancet* 1994; **344**: 999–1002.
7. Hawkins GC, Bonita R, Broad JB, Anderson NE. Inadequacy of clinical scoring systems to differentiate stroke subtypes in population-based studies. *Stroke* 1995; **26**: 1338–1342.
8. Hart RG, Boop BS, Anderson DC. Oral anticoagulants and intracranial haemorrhage. Facts and hypotheses. *Stroke* 1995; **26**: 1471–1477.

Chapter 6

1. Bamford J, Sandercock P, Dennis M et al. A prospective study of acute cerebrovascular disease in the community: the Oxfordshire Community

Stroke Project 1981–1986. 2. Incidence, case fatality rates and overall outcome at one year of cerebral infarction, primary intracerebral and subarachnoid haemorrhage. *J Neurol Neurosurg Psychiatry* 1990; **53**: 16–22.

2. Ross R. Atherosclerosis – an inflammatory disease. *N Engl J Med* 1999; **340**: 115–126.

3. Kullo IJ, Edwards WD, Schwartz RS. Vulnerable plaque: pathobiology and clinical implications. *Ann Intern Med* 1998; **129**: 1050–1060.

4. Danesh J, Whincup P, Walker M et al. Chlamydia pneumoniae IgG titres and coronary heart disease: prospective study and meta-analysis. *Br Med J* 2000; **321**: 208–213.

5. Rothwell PM, Villagra R, Gibson R et al. Evidence of a chronic systemic cause of instability of atherosclerotic plaques. *Lancet* 2000, **355**: 19–24.

6. George JN. Platelets. *Lancet* 2000; **355**: 1531–1539.

7. Topol EJ, Byzova TV, Plow EF. Platelet GPIIb-IIIa blockers. *Lancet* 1999; **353**: 223–227.

8. Furie B, Furie BC. Molecular and cellular biology of blood coagulation. *N Engl J Med* 1992; **326**: 800–806.

9. Broze GJ Jr. The role of tissue factor pathway inhibitor in a revised coagulation cascade. *Semin Haematol* 1992; **29**: 159–169.

10. Sandercock PAG, Warlow CP, Jones LN, Starkey I. Predisposing factors for cerebral infarction: the Oxfordshire Community Stroke Project. *Br Med J* 1989; **298**: 75–80.

11. EAFT (European Atrial Fibrillation Trial) Study Group: Secondary prevention in nonrheumatic atrial fibrillation and transient ischaemic attack or minor stroke. *Lancet* 1993; **342**: 1255–1262.

12. Freed LA, Levy D, Levine RA et al. Prevalence and clinical outcome of mitral-valve prolapse. *N Engl J Med* 1999; **341**: 1–7.

13. Gilon D, Buonanno FS, Joffe MM et al. Lack of evidence of an association between mitral valve prolapse and stroke in young patients. *N Engl J Med* 1999; **341**: 8–13.

14. Nishimura RA, McGoon MD. Perspectives on mitral-valve prolapse. *N Engl J Med* 1999; **341**: 48–50.

15. McGaw D, Harper R. Patent foramen ovale and cryptogenic cerebral infarction. *Intern Med J* 2001; **31**: 42–47.

16. Swannell AJ. Polymyalgia rheumatica and temporal arteritis: diagnosis and management. *Br Med J* 1997; **314**: 1329–1332.

17. Greaves M. Antiphospholipid antibodies and thrombosis. *Lancet* 1999; **353**: 1348–1353.

18. Dahlback B, Carlsson M, Svensson PJ. Familial thrombophilia due to a previously unrecognised mechanism characterised by poor anticoagulant response to activated protein C: Prediction of a cofactor to activated protein C. *Proc Natl Acad Sci USA* 1993; **90**: 1004.

19. Bertina RM, Koeleman BP, Koster T et al. Mutation in blood coagulation factor V associated with resistance to activated protein C in venous thrombophilia. *Nature* 1994; **369**: 64.

20. Bushnell CD, Goldstein LB. Diagnostic testing for coagulopathies in patients with ischemic stroke. *Stroke* 2000; **31**: 3067–3078.

Chapter 7

1. D'Agostino RB, Wolf PA, Belanger AJ, Kannel WB. Stroke risk profile: adjustment for antihypertensive medication. The Framingham Study. *Stroke* 1994; **25**: 40–43.
2. Truelsen T, Lindenstrom E, Boysen G. Comparison of probability of stroke between the Copenhagen City Heart Study and the Framingham Study. *Stroke* 1994; **25**: 802–807.
3. Collins R, MacMahon S. Blood pressure, antihypertensive drug treatment and the risks of stroke and of coronary heart disease. *Br Med Bull* 1994; **50**: 272–298.
4. Mulrow CD, Cornell JA, Herrera CR et al. Hypertension in the elderly. Implications and generalizability of randomised trials. *JAMA* 1994; **272**: 1932–1938.
5. Sandercock PAG, Warlow CP, Jones LN, Starkey I. Predisposing factors for cerebral infarction: the Oxfordshire Community Stroke Project. *Br Med J* 1989; **298**: 75–80.
6. Rose G. Strategy of prevention: lessons from cardiovascular disease. *Br Med J* 1981; **282**: 1847–1851.
7. MacMahon S, Peto R, Cutler J et al. Blood pressure, stroke, and coronary heart disease. Part 1. Prolonged differences in blood pressure: prospective observational studies corrected for the regression dilution bias. *Lancet* 1990; **335**: 765–774.
8. Eastern Stroke and Coronary Heart Disease Collaborative Research Group. Blood pressure, cholesterol and stroke in Eastern Asia. *Lancet* 1998; **352**: 1801–1807.
9. Prospective Studies Collaboration. Cholesterol, diastolic blood pressure, and stroke: 13,000 strokes in 450,000 people in 45 prospective cohorts. *Lancet* 1995; **346**: 1647–1653.
10. Fine-Edelstein JS, Wolf PA, OíLeary DH et al. Precursors of extracranial carotid atherosclerosis in the Framingham Study. *Neurology* 1994; **44**: 1046–1050.
11. Bamford J, Sandercock P, Dennis M et al. A prospective study of acute cerebrovascular disease in the community: the Oxfordshire Community Stroke Project-1981–1986. 2. Incidence, case fatality rates and overall outcome at one year of cerebral infarction, primary intracerebral and subarachnoid haemorrhage. *J Neurol Neurosurg Psychiatry* 1990; **53**: 16–22.
12. Hankey GJ. Smoking and risk of stroke. *J Cardiovasc Risk* 1999; **6**: 207–211.
13. Thrift AG, McNeil JJ, Donnan GA, for the Melbourne Risk Factor Study Group. The risk of intracerebral haemorrhage with smoking. *Cerebrovasc Dis* 1999; **9**: 34–39.
14. Burchfiel CM, Curb JD, Rodriguez BL et al. Glucose intolerance and 22 year stroke incidence. The Honolulu Heart program. *Stroke* 1994; **25**: 951–957.
15. Jorgensen HS, Nakayama H, Raaschou HO, Olsen TS. Stroke in patients with diabetes. The Copenhagen Stroke Study. *Stroke* 1994; **25**: 1977–1984.
16. Wolf PA, Abbott RD, Kannel WB. Atrial fibrillation as an independent risk factor for stroke: the Framingham Study. *Stroke* 1991; **22**: 983–988.

17. Atrial Fibrillation Investigators. Risk factors for stroke and efficacy of antithrombotic therapy in atrial fibrillation. Analysis of pooled data from five randomised controlled trials. *Arch Intern Med* 1994; **154**: 1449–1457.

18. Dennis M, Bamford J, Sandercock P, Warlow C. The prognosis of transient ischaemic attacks in the Oxfordshire community stroke project. *Stroke* 1990; **21**, 848–853.

19. Hankey GJ, Slattery JM, Warlow CP. The prognosis of hospital-referred transient ischaemic attacks. *J Neurol Neurosurg Psychiatry* 1991; **54**: 793–802.

20. Inzitari D, Eliasziw M, Gates P et al, for the North American Symptomatic Carotid Endarterectomy Trial Group. The causes and risk of stroke in patients with asymptomatic internal-carotid-artery stenosis. *N Engl J Med* 2000; **342**: 1693–1700.

21. European Carotid Surgery Trialists' Collaborative Group. Randomised trial of endarterectomy for recently symptomatic carotid stenosis: final results of the MRC European Carotid Surgery Trial (ECST). *Lancet* 1998; **351**: 1379–1387.

22. Barnett HJM, Taylor DW, Eliasziw M et al, for the North American Symptomatic Carotid Endarterectomy Trial collaborators. Benefit of carotid endarterectomy in patients with symptomatic moderate or severe carotid stenosis. *N Engl J Med* 1998; **339**: 1415–1425.

23. O'Leary DH, Polak JF, Kronmal A et al, on behalf of the CHS Collaborative Research Group. Distribution and correlates of sonographically detected carotid artery disease in the Cardiovascular Health Study. *Stroke* 1992; **23**: 1752–1760.

24. Leng GC, Fowkes FGR, Lee AJ et al. Use of ankle brachial pressure index to predict cardiovascular events and death: a cohort study. *Br Med J* 1996; **313**: 1440–1444.

25. Suh I, Jee SH, Kim HC et al. Low serum cholesterol and haemorrhagic stroke in men: Korea Medical Insurance Corporation Study. *Lancet* 2001; **357**: 922–925.

26. Di Mascio R, Marchioli R, Tognoni G. Cholesterol reduction and stroke occurrence: an overview of randomised clinical trials. *Cerebrovasc Dis* 2000; **10**: 85–92.

27. Byington RP, Davis PR, Plehn J et al. Reduction in stroke events with pravastatin: the Prospective Pravastatin Pooling (PPP) Project. *Circulation* 2001; **103**: 387–392.

28. Law MR, Wald NJ, Wu T et al. Systematic underestimation of association between serum cholesterol concentration and ischaemic heart disease in observational studies: data from the BUPA study. *Br Med J* 1994; **308**: 363–366.

29. Hokanson JE, Austin MA. Plasma triglyceride level is a risk factor for cardiovascular disease independent of high-density lipoprotein cholesterol level: a meta-analysis of population-based prospective studies. *J Cardiovasc Risk* 1996; **3**: 213–219.

30. Heart Outcomes Prevention Evaluation (HOPE) Study Investigators. Effects of an angiotensin- converting-enzyme inhibitor, ramipril, on

cardiovascular events in high-risk patients. *N Engl J Med* 2000; **342**: 145–153.

31. Ernst E, Resch KL. Fibrinogen as a cardiovascular risk factor: a meta-analysis and review of the literature. *Ann Intern Med* 1993; **118**: 956–963.

32. Macko RF, Kittner SJ, Epstein A et al. Elevated tissue plasminogen activator antigen and stroke risk. The stroke prevention in young women study. *Stroke* 1999; **30**: 7–11.

33. Eikelboom JW, Lonn E, Genest J Jr et al. Homocyst(e)ine and cardiovascular disease: a critical review of the epidemiologic evidence. *Ann Intern Med* 1999; **131**: 363–375.

34. Eikelboom JW, Hankey GJ, Anand SS et al. Association between high homocyst(e)ine and ischaemic stroke due to large- and small-artery disease but not other etiological subtypes of ischaemic stroke. *Stroke* 2000; **31**: 1069–1075.

35. Hankey GJ, Eikelboom JW. Homocysteine and vascular disease. *Lancet* 1999; **354**: 407–413.

36. Christen WG, Ajani UA, Glynn RJ, Hennekens CH. Blood levels of homocysteine and increased risks of cardiovascular disease: causal or casual? *Arch Intern Med* 2000; **160**: 422–434.

37. Homocysteine Lowering Trialist's Collaboration. Lowering blood homocysteine with folic acid based supplements: meta-analysis of randomised trials. *Br Med J* 1998; **316**: 894–898.

38. Byar DP, Corle DK. Hormone therapy for prostate cancer: results of the Veterans Administration Cooperative Urological Research Group Studies. *NCI Monographs* 1988; **7**, 165–170.

39. Heinemann LAJ, Lewis MA, Thorogood M et al and the Transnational Research Group on Oral Contraceptives and Health of Young Women. Case-control study of oral contraceptives and risk of thromboembolic stroke: results from international study on oral contraceptives and health of young women. *Br Med J* 1997; **315**: 1502–1504.

40. Gillum LA, Mamidipudi SK, Johnston SC. Ischemic stroke risk with oral contraceptives. A meta-analysis. *JAMA* 2000; **284**: 72–78.

41. Vandenbroucke JP. Cerebral sinus thrombosis and oral contraceptives. There are limits to predictability. *Br Med J* 1998; **317**: 483–484.

42. Viscoli CM, Brass LM, Kernan WN, Sarrell PM, Suissa S, Horwitz RI. A clinical trial of estrogen-replacement therapy after ischemic stroke. *N Engl J Med* 2001; **345**: 1243–1249.

43. Simon JA, Hsia J, Cauley JA et al. Postmenopausal hormone therapy and risk of stroke: the Heart and Estrogen-progestin Replacement Study (HERS). *Circulation* 2001; **103**: 638–642.

44. Vandenbroucke JP, Helmerhorst FM. Risk of venous thrombosis with hormone-replacement therapy. *Lancet* 1996; **348**: 972.

45. Thun MJ, Peto R, Lopez AD et al. Alcohol consumption and mortality among middle-aged and elderly US adults. *N Engl J Med* 1997; **337**: 1705–1714.

46. He J, Ogden LG, Vupputuri S et al. Dietary sodium intake and subsequent risk of cardiovascular disease in overweight adults. *JAMA* 1999; **282**: 2027–2034.

47. Hooper L, Summerbell CD, Higgins JPT et al. Dietary fat intake and prevention of cardiovascular disease: systematic review. *Br Med J* 2001; **322**: 757–763.
48. Walker SP, Rimm EB, Ascherio A et al. Body size and fat distribution as predictors of stroke among US men. *Am J Epidemiol* 1996; **144**: 1143–1150.
49. Lee I-M, Hennekens CH, Berger K et al. Exercise and risk of stroke in male physicians. *Stroke* 1999; **30**: 1–6.
50. Hu FB, Stampfer MJ, Colditz GA et al. Physical activity and risk of stroke in women. *JAMA* 2000; **283**: 2961–2967.
51. Everson SA, Kaplan GA, Goldberg DE et al. Anger expression and incident stroke: prospective evidence from the Kuopio ischaemic heart disease study. *Stroke* 1999; **30**: 523–528.
52. Natowicz M, Kelley RI. Mendelian aetiologies of stroke. *Ann Neurol* 1987; **22**: 175–192.
53. Liao D, Myers R, Hunt S et al. Familial history of stroke and stroke risk. The Family Heart Study. *Stroke* 1997; **28**: 1908–1912.
54. Rastenyte D, Tuomilehto J, Sarti C. Genetics of stroke – a review. *J Neurol Sci* 1998; **153**: 132–145.
55. Hademenos GJ, Alberts MJ, Awad I et al. Advances in the genetics of cerebrovascular disease and stroke. *Neurology* 2001; **56**: 997–1008.

Chapter 8

1. Hankey GJ, Warlow CP. Cost-effective investigation of patients with suspected transient ischaemic attacks. *J Neurol Neurosurg Psychiatry* 1992; **55**: 171–176.
2. Hankey GJ, Warlow CP. *Transient ischaemic attacks of the brain and eye.* London: WB Saunders; 1994.
3. Hankey GJ, Warlow CP, Sellar RJ. Cerebral angiographic risk in mild cerebrovascular disease. *Stroke* 1990; **21**: 209–222.
4. Hankey GJ, Warlow CP, Molyneux AJ. Complications of cerebral angiography for patients with mild carotid territory ischaemia being considered for carotid endarterectomy. *J Neurol Neurosurg Psychiatry* 1990b; **53**: 542–548.

Chapter 9

1. Dennis MS, Burn JP, Sandercock PAG et al. Long-term survival after first-ever stroke: the Oxfordshire community stroke project. *Stroke* 1993; **24**: 796–800.
2. Hankey GJ, Jamrozik K, Broadhurst RJ et al. Five year survival after first-ever stroke and related prognostic factors in the Perth Community Stroke Study. *Stroke* 2000; **31**: 2080–2086.
3. Bamford J, Sandercock PAG, Dennis M et al. A prospective study of acute cerebrovascular disease in the community: the Oxfordshire Community Stroke Project, 1981–1986. 2. Incidence, case fatality rates and overall outcome at one year of cerebral infarction, primary intracerebral and subarachnoid haemorrhage. *J Neurol Neurosurg Psychiatry* 1990; **53**: 16–22.

4. Hop JW, Rinkel GJE, Algra A, van Gijn J. Case-fatality rates and functional outcome after subarachnoid haemorrhage-a systematic review. *Stroke* 1997; **28**: 660–664.
5. Counsell C, Dennis M, McDowall M, Warlow CP. Predicting outcome after acute stroke: development and validation of new models. *Stroke* 2001; in press.
6. Hankey GJ, Jamrozik K, Broadhurst RJ et al. Long-term risk of recurrent stroke in the Perth Community Stroke Study. *Stroke* 1998; **29**: 2491–2500.
7. Dennis M, Bamford J, Sandercock P, Warlow C. The prognosis of transient ischaemic attacks in the Oxfordshire community stroke project. *Stroke* 1990; **21**: 848–853.
8. Hankey GJ, Slattery JM, Warlow CP. Transient ischaemic attacks: which patients are at high (and low) risk of serious vascular events? *J Neurol Neurosurg Psychiatry* 1992; **5**: 640–652.
9. Hankey GJ, Slattery JM, Warlow CP. Can the long-term outcome of patients with transient ischaemic attacks be predicted accurately? *J Neurol Neurosurg Psychiatry* 1993; **56**: 752–759.
10. Rothwell PM, Warlow CP. Prediction of benefit from carotid endarterectomy in individual patients: a risk-modelling study. *Lancet* 1999; **353**: 2105–2110.
11. Johnston SC, Gress DR, Browner WS, Sidney S. Short-term prognosis after emergency department diagnosis of TIA. *JAMA* 2000; **284**: 2901–2906.
12. Hijdra A, Vermeulen M, van Gijn J, van Crevel H. Rerupture of intracranial aneurysms: a clinicoanatomic study. *J Neurosurg* 1987; **67**: 29–33.
13. Hijdra A, van Gijn J, Nagelkerke NJD et al. Prediction of delayed cerebral ischaemia, rebleeding, and outcome after aneurysmal subarachnoid haemorrhage. *Stroke* 1988; **19**: 1250–1256.
14. Mast H, Young WL, Koennecke H-C et al. Risk of spontaneous haemorrhage after diagnosis of cerebral arteriovenous malformation. *Lancet* 1997; **350**: 1065–1068.
15. Duong DH, Young WL, Vang MC et al. Feeding artery pressure and venous drainage pattern are primary determinants of haemorrhage from cerebral arteriovenous malformations. *Stroke* 1998; **29**: 1167–1176.
16. Adams HP, Kassell NF, Torner JC, Haley EC. Predicting cerebral ischaemia after aneurysmal subarachnoid haemorrhage: influences of clinical condition, CT results, and antifibrinolytic therapy. A report of the Cooperative Aneurysm Study. *Neurology* 1987; **37**: 1586–1591.

Chapter 10
1. Stroke Unit Trialists' Collaboration. Organised inpatient (stroke unit) care for stroke (Cochrane Review). In: *The Cochrane Library*, Issue 4. Oxford: Update Software; 2001.

Chapter 11
1. Stroke Unit Trialists' Collaboration. Organised inpatient (stroke unit) care for stroke (Cochrane Review). In: *The Cochrane Library*, Issue 4. Oxford: Update Software; 2001.

2. Stegmayr B, Asplund K, Hulter-Asberg K et al. Stroke units in their natural habitat: can results of randomised trials be reproduced in routine clinical practice? For the Riks-Stroke Collaboration. *Stroke* 1999; **30**: 709–714.

3. Stroke Unit Trialists' Collaboration. How do stroke units improve patient outcomes? A collaborative systematic review of the randomised trials. *Stroke* 1997; **28**: 2139–2144.

4. Indredavik B, Bakke F, Slordahl SA et al. Treatment in a combined acute and rehabilitation stroke unit: which aspects are most important? *Stroke* 1999; **30**: 917–923.

5. Langhorne P, Tong BLP, Stott DJ. Association between physiological homeostasis and early recovery after stroke. *Stroke* 2000; **31**: 2526–2527.

6. Duncan PW. Synthesis of intervention trials to improve motor recovery following stroke. *Top Stroke Rehabil* 1997; **3**: 1–20.

7. Scheidtmann K, Fries W, Müller F, Koenig E. Effect of levodopa in combination with physiotherapy on functional motor recovery after stroke: a prospective, randomised, double-blind study. *Lancet 2001*; **358**: 787–790.

8. Walker MF, Gladman JRF, Lincoln NB et al. Occupational therapy for stroke patients not admitted to hospital: a randomised controlled trial. *Lancet* 1999; **354**: 278–280.

9. Gilbertson L, Langhorne P, Walker A et al. Domiciliary occupational therapy for patients with stroke discharged from hospital: a randomised controlled trial. *Br Med J* 2000; **320**: 603–606.

10. Walker MF, Drummond AE, Lincoln NB. Evaluation of dressing practice for stroke patients after discharge from hospital: a cross-over design. *Clin Rehab* 1996; **10**: 23–31.

Chapter 12

1. Nachtmann A, Siebler M, Rose G, et al. Cheyne-Strokes respiration in ischemic stroke. *Neurology* 1995; **45**: 820–821.

2. Ronning OM, Guldvog B. Should stroke victims routinely receive supplemental oxygen? A quasi-randomised controlled trial. *Stroke* 1999; **30**: 2033–2037.

3. Wallace JD, Levy LL. Blood pressure after stroke. *JAMA* 1981; **246**: 2177–2180.

4. Carlsson A, Britton M. Blood pressure after stroke. A 1 year follow up study. *Stroke* 1993; **24**: 195–199.

5. Bath FJ, Bath PMW. What is the correct management of blood pressure in acute stroke? The Blood Pressure in Acute Stroke Collaboration. *Cerebrovasc Dis* 1997; **7**: 205–213.

6. Potter JF. What should we do about blood pressure and stroke? *Q J Med* 1999; **92**: 63–66.

7. Blood Pressure in Acute Stroke Collaboration (BASC). Interventions for deliberately altering blood pressure in acute stroke (Cochrane Review). In: *The Cochrane Library*, Issue 4, 2001. Oxford: Update Software.

8. Reith J, Jorgensen HS, Pedersen PM, et al. Body temperature in acute stroke: relation to stroke severity, infarct size, mortality, and outcome. *Lancet* 1996; **347**: 422–425.

9. Schwab S, Schwarz S, Spranger M, et al. Moderate hypothermia in the treatment of patients with severe middle cerebral artery infarction. *Stroke* 1998; **29**: 2461–2466.

10. Dippel DWJ, van Breda EJ, van Gemert HMA et al. The effect of paracetamol (acetaminophen) on body temperature in acute ischaemic stroke. A double blind, randomised phase-II clinical trial. *Cerebrovasc Dis* 2001; **11**(suppl 4): 79.

11. Smithard DG, O'Neill PA, Park C, et al. Complications and outcome after stroke. Does dysphagia matter? *Stroke* 1996; **27**: 1200–1204.

12. Mann G, Hankey GJ, Cameron D. Swallowing dysfunction after acute stroke. Prognosis and prognostic factors at 6 months. *Stroke* 1999; **30**: 744–748.

13. Mann G, Hankey GJ, Cameron D. Swallowing disorders after acute stroke. Prevalence and diagnostic accuracy. *Cerebrovasc Dis* 2000; **10**: 380–386.

14. Smithard DG, O'Neill PA, Park C, et al. Can bedside assessment reliably exclude aspiration following acute stroke? *Age Ageing* 1999; **27**: 99–106.

15. Finestone HM. Safe feeding methods in stroke patients. *Lancet* 2000; **355**: 1662–1663.

16. Dennis MS. FOOD (Feed Or Ordinary Diet): a multicentre international randomised trial evaluating feeding policies for patients hospitalised with a recent stroke: introducing the concept of a family of trials [abstract]. *Age Ageing* 1998; **27** (suppl): 68.

17. Nakayama H, Jorgensen HS, Pedersen PM, et al. Prevalence and risk factors for incontinence after stroke. The Copenhagen stroke study. *Stroke* 1997; **28**: 58–62.

18. Nuffield Institute of Health. Effective health care. The prevention and treatment of pressure sores. *Effective Health Care* 1995; **2**: 1–16.

19. Warlow C, Ogston D, Douglas AS. Venous thrombosis following strokes. *Lancet* 1972; **I**: 1305–6.

20. Davenport RJ, Dennis MS, Wellwood I, Warlow CP. Complications after acute stroke. *Stroke* 1996; **27**: 415–420.

21. Langhorne P, Stott DJ, Robertson L et al. Medical complications after stroke. A multicenter study. *Stroke* 2000; **31**: 1223–1229.

22. Warlow C. Venous thromboembolism after stroke. *Am Heat J* 1978; **96**: 283–285.

23. Dromerick A, Reding M. Medical and neurological complications during inpatient stroke rehabilitation. *Stroke* 1994; **25**: 358–361.

24. Kalra L, Yu G, Wilson K, et al. Medical complications during stroke rehabilitation. *Stroke* 1995; **26**: 990–994.

25 McClatchie G. Survey of the rehabilitation outcomes of stroke. *Med J Aust* 1980; **1**: 649–651.

26. Wells PA, Lensing AWA, Hirsch J. Graduated pressure stockings in the prevention of postoperative venous thromboembolism: a meta analysis. *Arch Intern Med* 1994; **154**: 67–72.

27. Antiplatelet Trialists' Collaboration. Collaborative overview of randomised trials of antiplatelet therapy. III: Reduction in venous thrombosis and

pulmonary embolism by antiplatelet prophylaxis among surgical and medical patients. *Br Med J* 1994; **308**: 235–246.

28. Gubitz G, Counsell C, Sandercock P, et al. Anticoagulants in acute ischaemic stroke. (Cochrane Review). In: *The Cochrane Library*, Issue 4, 2001. Oxford: Update Software.

29. Scott JF, Gray CS, O'Connell JE, et al. Glucose and insulin therapy in acute stroke; why delay further? *Q J Med* 1998; **91**: 511–515.

30. Scott JF, Robinson GM, O'Connell JE, et al. Glucose potassium insulin (GKI) infusions in the treatment of acute stroke patients with mild to moderate hyperglycaemia: the Glucose, Insulin in Stroke Trial (GIST). *Stroke* 1999; **30**: 793–799.

31. Van Gijn J, Rinkel GJE. Subarachnoid haemorrhage: diagnosis, causes and management. *Brain* 2001; **124**: 249–278.

Chapter 13

1. Lee JM, Zipfel GJ, Choi DW. The changing landscape of ischaemic brain injury mechanisms. *Nature* 1999; **399**(Suppl): A7–A14.

2. Klijn CJM, Hankey GJ. Management of acute ischaemic stroke: new guidelines from the American Stroke Association and European Stroke Initiative. *Lancet Neurology* 2003; **2**: 698–701.

3. Wardlaw JM, del Zoppo G, Yamaguchi T. Thrombolysis for acute ischaemic stroke. In: *The Cochrane Library*, Issue 4. Oxford: Update Software; 2001.

4. Kalafut MA, Schriger DL, Saver JL, Starkman S. Detection of early CT signs of >1/3 middle cerebral artery infarctions. Interrater reliability and sensitivity of CT interpretation by physicians involved in acute stroke care. *Stroke* 2000; **31**: 1667–1671.

5. Barber PA, Demchuk AM, Zhang J, Buchan AM. Validity and reliability of a quantitative computed tomography score in predicting outcome of hyperacute stroke before thrombolytic therapy. *Lancet* 2000; **355**: 1670–1674.

6. Nawashiro H, Fukui S. Intra-arterial thrombolysis for hyperacute stroke. *Lancet* 2000; **356**: 1111–1112.

7. Albers GW. Expanding the window for thrombolytic therapy in acute stroke. The potential role of acute MRI for patient selection. *Stroke* 1999; **30**: 2230–2237.

8. National Institute of Neurological Disorders and Stroke rt-PA Stroke Study Group. A systems approach to immediate evaluation and management of hyperacute stroke: experience at eight centers and implications for community practice and patient care. *Stroke* 1997; **28**: 1530–1540.

9. Buchan AM, Barber PA, Newcommon N et al. Effectiveness of t-PA in acute ischaemic stroke. Outcome relates to appropriateness. *Neurology* 2000; **54**: 679–684.

10. Adams HP, Brott TG, Furlan AJ et al. Guidelines for thrombolytic therapy for acute stroke: a supplement to the guidelines for the management of patients with acute ischemic stroke. *Circulation* 1996; **94**: 1167–1174.

11. Hankey GJ. Thrombolysis for acute ischaemic stroke. *J Clin Neurosci* 2001; **8**: 103–105.

12. Chinese Acute Stroke Trial Collaborative Group. CAST: randomised placebo- controlled trial of early aspirin use in 20 000 patients with acute ischaemic stroke. *Lancet* 1997; **349**: 1641–1649.

13. International Stroke Trial Collaborative Group. The International Stroke Trial (IST): a randomised trial of aspirin, subcutaneous heparin, both, or neither among 19 435 patients with acute ischaemic stroke. *Lancet* 1997; **349**: 1569–1581.

14. Chen Z, Sandercock P, Pan H et al. Indications for early aspirin use in acute ischaemic stroke. A combined analysis of 40,000 randomized patients from the Chinese Acute Stroke Trial and the International Stroke Trial. *Stroke* 2000; **31**: 1240–1249.

15. Gubitz G, Sandercock P, Counsell C, Signorini D. Anticoagulants for acute ischaemic stroke (Cochrane Review). In: *The Cochrane Library*, Issue 4. Oxford: Update Software; 2001.

16. Gubitz G, Sandercock P, Counsell C. Antiplatelet therapy for acute ischaemic stroke (Cochrane Review). In: *The Cochrane Library*, Issue 4. Oxford: Update Software; 2001

17. Antiplatelet Trialists' Collaboration. Collaborative overview of randomised trials of anti platelet therapy – I: Prevention of death, myocardial infarction and stroke by prolonged antiplatelet therapy in various categories of patients. *Br Med J* 1994; **308**: 81–106.

18. Roderick PJ, Wilkes HC, Meade TW. The gastrointestinal toxicity of aspirin: an overview of randomised controlled trials. *Br J Clin Pharmacol* 1993; **35**: 241–249.

19. Slattery J, Warlow CP, Shorrock CJ, Langman MJS. Risks of gastrointestinal bleeding during secondary prevention of vascular events with aspirin – analysis of gastrointestinal bleeding during the UK-TIA trial. *Gut* 1995; **37**: 509–511.

20. Bath PMW, Iddenden R, Bath FJ. Low-molecular-weight heparins and heparinoids in acute ischaemic stroke. A meta-analysis of randomised controlled trial. *Stroke* 2000; **31**: 1770–1778.

21. Berge E, Abdelnoor M, Nakstad PH, Sandset PM, on behalf of the HAEST Study Group. Low molecular-weight heparin versus aspirin in patients with acute ischaemic stroke and atrial fibrillation: a double-blind randomised study. *Lancet* 2000; **355**: 1205–1210.

22. Pulmonary Embolism Prevention Trial Collaborative Group. Prevention of pulmonary embolism and deep vein thrombosis with low-dose aspirin: Pulmonary Embolism Prevention (PEP) trial. *Lancet* 2000; **355**: 1295–1302.

23. Sandercock P, Dennis M. Venous thromboembolism after acute stroke. *Stroke* 2001; **32**: 1445.

24. Lees KR. Does neuroprotection improve stroke outcome? *Lancet* 1998; **351**: 1447–1448.

25. Morfis L, Schwartz RS, Poulos R, Howes LG. Blood pressure changes in acute cerebral infarction and haemorrhage. *Stroke* 1997; **28**: 1401–1405.

26. Blood Pressure in Acute Stroke Collaboration. Interventions for deliberately altering blood pressure in acute stroke. In: *The Cochrane Library*, Issue 2. Oxford: Update Software; 2001.

27. Horn J, Orgogozo JM, Limburg M. Review on calcium antagonists in ischaemic stroke: mortality data. *Cerebrovasc Dis* 1998; **8**(Suppl 4): 27.

28. Broderick JP, Adams HP Jr, Barsan W et al. Guidelines for the management of spontaneous intracerebral hemorrhage. *Stroke* 1999; **30**: 905–915.

29. Hankey GJ, Hon C: Surgery for primary intracerebral haemorrhage: is it safe and effective? A systematic review of case series and randomised trials. *Stroke* 1997; **28**: 2126–2132.

30. Gerritsen van der Hoop R, Vermeulen M, van Gijn J. Cerebellar haemorrhage: diagnosis and treatment. *Surg Neurol* 1988; **29**: 6–10.

31. Van Gijn J, Rinkel GJE. Subarachnoid haemorrhage: diagnosis, causes and management. *Brain* 2001; **124**: 249–278.

32. Roos YBWEM, Rinkel GJE, Vermeulen M et al. Antifibrinolytic therapy for aneurysmal subarachnoid haemorrhage (Cochrane Review). In: *The Cochrane Library*, Issue 4. Oxford: Update Software; 2001

33. Feigin VL, Rinkel GJE, Algra A et al. Calcium antagonists for aneurysmal subarachnoid haemorrhage (Cochrane Review). In: *The Cochrane Library*, Issue 2. Oxford: Update Software; 2001

Chapter 14

1. PROGRESS Collaborative Group. Randomised trial of a perindopril-based blood-pressure-lowering regimen among 6105 individuals with previous stroke or transient ischaemic attack. *Lancet* 2001; **358**: 1033–1041.

2. INDANA (Individual Data Analysis of Antihypertensive intervention trials) Project Collaborators. Effect of antihypertensive treatment in patients having already suffered from stroke. Gathering the evidence. *Stroke* 1997; **28**: 2557–2562.

3. Rodgers A, Neal B, MacMahon S. The effects of blood pressure lowering in cerebrovascular disease. *Neurol Rev Int* 1997, **2**: 12–15.

4. PATS Collaborating Group. Post-stroke antihypertensive treatment study: a preliminary result. *Chinese Med J* 1995; **108**: 710–717.

5. Hankey GJ, Jamrozik K, Broadhurst RJ et al. Long-term risk of recurrent stroke in the Perth Community Stroke Study. *Stroke* 1998; **29**: 2491–2500.

6. Hankey GJ, Warlow CP: Treatment and secondary prevention of stroke: evidence, costs, and effects on individuals and populations. *Lancet* 1999; **354**: 1457–1463.

7. Rodgers A, MacMahon S, Gamble G et al, for the United Kingdom Transient Ischaemic Attack Collaborative Group. Blood pressure and risk of stroke in patients with cerebrovascular disease. *Br Med J* 1996; **313**: 147.

8. Neal B, Clark T, MacMahon S et al, on behalf of the Antithrombotic Trialists' Collaboration. Blood pressure and the risk of recurrent vascular disease. *Am J Hypertension* 1998; **11**: 25A–26A.

9. Antithrombotic Trialists' Collaboration. Collaborative meta-analysis of randomised trials of antiplatelet therapy for prevention of death, myocardial infarction, and stroke in high risk patients. *BMJ* 2002; **324**: 71–86.

10. Blood Pressure Lowering Treatment Trialists' Collaboration. Effects of ACE inhibitors, calcium antagonists, and other blood-pressure-lowering

drugs: results of prospectively designed overviews of randomised trials. *Lancet* 2000; **355**: 1955–1964.

11. He J, Whelton PK. Selection of initial antihypertensive drug therapy. *Lancet* 2000; **356**: 1942–1943.

12. Collins R, Peto R, MacMahon S et al. Blood pressure, stroke, and coronary heart disease. Part 2, short-term reductions in blood pressure: overview of randomised drug trials in their epidemiological context. *Lancet* 1990; **335**: 827–839.

13. Eastern Stroke and Coronary Heart Disease Collaborative Research Group. Blood pressure, cholesterol, and stroke in eastern Asia. *Lancet* 1998; **352**: 1801–1807.

14. Arnolda L. Containing the costs of managing hypertension. *Med J Aust* 2001; **174**: 556–557.

15. Nelson MR, McNeil JJ, Peeters A et al. PBS. RPBS cost implications of trends and guideline recommendations in the pharmacological management of hypertension in Australia 1994–1998. *Med J Aust* 2001; **174**: 565–568.

16. Heart Outcomes Prevention Evaluation (HOPE) Study Investigators. Effects of an angiotensin-converting-enzyme inhibitor, ramipril, on cardiovascular events in high-risk patients. *N Engl J Med* 2000; **342**: 145–153.

17. Hankey GJ. Angiotensin-converting enzyme inhibitors for stroke prevention: Is there HOPE for PROGRESS after LIFE? *Stroke* 2003; **34**: 354–356.

18. Hankey GJ. Role of lipid-modifying therapy in the prevention of initial and recurrent stroke. *Curr Op Lipidology* 2002; **13 (6)**: 645–651.

19. Manktelow B, Gillies C, Potter JF. Interventions in the management of serum lipids for preventing stroke recurrence (Cochrane Review). In: *The Cochrane Library*, Issue 3 2003; Oxford: Update Software.

20. Plehn JF, Davis BR, Sacks FM, Rouleau JL, Pfeffer MA, Bernstein V, Cuddy TE, Moyé LA, Piller LB, Rutherford JD, Simpson LM, Braunwald E. Reduction of stroke incidence after myocardial infarction with pravastatin: the Cholesterol and recurrent Events (CARE) study. The CARE Investigators. *Circulation* 1999; **99**: 216–223.

21. White HD, Simes RJ, Anderson NE, Hankey GJ, Watson JDG, Hunt D, Colquhoun DM, Glasziou P, MacMahon SR, Kirby AC, West MJ, Tonkin AM. Pravastatin therapy and the risk of stroke. *N Engl J Med* 2000; **343**: 317–326.

22. Heart Protection Study Collaborative Group. MRC/BHF Heart Protection Study of cholesterol lowering with simvastatin in 20 536 high-risk individuals: a randomised placebo-controlled trial. *Lancet* 2002; **360**: 7–22.

23. Cholesterol Treatment Trialists' (CTT) Collaboration. Protocol for a prospective collaborative overview of all current and planned randomised trials of cholesterol treatment regimens. *AM J Cardiol* 1995; **75**: 1130–1134.

24. Hankey GJ. Smoking and risk of stroke. *J Cardiovasc Risk* 1999; **6**: 207–211.

25. Sandercock P. Statins for stroke prevention? *Lancet* 2001; **357**: 1548–1549.

26. Algra A, van Gijn J. Cumulative meta-analysis of aspirin efficacy after cerebral ischaemia of arterial origin. *J Neurol Neurosurg Psychiatry* 1999; **66**: 255.

27. Taylor DW, Barnett HJM, Haynes RB et al. Low- dose and high-dose acetylsalicyclic acid for patients undergoing carotid endarterectomy: a randomised controlled trial. *Lancet* 1999; **353**: 2179–2184.

28. Dutch TIA Trial Study Group. A comparison of two doses of aspirin (30mg vs 283mg a day) in patients after a transient ischemic attack or minor ischemic stroke. *N Engl J Med* 1991; **325**: 1261–1266.

29. He J, Whelton PK, Vu B, Klag MJ. Aspirin and risk of hemorrhagic stroke. A meta-analysis of randomised controlled trials. *JAMA* 1998; **280**: 1930–1935.

30. Roderick PJ, Wilkes HC, Meade TW. The gastrointestinal toxicity of aspirin: an overview of randomised controlled trials. *Br J Clin Pharmacol* 1993; **35**: 241–249.

31. UK-TIA Study Group. The United Kingdom transient ischaemic attack (UK-TIA) aspirin trial: final results. *J Neurol Neurosurg Psychiatry* 1991; **54**: 1044–1054.

32. Kelly JP, Kaufman DW, Jurgelon JM et al. Risk of aspirin-associated major upper-gastrointestinal bleeding with enteric-coated or buffered product. *Lancet* 1996; **348**: 1413–1416.

33. Patrono C. Aspirin as an antiplatelet drug. *N Engl J Med* 1994; **330**: 1287–1293.

34. Hankey GJ, Sudlow CLM, Dunbabin DW. Thienopyridines or aspirin to prevent stroke and other serious vascular events in patients at high risk of vascular disease. *Stroke* 2000; **31**: 1779–1784.

35. Steinhubl SR, Tan WA, Foody JM, Topol EJ, for the EPISTENT investigators. Incidence and clinical course of thrombotic thrombocytopenic purpura due to ticlopidine following coronary stenting. *JAMA* 1999; **281**: 806–810.

36. Torok TJ, Holman RC, Chorba TL. Increasing mortality from thrombotic thrombocytopenic purpura in the United States: an analysis of national mortality data, 1968–1991. *Am J Haematol* 1995; **50**: 84–90.

37. Gent M, Beaumont D, Blanchard J et al. A randomised, blinded, trial of clopidogrel versus aspirin in patients at risk of ischaemic events (CAPRIE). *Lancet* 1996; **348**: 1329–1338.

38. Bennett CL, Connors JM, Carwile JM et al. Thrombotic thrombocytopenic purpura associated with clopidogrel. *N Engl J Med* 2000; **342**: 1773–1777.

39. Hankey GJ. Clopidogrel and thrombotic thrombocytopenic purpura. *Lancet* 2000; **356**: 269–270.

40. Hankey GJ. One year after CAPRIE, IST and ESPS 2: any changes in concepts? *Cerebrovasc Dis* 1998; **8**(Suppl 5): 1–7.

41. Wilterdink JL, Easton JD. Dipyridamole plus aspirin in cerebrovascular disease. *Arch Neurol* 1999; **56**: 1087–1092.

42. Diener HC, Cunha L, Forbes C et al. European stroke prevention study 2. Dipyridamole and acetylsalicyclic acid in the secondary prevention of stroke. *J Neurol Sci* 1996; **143**: 1–13.

43. De Schryver ELLM, on behalf of the European/Australian Stroke Prevention in Reversible Ischaemia Trial (ESPRIT) Group. Design of ESPRIT: an international randomised trial for secondary prevention after non disabling cerebral ischaemia of arterial origin. *Cerebrovasc Dis* 2000; **10**: 147–150.

44. Topol EJ. Toward a new frontier in myocardial reperfusion therapy. Emerging platelet preeminence. *Circulation* 1998; **97**: 211–218.

45. Heeschen C, Hamm CW. Difficulties with oral platelet glycoprotein IIb/IIIa receptor antagonists. *Lancet* 2000; **355**: 330–331.

46. Hankey GJ. Warfarin-Aspirin Recurrent Stroke Study (WARSS) trial: Is warfarin really a reasonable therapeutic alternative to aspirin for preventing recurrent noncardioembolic ischaemic stroke? *Stroke* 2002; **33**: 1723–1726.

47. The Stroke Prevention in Reversible Ischaemia Trial (SPIRIT) Study Group. A randomized trial of anticoagulants versus aspirin after cerebral ischaemia of presumed arterial origin. *Ann Neurol* 1997, **42**: 857–865.

48. European Carotid Surgery Trialists' Collaborative Group. Randomised trial of endarterectomy for recently symptomatic carotid stenosis: final results of the MRC European Carotid Surgery Trial (ECST). *Lancet* 1998; **351**: 1379–1387.

49. Barnett HJM, Taylor DW, Eliasziw M, for the North American Symptomatic Carotid Endarterectomy Trial collaborators. Benefit of carotid endarterectomy in patients with symptomatic moderate or severe carotid stenosis. *N Engl J Med* 1998; **339**: 1415–1425.

50. Cina C, Clase C, Haynes BR. Carotid endarterectomy for symptomatic carotid stenosis. In: *The Cochrane Library*, Issue 4. Oxford: Update Software; 2001.

51. Alamowitch S, Eliasziw M, Algra A et al, for the North American Symptomatic Carotid Endarterectomy Trial (NASCET) Group. Risk, causes, and prevention of ischaemic stroke in elderly patients with symptomatic internal-carotid-artery stenosis. *Lancet* 2001; **357**: 1154–1160.

52. Rothwell PM. Carotid endarterectomy and prevention of stroke in the very elderly. *Lancet* 2001; **357**: 1142–1143.

53. Rothwell PM, Warlow CP. Prediction of benefit from carotid endarterectomy in individual patients: a risk- modelling study. *Lancet* 1999; **353**: 2105–2110.

54. Hankey GJ. 'You need an operation'. *Lancet* 1999; **353**(Suppl 1): 35–36.

55. Rothwell PM, Warlow CP. Is self-audit reliable? *Lancet* 1995; **346**: 1623.

56. Rothwell PM, Warlow CP, on behalf of the European Carotid Surgery Trialists' Collaborative Group. Interpretation of operative risks of individual surgeons. *Lancet* 1999; **353**: 1325.

57. Rothwell P, Slattery J, Warlow C. Clinical and angiographic predictors of stroke and death from carotid endarterectomy: systematic review. *Br Med J* 1997; **315**: 1571–1577.

58. CAVATAS investigators. Endovascular versus surgical treatment in patients with carotid artery stenosis in the Carotid and Vertebral Artery Transluminal Angioplasty Study (CAVATAS): a randomised trial. *Lancet* 2001; **357**: 1729–1737.

59. Benavente O, Moher D, Pham B. Carotid endarterectomy for asymptomatic carotid stenosis: a meta- analysis. *Br Med J* 1998; **317**: 1477–1480.

60. Whitty C, Sudlow C, Warlow C. Investigating individual subjects and screening populations for asymptomatic carotid stenosis can be harmful. *J Neurol Neurosurg Psychiatry* 1998; **64**: 619–623.

61. Falk RH. Atrial fibrillation. *N Engl J Med* 2001; **344**: 1067–1078.

62. Hart RG, Benavente O, McBride R, Pearce LA. Antithrombotic therapy to prevent stroke in patients with atrial fibrillation: a meta-analysis. *Ann Intern Med* 1999; **131**: 492–501.

63. European Atrial Fibrillation Trial Study Group. Secondary prevention in non-rheumatic atrial fibrillation after transient ischaemic attack or minor stroke. *Lancet* 1993; **342**: 1255–1262.

64. Cannegieter SC, Rosendal FR, Wintzen AR et al. Optimal oral anticoagulant therapy in patients with mechanical heart valves. *N Engl J Med* 1995; **333**: 11–17.

65. Hylek EM, Skates SJ, Sheehan MA, Singer DE. An analysis of the lowest effective intensity of prophylactic anticoagulation for patients with non-rheumatic atrial fibrillation. *N Engl J Med* 1996; **335**: 540–546.

66. Hacke W. The dilemma of reinstituting anticoagulation for patients with cardioembolic sources and intracranial hemorrhage. *Arch Neurol* 2000; **57**: 1682–1684.

67. Crawley F, Bevan D, Wren D. Management of intracranial bleeding associated with anticoagulation: balancing the risk of further bleeding against thromboembolism from prosthetic heart valves. *J Neurol Neurosurg Psychiatry* 2000; **69**: 396–398.

68. Gallus AS, Baker RI, Chong BH et al. Consensus guidelines for warfarin therapy. Recommendations from the Australasian Society of Thrombosis and Haemostasis. *Med J Aust* 2000; **172**: 600–605.

69. McGaw D, Harper R. Patent foramen ovale and cryptogenic cerebral infarction. *Intern Med J* 2001; **31**: 42–47.

Chapter 15

1. Gautier JC. Stroke-in-progression. *Stroke* 1985; **16**: 729–733.

2. Asplund K. Any progress on progressing stroke? *Cerebrovasc Dis* 1992; **2**: 317–319.

3. Berger C, Fiorelli M, Steiner T et al. Hemorrhagic transformation of ischemic brain tissue. Asymptomatic or symptomatic? *Stroke* 2001; **32**: 1330–1335.

4. Molina CA, Montaner J, Abilleira S et al. Timing of spontaneous recanalisation and risk of hemorrhagic transformation in acute cardioembolic stroke. *Stroke* 2001; **32**: 1079–1084.

5. Schwartz S, Schwab S, Bertram M et al. Effects of hypertonic saline hydroxyethyl starch solution and mannitol in patients with increased intracranial pressure after stroke. *Stroke* 1998; **29**: 1550–1555.

6. Schwab S, Steiner T, Aschoff A et al. Early hemicraniectomy in patients with complete middle cerebral artery infarction. *Stroke* 1998; **29**: 1888–1893.

7. Davenport RJ, Dennis MS, Wellwood I, Warlow CP. Complications following acute stroke. *Stroke* 1996; **27**: 415–420.

8. Kilpatrick CJ, Davis SM, Tress BM et al. Epileptic seizures in acute stroke. *Arch Neurol* 1990; **47**: 157–160.

9. So EL, Annegers JF, Hauser WA et al. Population-based study of seizure disorders after cerebral infarction. *Neurology* 1996; **46**: 350–355.

10. Burn J, Dennis M, Bamford J et al. Epileptic seizures after a first stroke: the Oxfordshire community stroke project. *Br Med J* 1997; **315**: 1582–1587.

11. Brodie MJ, Overstall PW, Giorgi L, and the UK Lamotrigine Elderly Study Group. Multicentre, double-blind, randomised comparison between lamotrigine and carbamazepine in elderly patients with newly diagnosed epilepsy. *Epilepsy Res* 1999; **37**: 81–87.

12. Brodie MJ, French JA. Management of epilepsy in adolescents and adults. *Lancet* 2000; **356**: 323–329.

13. Burvill PW, Johnson GA, Jamrozik KD et al. Prevalence of depression after stroke: the Perth Community Stroke Study. *Br J Psychiatry* 1995; **166**: 320–327.

14. Carson AJ, MacHale S, Allen K et al. Depression after stroke and lesion location: a systematic review. *Lancet* 2000; **356**: 122–126.

15. Beekman ATF, Penninx BWJH, Deeg DJH et al. Depression in survivors of stroke: a community-based study of prevalence, risk factors and consequences. *Soc Psychiatry Psychiatr Epidemiol* 1998; **33**: 463–470.

16. Hermann N, Black SE, Lawrence J et al. The Sunnybook Stroke Study: a prospective study of depressive symptoms and functional outcome. *Stroke* 1998; **29**: 618–624.

17. Pohjasvaara T, Leppävuori A, Siira I et al. Frequency and clinical determinants of poststroke depression. *Stroke* 1998; **29**: 2311–2317.

18. Van de Weg FB, Kuik DJ, Lankhorst GJ. Post-stroke depression and functional outcome: a cohort study investigating the influence of depression on functional recovery from stroke. *Clin Rehab* 1999; **13**: 268–272.

19. House A, Knapp P, Bamford J, Vail A. Mortality at 12 and 24 months after stroke may be associated with depressive symptoms at 1 month. *Stroke* 2001; **32**: 696–701.

20. Lipsey JR, Robinson RG, Pearlson GD et al. Nortriptyline treatment of post-stroke depression: a double-blind study. *Lancet* 1984; **1**: 297–300.

21. Andersen G, Vestergaard K, Lauritzen L. Effective treatment of poststroke depression with selective serotonin reuptake inhibitor citalopram. *Stroke* 1994; **25**: 1099–1104.

22. Wiart L, Petit H, Joseph PA et al. Fluoxetine in early poststroke depression: a double-blind placebo-controlled study. *Stroke* 2000; **31**: 1829–1832.

23. Kelly J, Rudd A, Lewis R, Hunt BJ. Venous thromboembolism after acute stroke. *Stroke* 2001; **32**: 262–267.

24. Lensing AWAA, Prandoni P, Prins MH, Büller HR. Deep-vein thrombosis. *Lancet* 1999; **353**: 479–485.

25. Austroads. *Assessing fitness to drive. Guidelines and standards for health professionals in Australia*, 2nd ed. Sydney: National Library of Australia; 2001.

26. Hamad A, Hamad A, Sokrab T-EO et al. Poststroke sexual function. *Stroke* 1999; **30**: 2238.

27. Korpelainen JT, Nieminen P, Myllylä VV. Sexual functioning among stroke patients and their spouses. *Stroke* 1999; **30**: 715–719.

28. Simpson DM, Alexander DN, O'Brien CF et al. Botulinum toxin type A in the treatment of upper extremity spasticity: a randomised, double-blind, placebo-controlled trial. *Neurology* 1996; **46**: 1306–1310.

Chapter 16

1. Lanthier S, Carmant L, David M et al. Stroke in children. The coexistence of multiple risk factors predict poor outcome. *Neurology* 2000; **54**: 371–378.
2. Grosset DG, Ebrahim S, Bone I, Warlow CP. Stroke in pregnancy and the puerperium: what magntude of risk? *J Neurol Neurosurg Psychiatry* 1995; **58**: 129–131.
3. Garg RK. Posterior leukoencephalopathy syndrome. *Postgrad Med J* 2001; **77**: 24–28.
4. Mas J-L, Lamy C. Stroke in pregnancy and the puerperium. *J Neurol* 1998; **245**: 305–313.

GLOSSARY

ACA – anticardiolipin antibody

ACE – angiotensin-converting enzyme

ADP – adenosine diphosphate

AF – atrial fibrillation

APA – antiphospholipid protein antibody

APCR – resistance to activated protein C

APLAb – antiphospholipid antibody

APTT – activated partial thromboplastin time

ARI – absolute risk increase

ARR – absolute risk reduction

AVM – arteriovenous malformation

BP – blood pressure

CI – confidence interval

CNS – central nervous system

CSF – cerebrospinal fluid

CT – computed tomography

dPT – dilute prothrombin time

dRVVT – dilute Russell viper venom time

DVT – deep vein thrombosis

DWI – diffusion weighted (MRI) imaging

ECA – external carotid artery

ECG – electrocardiogram/electrocardiography

EEG – electroencephalogram/electroencephalography

ELISA – enzyme-linked immunosorbent assay

ESR – erythrocyte sedimentation rate

FLAIR – fluid-attenuated inversion recovery

Gp – glycoprotein

GP – general practitioner

HIV – human immunodeficiency virus

HTI – haemorrhagic transformation

IA-DSA – intra-arterial digital subtraction angiography

ICA – internal carotid artery

INR – international normalised ratio

KCT – kaolin clotting time

LA – lupus anticoagulant

LACI – lacunar infarction

LACS – lacunar syndrome

LDL – low-density lipoprotein

MCA – middle cerebral artery

MELAS – mitochondrial encephalomyopathy with lactic acidosis and stroke-like episodes

MI – myocardial infarction

MRA – magnetic resonance angiography

MRI – magnetic resonance imaging

NIH – National Institutes of Health

NNH – number of patients needed to treat for 1 year to cause harm to one each year

NNT – number of patients needed to treat for 1 year to prevent one event each year

OR – odds ratio

PACI – partial anterior circulation infarction

PACS – partial anterior circulation syndrome

PCA – posterior cerebral artery

PCR – polymerase chain reaction

PFO – patent foramen ovale

PICH – primary intracerebral haemorrhage

POCI – posterior circulation infarction

POCS – posterior circulation syndrome

PWI – perfusion weighted (MRI) imaging

RIA – radioimmunoassay

RPR – rapid plasma reagin

RRI – relative risk increase

RRR – relative risk reduction

r-tPA – recombinant tissue plasminogen activator

SAH – subarachnoid haemorrhage

SD – standard deviation

SLE – systemic lupus erythematosus

TACI – total anterior circulation infarction

TACS – Total anterior circulation syndrome

TF – tissue factor

TFPI – tissue factor pathway inhibitor

tHcy – total homocysteine

TIA – transient ischaemic attack of the brain or eye

TMB – transient monocular blindness

tPA – tissue plasminogen activator

VBA – vertebrobasilar artery

VDRL – Venereal Disease Research Laboratories

vWF – von Willebrand factor

VTE – venous thromboembolism

LIST OF PATIENT QUESTIONS

INDEX

Numbers in bold refer to figures or tables

H

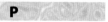

O

P

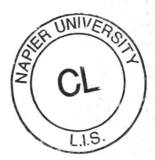